T0263499

Medical and Surgical Management of Crohn's Disease

Editor

SUNANDA V. KANE

GASTROENTEROLOGY CLINICS OF NORTH AMERICA

www.gastro.theclinics.com

Consulting Editor
ALAN L. BUCHMAN

June 2022 • Volume 51 • Number 2

ELSEVIER

1600 John F. Kennedy Boulevard ● Suite 1800 ● Philadelphia, Pennsylvania, 19103-2899
http://www.theclinics.com

**GASTROENTEROLOGY CLINICS OF NORTH AMERICA Volume 51, Number 2
June 2022 ISSN 0889-8553, ISBN-13: 978-0-323-89770-9**

Editor: Kerry Holland
Developmental Editor: Hannah Almira Lopez

Gastroenterology Clinics of North America (ISSN 0889-8553) is published quarterly by Elsevier Inc., 360 Park Avenue South, New York, NY 10010-1710. Months of issue are March, June, September, and December. Business and Editorial Offices: 1600 John F. Kennedy Blvd., Suite 1800, Philadelphia, PA 19103-2899. Customer Service Office: 6277 Sea Harbor Drive, Orlando, FL 32887-4800. Periodicals postage paid at New York, NY and additional mailing offices. Subscription prices are $368.00 per year (US individuals), $100.00 per year (US students), $973.00 per year (US institutions), $395.00 per year (Canadian individuals), $100.00 per year (Canadian students), $1002.00 per year (Canadian institutions), $468.00 per year (international individuals), $220.00 per year (international students), and $1002.00 per year (international institutions). Foreign air speed delivery is included in all *Clinics* subscription prices. All prices are subject to change without notice. **POSTMASTER**: Send address changes to *Gastroenterology Clinics of North America*, Elsevier Health Sciences Division, Subscription Customer Service, 3251 Riverport Lane, Maryland Heights, MO 63043. **Telephone: 1-800-654-2452 (U.S. and Canada); 314-447-8871 (outside U.S. and Canada). Fax: 314-447-8029. E-mail: journalscustomerservice-usa@elsevier.com (for print support); journalsonlinesupport-usa@elsevier.com (for online support).**

Reprints. For copies of 100 or more, of articles in this publication, please contact the Commercial Reprints Department, Elsevier Inc., 360 Part Avenue South, New York, New York 10010-1710. Tel. 212-633-3874, Fax: 212-633-3820, E-mail: reprints@elsevier.com.

Gastroenterology Clinics of North America is also published in Italian by Il Pensiero Scientifico Editore, Rome, Italy; and in Portuguese by Interlivros Edicoes Ltda., Rua Commandante Coelho 1085, 21250 Cordovil, Rio de Janeiro, Brazil.

Gastroenterology Clinics of North America is covered in *MEDLINE/PubMed (Index Medicus)*, *Excerpta Medica*, *Current Contents/Clinical Medicine*, *Science Citation Index*, *ISI/BIOMED*, and *BIOSIS*.

Contributors

CONSULTING EDITOR

ALAN L. BUCHMAN, MD, MSPH, FACP, FACN, FACG, AGAF
Professor of Clinical Surgery, Medical Director, Intestinal Rehabilitation and Transplant
Center, The University of Illinois at Chicago/UI Health, Chicago, Illinois, USA

EDITOR

SUNANDA V. KANE, MD, MSPH
Professor of Medicine, Division of Gastroenterology and Hepatology, Mayo Clinic,
Rochester, Minnesota

AUTHORS

JESSICA R. ALLEGRETTI, MD, MPH
Division of Gastroenterology, Hepatology, and Endoscopy, Brigham and Women's
Hospital, Chestnut Hill, Massachusetts; Harvard Medical School, Boston, Massachusetts

ADAM S. CHEIFETZ, MD
Division of Gastroenterology, Center for Inflammatory Bowel Diseases, Beth Israel
Deaconess Medical Center, Harvard Medical School, Boston, Massachusetts

RISHIKA CHUGH, MD
Section of Digestive Diseases, Department of Medicine, Yale School of Medicine, Yale
University, New Haven, Connecticut; Gastroenterology, Department of Medicine,
University of California, San Francisco, San Francisco, California

PARAKKAL DEEPAK, MBBS, MS
Division of Gastroenterology, Inflammatory Bowel Diseases Center, Washington
University School of Medicine, St Louis, Missouri

PARAMBIR S. DULAI, MBBS
Assistant Professor of Clinical Medicine, Division of Gastroenterology, University of
California, San Diego, La Jolla, California

FRANCIS A. FARRAYE, MD, MSc
Division of Gastroenterology and Hepatology, Inflammatory Bowel Disease Center, Mayo
Clinic, Jacksonville, Florida

LINDA A. FEAGINS, MD
Department of Medicine, Director, Center for Inflammatory Bowel Diseases, Associate
Professor of Medicine, University of Texas at Austin, Dell Medical School, Austin, Texas

SCOTT FRIEDBERG, MD
University of Chicago Medicine Inflammatory Bowel Disease Center, Section of
Gastroenterology, Hepatology, and Nutrition, University of Chicago Medical Center,
Chicago, Illinois

JILL K.J. GAIDOS, MD, FACG
Section of Digestive Diseases, Department of Medicine, Director of Clinical Research,
Yale School of Medicine, Yale University, Associate Professor, Yale Inflammatory Bowel
Disease Program, New Haven, Connecticut

JONATHAN GALATI, MD
Division of Gastroenterology and Hepatology, Inflammatory Bowel Disease Center, NYU
Langone Health, New York, New York

MATÉ GERGELY, MD
Division of Gastroenterology, Inflammatory Bowel Diseases Center, Washington
University School of Medicine, St Louis, Missouri

LAURIE B. GROSSBERG, MD
Division of Gastroenterology, Center for Inflammatory Bowel Diseases, Beth Israel
Deaconess Medical Center, Harvard Medical School, Boston, Massachusetts

PHILLIP GU, MD
Gastroenterology Fellow, Division of Digestive and Liver Diseases, UT Southwestern
Medical Center, Dallas, Texas

SANCHIT GUPTA, MD, MS
Division of Gastroenterology, Hepatology, and Endoscopy, Brigham and Women's
Hospital, Chestnut Hill, Massachusetts; Harvard Medical School, Boston, Massachusetts

JANA G. HASHASH, MD, MSc
Division of Gastroenterology and Hepatology, Inflammatory Bowel Disease Center, Mayo
Clinic, Jacksonville, Florida

SIMON J. HONG, MD
Assistant Professor of Medicine, Division of Gastroenterology and Hepatology,
Inflammatory Bowel Disease Center, NYU Langone Health, New York, New York

SUNANDA V. KANE, MD, MSPH
Professor of Medicine, Division of Gastroenterology and Hepatology, Mayo Clinic,
Rochester, Minnesota

SEYMOUR KATZ, MD
Division of Gastroenterology and Hepatology, Inflammatory Bowel Disease Center, NYU
Langone Health, New York, New York

AMY L. LIGHTNER, MD
Department of Colorectal Surgery, Director, Center for Regenerative Medicine and
Surgery, Associate Professor of Colorectal Surgery, Digestive Disease and Surgery
Institute, Associate Professor of Inflammation and Immunity, Lerner Research Institute,
Core Member, Center for Immunotherapy, Cleveland Clinic, Cleveland, Ohio

ELANA B. MITCHEL, MD, MSCE
Children's Hospital of Philadelphia, Philadelphia, Pennsylvania

KONSTANTINOS PAPAMICHAEL, MD, PhD
Division of Gastroenterology, Center for Inflammatory Bowel Diseases, Beth Israel
Deaconess Medical Center, Harvard Medical School, Boston, Massachusetts

STACEY ROLAK, MD, MPH
Department of Internal Medicine, Mayo Clinic College of Medicine and Science,
Rochester, Minnesota

JOEL R. ROSH, MD
Goryeb Children's Hospital, Atlantic Children's Health, Morristown, New Jersey

DAVID T. RUBIN, MD
University of Chicago Medicine Inflammatory Bowel Disease Center, Section of
Gastroenterology, Hepatology, and Nutrition, University of Chicago Medical Center,
Chicago, Illinois

JENNIFER SEMINERIO, MD
Director of Inflammatory Bowel Disease, Assistant Professor of Medicine, University of
South Florida, The Carol and Frank Morsani Center, Tampa, Florida

CHUNG SANG TSE, MD
Inflammatory Bowel Disease Preceptorship, Division of Gastroenterology, University of
California, San Diego, La Jolla, California

VALERY VILCHEZ, MD
Department of Colorectal Surgery, Digestive Disease and Surgery Institute, Cleveland
Clinic, Cleveland, Ohio

Contents

Foreword   xiii

Alan L. Buchman

Preface: Some Thoughts About Crohn's Disease   xv

Sunanda V. Kane

Tools for the Diagnosis and Management of Crohn's Disease   213

Maté Gergely and Parakkal Deepak

Numerous tools have emerged over recent decades to aid in the increasingly complex management of patients with Crohn's disease (CD) beyond endoscopy, including video capsule endoscopy, magnetic resonance enterography, computed tomography enterography, a variety of biomarkers, and even wearable biosensors and smartphone applications. These tools have allowed for a more sophisticated and less invasive complementary approach to the evaluation of disease activity and treatment response in patients with CD. This article details the characteristics, practical application, and limitations of these various modalities and discusses how updated guidelines are now incorporating many of them into a treat-to-target strategy.

Mimics of Crohn's Disease   241

Sanchit Gupta and Jessica R. Allegretti

Crohn's disease is a chronic inflammatory disease that can affect any portion of the gastrointestinal tract. Associated symptoms can vary based on the severity of disease, extent of involvement, presence of extraintestinal manifestations, and development of complications. Diagnosis is based on a constellation of findings. Many diseases can mimic Crohn's disease and lead to diagnostic conundrums. These include entities associated with the gastrointestinal luminal tract, vascular disease, autoimmune processes, various infections, malignancies and complications, drug- or treatment-induced conditions, and genetic diseases. Careful consideration of possible causes is necessary to establish the correct diagnosis.

Conventional Therapies for Crohn's Disease   271

Stacey Rolak and Sunanda V. Kane

Crohn's disease is a chronic and progressive immune-mediated disease with increasing incidence worldwide. There are no curative therapies. The primary agents used in the treatment of Crohn's disease are aminosalicylates, corticosteroids, immunomodulators, and biologics. Each agent has different roles in the induction and maintenance of remission of disease. The biologics available include anti-TNF agents, anti-integrins, and anti-interleukins. The choice of initial biologic therapy should be determined through shared decision-making between the patient and provider.

Dual Advanced Therapies and Novel Pharmacotherapies for Moderately to Severely
Active Crohn's Disease   283

Chung Sang Tse and Parambir S. Dulai

Over the past 2 decades, there have been incredible advances in the phar-
macotherapeutic options for the treatment of patients with moderately to
severely active Crohn's disease. Despite the leaps and strides in safety, efficacy, and mechanistic specificity of treatment targets, a significant
portion (up to ~20–50%) of patients have refractory Crohn's disease ±
concomitant rheumatologic disease/extraintestinal manifestations for
which existing biologic and small molecule therapies are ineffective. In
this review, we will explore the available evidence for the use of dual
advanced therapies (combination of biologic and/or small molecule therapies) and novel pharmacotherapies in phase 2 to 3 clinical trials.

Therapeutic Drug Monitoring of Biologics in Crohn's Disease   299

Laurie B. Grossberg, Adam S. Cheifetz, and Konstantinos Papamichael

Reactive therapeutic drug monitoring (TDM) is considered the standard of
care for optimizing biologics in inflammatory bowel disease (IBD) including
Crohn's disease (CD). Preliminary data show that proactive TDM is associated with positive outcomes in IBD and can be also used to efficiently
guide therapeutic decisions in specific clinical scenarios. Higher biological
drug concentrations are associated with favorable therapeutic outcomes
in specific IBD populations or phenotypes including pediatric CD, perianal
fistulizing CD, small bowel CD, and following an ileocolonic resection for
CD. Future perspectives of TDM include the use of rapid testing, pharmacogenomics, and pharmacokinetic dashboards toward individualized
therapy.

Diet in the Pathogenesis and Management of Crohn's Disease   319

Phillip Gu and Linda A. Feagins

Crohn's disease (CD) is chronic immune-related disease of the gastrointestinal tract hypothesized to be caused by an interplay of genetic predis-
position and environmental exposures. With the global incidence
increasing, more patients are exploring dietary exposures to explain and
treat CD. However, most patients report minimal nutritional education
from their provider, and providers report few nutritional resources to
help them educate patients. This highlights the previous deficit of literature
describing the role and influence of diet in CD. To address this need, this
article reviews available literature on the possible roles of diet in the pathogenesis, exacerbation, and treatment of CD.

Complementary and Alternative Medicine in Crohn's Disease   337

Jennifer Seminerio

Complementary and alternative medicine (CAM) is a growing entity within
inflammatory bowel disease (IBD). CAM includes mind-based therapies,
body-based therapies, supplements, vitamins, and probiotics. Limitations
currently exist for health care providers as it pertains to IBD and CAM that
stem from knowledge gaps, conflicting reports, limited oversight, and a
lack of well-organized clinical data. Even without well-described data,

patients are turning to these forms of therapy at increasing rates. It is imperative that the ongoing review of CAM therapies is performed, and future trials are performed to better understand efficacy as well as adverse effects related to these therapies.

Surgical Management of Crohn's Disease   353

Valery Vilchez and Amy L. Lightner

Treatment of Crohn's disease (CD) focuses on providing acceptable quality of life for the affected individual by optimizing medical therapy, endoscopic procedures, and surgical intervention. Biologics have changed the medical management of moderate to severe CD. However, despite their introduction, the need for surgical resection in CD has not drastically changed, with two-thirds of the patients still requiring an intestinal resection. Patient outcomes are optimized by focusing on preoperative management and intraoperative technical aspects to maximize bowel preservation. This article reviews some of the important principles of Crohn's surgery to help guide surgeons when approaching this challenging patient population.

Intestinal Cancer and Dysplasia in Crohn's Disease   369

Scott Friedberg and David T. Rubin

Crohn's disease is associated with an increased risk of adenocarcinoma of the involved portions of the small bowel and colorectum and has similar risk factors to those described in ulcerative colitis, most significantly, extent of bowel involvement, PSC, and duration of unresected disease. Prevention strategies include risk stratification and secondary prevention with colonoscopic screening and surveillance to identify dysplasia or early-stage cancers, with surgery when needed. There is emerging information to suggest that control of inflammation may provide primary prevention of neoplasia, but further studies are required to test this strategy.

Fertility and Pregnancy in Crohn's Disease   381

Rishika Chugh and Jill K.J. Gaidos

The prevalence of inflammatory bowel disease is continuing to increase worldwide and is more commonly diagnosed in women of reproductive age. Individuals with Crohn's disease may have inaccurate perceptions regarding the rate of infertility, heritability, and the safety of taking therapies for Crohn's disease during pregnancy, all of which greatly affect their decisions surrounding family planning. Given this area of need for both patients and providers, in this article, we have included the latest evidence on the impact of Crohn's disease on fertility, heritability, pregnancy outcomes, and the safety of medications for Crohn's disease during pregnancy and lactation.

Pediatric Management of Crohn's Disease   401

Elana B. Mitchel and Joel R. Rosh

Pediatric Crohn's disease is often more severe, requires higher levels of immunosuppression, and is associated with greater morbidity compared with adult Crohn's disease. Unique considerations in pediatric Crohn's disease include growth impairment, pubertal delay, bone disease, longevity of disease burden, and psychosocial impact. Treatment options are limited, requiring off-label use of therapy in this challenging patient population. Understanding the medications available, the existing evidence supporting their use, and side effects is important. There is tremendous potential for growth and improvement in this field and it is essential that all gastroenterologists have an understanding of this complex and unique patient population.

Crohn's Disease of the Elderly: Unique Biology and Therapeutic Efficacy and Safety   **425**

Simon J. Hong, Jonathan Galati, and Seymour Katz

The incidence and prevalence of inflammatory bowel disease (IBD) is increasing in the elderly population. Compared with patients with onset during younger years, patients with elderly-onset IBD have a distinct clinical presentation, disease phenotype, and natural history. Genetics contribute less to pathogenesis of disease, whereas aging-related biological changes, such as immunosenescence and dysbiosis, are associated with elderly-onset IBD. Frailty is an increasingly recognized predictor of adverse outcomes. As an increasingly wider array of biologic and small molecule therapeutic options becomes available, data regarding efficacy and safety of these agents in patients are paramount given the unique characteristics of this population.

Health Care Maintenance in Patients with Crohn's Disease   **441**

Jana G. Hashash and Francis A. Farraye

Health care maintenance is critical for patients with inflammatory bowel disease (IBD), particularly for those receiving immunosuppressive medications. Vaccination recommendations for potentially preventable diseases, cancer prevention recommendations, and assessment of bone health and mood disorders are discussed in this article. Staying up to date with health care maintenance is of utmost importance, and all gastroenterologists caring for patients with IBD should be able to make recommendations regarding preventative care of these patients.

GASTROENTEROLOGY
CLINICS OF NORTH AMERICA

FORTHCOMING ISSUES

September 2022
Diagnosis and Treatment of Gastrointestinal Cancers
Marta L. Davila and Raquel E. Davila, *Editors*

December 2022
Psychogastroenterology
Laurie Keefer, *Editor*

March 2023
Management of Obesity, Part I: Overview and Basic Mechanisms
Lee M. Kaplan, *Editor*

RECENT ISSUES

March 2022
Pelvic Floor Disorder
Darren M. Brenner, *Editor*

December 2021
Diseases of the Esophagus
John O. Clarke, *Editor*

September 2021
Irritable Bowel Syndrome
William D. Chey, *Editor*

SERIES OF RELATED INTEREST

Gastrointestinal Endoscopy Clinics of North America
(Available at: https://www.giendo.theclinics.com)
Clinics in Liver Disease
(Available at: https://www.liver.theclinics.com)

Foreword

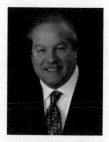

Alan L. Buchman, MD, MSPH
Consulting Editor

Some 20 years ago, Britney Spears sang "I cannot hold it! I cannot control it!" in the chorus of "I'm a Slave for You." That was largely the case for Crohn's disease at the time as well. We have learned so much, and we have come so far. We can now hold it, and we can control it—to some extent at least.

As Dr Kane points out in her preface, the true game-changer in the management of Crohn's disease was the development of biological therapies. A heightened index of suspicion for the disease and greater social awareness, coupled with new diagnostic modalities, now assists us in the earlier diagnosis of patients. We have learned though that the disease cannot be cured by surgery, and our goal is to preserve the bowel rather than remove all diseased bowel.

As much as we have learned in the past 20 years, we have that much more to learn. With greater knowledge comes additional questions and concerns. Our panacea, the biologic therapies, as game-changing as they may be, have finite lifespans, as inflammation adapts to their use over time. It is challenging to keep treatment development a step in front of treatment resistance.

We are finding that Crohn's disease is not one disease, but many—all of which historically we have treated all the same, with disparate results. Someday treatments will be tailored to individual patients with their unique cytokine patterns, and their individual Crohn's-like disease.

For many years it has been postulated that diet has had a significant role in the development as well as the treatment of Crohn's disease. Many think, as well as seemingly want, diet to be the cause, rather than the result of their disease, and manipulation to be the cure. That information is being refined, much like our diet, although there currently may be more that is not so that is so.

We've discovered Crohn's disease in areas of the world where it was previously unknown, even if it was not really unknown, but only unknown to us. Perhaps it was simply the result of a revolution in the availability and positioning of the endoscope and other imaging modalities rather than a change to the developed world's diet.

Gastroenterol Clin N Am 51 (2022) xiii–xiv
https://doi.org/10.1016/j.gtc.2022.04.002
0889-8553/22/© 2022 Published by Elsevier Inc.

We recognize that Crohn's has important and varied effects before and during pregnancy, where the health of the mother is of utmost importance. These effects are not limited to the mother but affect growth and development of the child.

We have learned that chronic inflammation and the constant need for healing may eventually result in uncontrolled cell growth, dysplasia, and malignancy.

Despite all of our gains in knowledge, Crohn's still remains a chronic and uncurable disease. As such, it has attracted a significant following in alternative medical therapy; some of which may be helpful and much of which is not, all of which however should be subject to the rigors of evidence-based medicine, something Western medicine aspires to but not infrequently fails itself to achieve.

All that being said, Dr Kane has assembled an outstanding group of authors that provides us with comprehensive up-to-date reviews of all contemporary diagnostic and treatment modalities and concerns for Crohn's disease, which of course are subject to continuous evolution as we unlearn what we find is not true and answer new questions on the basis of well-designed studies.

Alan L. Buchman, MD, MSPH
Intestinal Rehabilitation and Transplant Center
Department of Surgery/UI Health
University of Illinois at Chicago
840 South Wood Street
Suite 402 (MC958)
Chicago, IL 60612, USA

E-mail address:
a.buchman@hotmail.com

Preface
Some Thoughts About Crohn's Disease

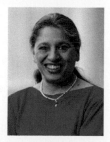

Sunanda V. Kane, MD, MSPH
Editor

The diagnosis, natural history, and management of Crohn's disease have changed substantially just during my career. We used to have only steroids, thiopurines, and surgery. The development of new imaging modalities, including enterography and video capsule, along with balloon endoscopy for tissue acquisition has advanced the way we diagnose and monitor patients with disease limited to the small bowel. The obvious game changer has been the introduction of biologics to our treatment strategies. It was a pipe dream to think that we could heal mucosa, and now we consider that standard of care. Surgical resection is performed less often, and length of stay after a surgery is now down to 2 to 3 days.

Within this issue, we explore the most up-to-date topics with regard to diagnosis, management, and monitoring. We understand so much more now in terms of the implications of our drug choices early on in diagnosis, how to avoid complications, and how to treat extraintestinal manifestations. In this issue, I have invited top experts in a variety of areas to review the latest literature and provide clinically useful and practical information.

Sunanda V. Kane, MD, MSPH
Division of Gastroenterology and Hepatology
Mayo Clinic Rochester
200 First Street SW
Rochester, MN 55905, USA

E-mail address:
Kane.sunanda@mayo.edu

Gastroenterol Clin N Am 51 (2022) xv
https://doi.org/10.1016/j.gtc.2022.04.001
0889-8553/22/© 2022 Published by Elsevier Inc.

Tools for the Diagnosis and Management of Crohn's Disease

Maté Gergely, MD, Parakkal Deepak, MBBS, MS*

KEYWORDS

- Treat-to-target • Endoscopy • Enterography • Small bowel Crohn's disease
- Biomarker

KEY POINTS

- Endoscopy remains a key tool in the initial diagnosis, prognostication, and longitudinal follow-up as part of a treat-to-target strategy in Crohn's disease.
- Cross-sectional imaging, using MR enterography, CT enterography and to a more limited extent bowel ultrasound, is an important complementary tool for the initial evaluation of disease activity and severity, and to monitor therapeutic response and assess radiologic healing in small bowel Crohn's disease.
- Biomarkers, where elevated at baseline, may play a limited complementary role in the serial noninvasive assessment of response to therapy in a treat-to-target approach in Crohn's disease.
- Video capsule endoscopy may be a useful adjunct to cross-sectional imaging, especially for the detection and longitudinal follow-up of proximal small bowel Crohn's disease.

INTRODUCTION

The management of Crohn's disease (CD) has become increasingly complex over recent years with the emergence of novel therapeutic agents. With the periodic requirement of dose and frequency adjustment of biologics or necessity of switching to a new mechanism because of the presence of drug antibodies, surveillance of response to these changes has become of utmost importance. Although endoscopic evaluation is the gold standard in the diagnosis and surveillance of CD, it is expensive and invasive. As a result of significant technological advances in the field within the past decades, many tools have emerged to aid in the management of these patients. Such tools include video capsule endoscopy (VCE), radiological tests such as magnetic resonance enterography (MRE) and computed tomography enterography

Division of Gastroenterology, Inflammatory Bowel Diseases Center, Washington University School of Medicine, 600 South Euclid Avenue, Campus Box 8124, Saint Louis, MO 63110, USA
* Corresponding author.
E-mail address: deepak.parakkal@wustl.edu

Gastroenterol Clin N Am 51 (2022) 213–239
https://doi.org/10.1016/j.gtc.2021.12.003
0889-8553/22/© 2021 Elsevier Inc. All rights reserved.

gastro.theclinics.com

(CTE), serum and stool biomarkers, and even emerging smartphone applications and wearable biosensors. These tools each have their unique advantages and limitations, and as such, are most effectively used in conjunction with one another. The focus of this article will be to discuss the unique characteristics, indications, limitations, and practical application of these various modalities.

ENDOSCOPY

Endoscopy has been integral to the diagnosis, management, and dysplasia surveillance in CD for many years. It can serve to (1) ensure a proper diagnosis while ruling out other disease processes, (2) monitor disease activity, (3) surveil for colon cancer, (4) manage strictures, and (5) assess for postsurgical complications. Moreover, endoscopic healing is an important long-term target in CD. With the advent of capsule endoscopy and various small bowel enteroscopy (SBE) techniques, the indications for endoscopy in CD are continuing to expand.

Colonoscopy with Ileoscopy

When inflammatory bowel disease (IBD) is suspected, colonoscopy with terminal ileal intubation should be performed in the initial phase of the evaluation.[1] This allows for direct visualization of the mucosa and for biopsy specimens to be obtained for a pathologist to review. A prospective study from 2008 demonstrated that colonoscopy was safe in patients with diagnosed or suspected IBD, with a major complication rate of less than 1%.[2] Relative contraindications to performing colonoscopy in this patient cohort are toxic megacolon and severe colitis. Nonsteroidal anti-inflammatory drugs (NSAIDs) and sodium-phosphate–based bowel preparation should be ideally avoided before performing ileocolonoscopy, because of the potential for causing mucosal changes which can mimic active IBD.[3,4] Biopsies should be obtained from both normal and affected mucosa, consisting of 2 biopsy specimens from at least 5 separate sites including the ileum and rectum.[5] Specimens from different locations should be submitted separately. It is crucial to perform colonoscopy before initiating a new treatment for IBD if possible. Once treatment is initiated, features of CD and ulcerative colitis (UC) can often be difficult to distinguish from one another. The most characteristic findings of CD on endoscopy include cobblestoned mucosa, aphthous ulcers, and discontinuous "skip lesions." The diagnostic accuracy of initial colonoscopy for differentiating between these 2 diseases was 89% in a prospective study.[6] On ileoscopy, up to 25% of patients with ulcerative pancolitis can have "backwash ileitis." Although this is best distinguished from CD histologically, findings favoring backwash ileitis include a short and continuous pattern of inflammation in the absence of stenosis, ulcerations, or strictures.[7]

Achievement of endoscopic mucosal healing as a treatment target has been associated with sustained remission and resection-free survival.[8] Even in the absence of clinical symptoms, mucosal inflammation is associated with long-term disease progression.[9] Although several endoscopic scoring systems exist, perhaps the 2 most commonly used are the SES-CD (simple endoscopic score in CD) and CDEIS (CD endoscopic index of severity).[10,11] Both have been used widely as end-points in clinical trials, though SES-CD is simpler to calculate and more suitable for practical application. It assesses across both inflammatory and stricturing phenotypic features in the ileum and colonic segments, assigning a score of 0 to 12 for each segment of bowel traversed (**Table 1**). Using these scoring systems, endoscopic response has been defined as greater than 50% decrease in the SES-CD, whereas endoscopic remission is classified as SES-CD ≤2 points and lack of ulceration.[12]

Table 1
Simple endoscopic score in Crohn's disease (SES-CD)

Variable	0	1	2	3
Presence and size of ulcers	None	Aphthous ulcers (0.1–0.5 cm)	Large ulcers (0.5–2 cm)	Very large ulcers (>2 cm)
Extent of ulcerated surface	None	<10%	10%–30%	>30%
Extent of affected surface	Unaffected segment	<50%	50%–75%	>75%
Presence, number, and type of stenosis	None	Single, can be passed	Multiple, can be passed	Cannot be passed
Score = total of 5 segments	Ileum Right colon Transverse colon Left colon Rectum	SES-CD score interpretation	Inactive = 0–2 Mild activity = 3–6 Moderate activity = 7–15 Severe activity = ≥16	

Patients with CD who undergo ileocolonic or partial colonic resection are recommended to have a repeat colonoscopy in 6 to 12 months after surgery for evaluation of CD recurrence and anastomotic healing.[13] CD most often recurs at the surgical anastomosis and neoterminal ileum.[14] The Postoperative Crohn's Endoscopic Recurrence (POCER) randomized trial showed that postoperative endoscopic monitoring at 6 months after surgery with escalated therapy (in the event of endoscopic recurrence) proved superior to continued pharmacologic therapy in decreasing clinical and endoscopic recurrence rates.[15] The most significant factor in predicting postoperative

Table 2
Rutgeerts' score for the assessment of postoperative recurrence in CD

Score	Endoscopic Findings	Risk of Symptomatic Recurrence at 5 y
i0	No lesions in neo-TI	6%
i1	< 5 aphthous lesions in neo-TI	6%
i2	>5 aphthous lesions with normal mucosa, skip areas with larger lesions, anastomotic lesions	27%
i3	Diffuse aphthous ileitis	63%
i4	Diffuse inflammation with ulcer, nodules, and/or stenosis	100%

Abbreviations: CD, Crohn's disease; neo-TI, neoterminal ileum.

recurrence is active tobacco smoking. The Rutgeerts' score (not validated) assesses postsurgical risk of CD recurrence in the neoterminal ileum in patients who have undergone ileocolonic resection with anastomosis (**Table 2**) but does not measure colonic disease activity.[16]

Surveillance colonoscopy for prevention of colorectal cancer (CRC) is recommended starting at 8 years for patients with at least 30% colonic involvement.[17] The exception is IBD patients with coexistent primary sclerosing cholangitis (PSC), in whom yearly surveillance should be initiated at the time of PSC diagnosis regardless of disease distribution. The AGA Clinical Practice Update best practice advice recommends virtual chromoendoscopy as a suitable alternative to dye spray chromoendoscopy (DCE) for dysplasia detection for surveillance when using high-definition white light endoscopy (HD-WLE), whereas DCE maybe suggested when working with standard definition WLE (SD-WLE).[17] Extensive nontargeted biopsies (roughly 4 adequately spaced biopsies every 10 cm) are recommended when using HD-WLE is used without DCE or virtual chromoendoscopy or if there is a history of dysplasia or PSC.[17]

After a negative screening colonoscopy, surveillance colonoscopy should be performed every 1 to 5 years based on risk factors for CRC as shown in **Table 3**.[17]

Table 3
Timing of next surveillance colonoscopy when no dysplasia detected at present colonoscopy

Risk Stratification	Characteristics	Next Surveillance Interval (y)
Higher Risk	• Moderate or severe inflammation (any extent) • Family history of CRC in first degree relative age <50 y • Dense pseudopolyposis • History of invisible dysplasia or higher-risk visible dysplasia < 5 y ago • History of PSC	1
Intermediate Risk	• Mild inflammation (any extent) • Strong family history of CRC (but no first degree relative < age 50 y) • Features of prior severe colitis (moderate pseudopolyposis, extensive mucosal scarring) • History of invisible dysplasia or higher-risk visible dysplasia >5 y ago • History of lower risk visible dysplasia < 5 y ago	2–3
Lower Risk	Continuous disease remission since last colonoscopy with mucosal healing on current examination, plus either of: • ≥ 2 consecutive examinations without dysplasia • Minimal historical colitis extent (ulcerative proctitis or < 1/3 of colon in CD)	5

Guidance for endoscopic severity, Simple Endoscopic Score for Crohn's (SES-CD). Moderate-Severe: SES-CD ≥ 7; Mild: SES-CD 3 to 6; No active disease: SES-CD 0 to 2.
Abbreviations: CD, Crohn's disease; CRC, colorectal cancer; PSC, primary sclerosing cholangitis.

Flexible Sigmoidoscopy

Flexible sigmoidoscopy is inadequate for evaluation of the proximal colon but may be used preferentially in patients with severe CD of the colon who are considered high-risk for a full colonoscopy. It can also be useful to rule out a superimposed etiology of colitis (eg, *Clostridium difficile*, cytomegalovirus, or ischemic colitis) in patients who have persistent or progressive disease not responding to medical therapy.[1]

Esophagogastroduodenoscopy

Upper GI tract involvement can occur in up to 16% of patients with CD.[18] Esophago-gastroduodenoscopy (EGD) is not recommended routinely in the diagnostic evaluation of CD unless patients specifically have upper GI complaints.[19] Endoscopic findings include aphthous lesions, ulcers, strictures, erythema, and fistulas.[18] A minimum of 2 biopsies from the esophagus, stomach, and duodenum should be obtained for suspected CD.[20] EGD can be useful for balloon dilation of isolated short segment (≤5 cm) fibrostenotic strictures without adjacent fistulization or perforation and should be considered as first-line therapy.[21] It is most effective in short strictures with minimal inflammation, straight angle, and related to a single surgical anastomosis.[22]

Video Capsule Endoscopy

Up to 20% of patients have small bowel (SB) disease not reachable by ileocolono-scopy.[23] Wireless VCE is a noninvasive tool, which was approved in 2001, and is an effective modality for evaluating the SB. A recent meta-analysis showed that its overall diagnostic yield in detecting active SB CD is similar to an MRE but superior in detecting proximal SB disease.[24] Its diagnostic yield has been found to be significantly higher for detecting suspected or known CD compared with a CTE.[25] Findings on VCE, which suggest CD, include erythema, erosions, ulceration, strictures, and villous

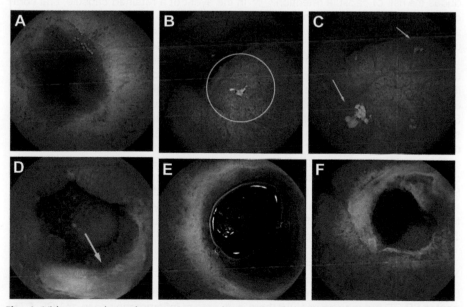

Fig. 1. Video capsule endoscopy images diagnostic of small bowel Crohn's disease. (*A*) Villous atrophy in the jejunum. (*B*) Aphthous ulcer. (*C*) Multiple aphthous ulcers. (*D*) Ulceration. (*E*) Circumferential stenosis that was traversed. (*F*) Circumferential stenosis with ulceration.

Table 4
Lewis score

	Number	Extent	Descriptors
Villous appearance (worst-affected tertile)	• Normal - 0 • Edematous - 1	• ≤10% - 8 • 11% to 50% - 12 • >50% - 20	• Single - 1 • Patchy - 14 • Diffuse - 17
Ulcer (worst-affected tertile)	• None - 0 • Single - 3 • 2 to 7 - 5 • ≥810	• ≤10% - 5 • 11% to 50% - 10 • >50% - 15	• < 1/4 - 9 • 1/4 to 1/2 - 12 • >1/2 – 18 (% *Frame occupied by largest ulcer*)
Stenosis (entire study)	• None - 0 • Single - 14 • Multiple - 20	• Nonulcerated - 2 • Ulcerated - 24	• Traversed - 7 • Not traversed - 10

atrophy (**Fig. 1**).[26] Its major limitations include the potential for capsule retention, inability to obtain tissue samples or perform therapeutic intervention, and the lack of standardized diagnostic criteria for diagnosing CD on VCE.[1] Multiple etiologies can mimic the appearance of SB CD, including NSAID enteropathy, SB ischemia, infectious enteritis, and radiation injury.[26] To limit misdiagnosis, NSAID use is recommended to be discontinued 1 to 2 months before performing VCE.[27] Capsule retention due to strictures can occur in up to 3.5% (95% confidence interval [CI], 2.7%–4.5%) of adult patients with CD.[28] A patency capsule or SB imaging study (MRE, CTE, or SB follow-through) is recommended before VCE in patients with diagnosed CD, which reduces the risk of capsule retention.[27,28] In the event of a retained capsule, oral corticosteroids can be tried, failing which a balloon-assisted enteroscopy (BAE) may be attempted, though surgery may ultimately be required if these efforts are unsuccessful.[1]

Two scoring systems have emerged that aim to standardize the description of lesions using VCE: the Lewis Score and the Capsule Endoscopy Crohn's Disease Activity Index (CECDAI). The Lewis score (**Table 4**) has been validated for clinical practice[29] and a software is now available for its automated calculation. It consists of dividing the SB into 3 equal parts (tertiles) based on SB capsule transit time and assigning a subscore to each tertile based on the degree of edema or ulceration. The sum of the worst affected tertile is then added to a stenosis score, which takes into consideration the entire examined SB.[30] The CECDAI or Niv score (**Box 1**) is another prospectively validated scoring system,[31] which sums up the score in the proximal and distal portions of SB (based on transit time) across the 3 parameters of inflammation, disease extent, and strictures.[32] Although no clear cut-off for inflammatory severity has been validated for the CECDAI score, the values of 3.8 and 5.8 correlate approximately to the 135 and 790 cut-offs of the Lewis score, respectively.

Small Bowel Enteroscopy

SBE with push or BAE is not recommended for routine evaluation of patients with suspected SB CD but may be useful if there is an area of inflammation seen on VCE, CTE, or MRE, which cannot be sampled by traditional EGD or colonoscopy, or for the purposes of SB stricture dilation or retrieval of an impacted VCE.[33,34] Using a retrograde approach, a modification of the SES-CD has been developed for the SB, known as the

---

Box 1
Capsule endoscopy Crohn's disease activity index

A. Inflammation Score
    0 = None
    1 = Mild to moderate edema/hyperemia/denudation
    2 = Severe edema/hyperemia/denudation
    3 = Bleeding, exudate, aphthae, erosion, small ulcer (<0.5 cm)
    4 = Moderate ulcer (0.5–2 cm), pseudopolyp
    5 = Large ulcer (>2 cm)

B. Extent of Disease Score
    0 = No disease (normal examination)
    1 = Focal disease (single segment involved)
    2 = Patchy disease (2–3 segments involved)
    3 = Diffuse disease (>3 segments involved)

C. Stricture Score
    0 = None
    1 = Single (traversed)
    2 = Multiple (traversed)
    3 = Obstruction (nontraversed)

Segmental score (proximal or distal) = (A x B) + C.

Total score = proximal ([A x B] + C) + distal ([A x B] + C)

Simple Endoscopic Active Score for CD (SES-CDa).[35] The SB is divided into 3 segments: terminal ileum; proximal ileum; and jejunum, where the length of SB is measured using the number of strokes of the overtube. The terminal ileum is defined as the segment ≤10 cm, proximal ileum 10 to 300 cm, and jejunum greater than 300 cm from the ileocecal valve. Using the SES-CDa, 139 patients with CD were prospectively followed after BAE and MRE procedures, demonstrating that MRE is a valid and reliable noninvasive examination both for cross-sectional evaluations and prognostic prediction (longitudinal responsiveness kappa coefficient BAE vs MRE 0.754 [95% CI, 0.658–0.850] for clinical relapse and 0.783 [95% CI, 0.701–0.865] for serologic relapse).[35]

HISTOLOGY

Mucosal biopsies from patients with CD demonstrate patchy or focal inflammation with possible crypt distortion. Granulomatous inflammation is seen in only approximately 50% of CD patients[36] and upper GI specimens are more likely to contain granulomas (40%–68%) than colonic specimens.[37] There can be challenges in distinguishing CD and UC, as patients with UC can have "backwash ileitis," cryptolytic granulomas, and patchy inflammation in partially treated disease.[19,36] In addition, presentation of other colitides can mimic that of IBD. These entities include infectious colitis, ischemic colitis, drug-induced colitis, and segmental colitis associated with diverticulosis.[38] Histology provides an important means of differentiating these disease processes.

The development of validated histologic scoring systems in CD has been challenging in part due to the segmental, transmural nature of inflammation in CD giving rise to the possibility of sampling error. In addition, limited data exist for determining which histologic features serve best to assess active inflammation and whether this correlates with clinical outcomes compared with endoscopy.[39,40] The STRIDE II initiative currently recommends against using histologic remission as a formal treatment target in CD for various reasons: a lack of reliable and well-validated tools to assess histology, insufficient data to rationalize intensifying therapy based on this goal, and current medical therapies having limited efficacy at achieving histologic remission.[12]

RADIOLOGY
Plain Film Radiography

The role of abdominal x-ray is very limited in the evaluation of CD given that it lacks the sensitivity required to evaluate disease severity and does not provide information regarding mural changes or extramural complications.[41] It continues to serve a role, however, in the first-line evaluation of acute pathology such as intestinal obstruction, characterized by dilated bowel loops with air-fluid levels, or perforation, evidenced by the presence of free air.[41] For evaluation of a perforation, both upright and supine views are recommended; in patients who cannot stand upright, the left lateral decubitus view is most optimal. Plain film can also be useful in identifying toxic megacolon, which is more commonly seen in UC than CD, and can be identified by colonic dilation greater than 6 cm accompanied by clinical signs of toxicity.

SB Enteroclysis

SB enteroclysis was previously a key technique in detecting stenosis and wall thickening in CD. The traditional fluoroscopic technique requires overnight fasting followed by an orally administered contrast administered through a nasojejunal tube.[42] Its use has significantly declined because of lower sensitivity when compared with CTE and MRE. CT enteroclysis has an increased sensitivity at detecting subtle partial obstruction compared with CTE. It is useful if CTE is negative and there remains a high clinical suspicion for obstruction secondary to adhesive disease.[43]

Computed Tomography and Magnetic Resonance Enterography

CTE and MRE are widely used in the evaluation of SB CD. CTE and MRE have a reported sensitivity and specificity greater than 90% for detecting lesions associated with CD (**Table 5**).[41] Characteristic features of active inflammation on CTE or MRE include various bowel wall features, penetrating complications, and mesenteric findings (**Table 6** and **Fig. 2**).[44,45] Given the similar sensitivity and specificity of CTE and MRE across the detection of inflammation and complications of CD (as shown in **Table 5**), MRE is preferred over CTE in patients younger than 35 years and in patients who will likely require serial imaging studies.[46] Such patients include those with persistently active SB CD, active smoking, elevated C-reactive protein (CRP) in the absence

Table 5
Performance characteristics of CT and MR enterography in Crohn's disease

	CT Enterography		MR Enterography	
	Sensitivity	Specificity	Sensitivity	Specificity
Inflammation	>90%	>90%	>90%	>90%
Stricture	85%–93%	100%	75%–100%	91%–100%
Internal penetrating disease	70%	97%	76%	96%
Intraabdominal abscess	85%	87.5%–95%	86%	93%

Abbreviations: CT, computed tomography; MR, magnetic resonance.

Table 6 Enterography features of small bowel Crohn's disease		
Bowel wall features	Segmental mural hyperenhancement	Asymmetric Stratified (bilaminar or trilaminar) Homogeneous, symmetric
	Wall thickening	Mild (3–5 mm) Moderate (6–9 mm) Severe (>10 mm)
	Stricture	Probable stricture without upstream dilation (<3 cm) Stricture with mild upstream dilation (3–4 cm) Stricture with moderate to severe upstream dilation (>4 cm)
	Intramural edema Ulcerations Restricted diffusion Sacculations Diminished motility	
Penetrating disease	Sinus tract	
	Fistula	Simple[a] Complex[b]
	Inflammatory mass Abscess Free perforation	
Mesentery findings	Perienteric edema and/or inflammation Engorged vasa recta Fibrofatty proliferation Mesenteric venous thrombosis and/or occlusion Lymphadenopathy	

Abbreviation: CD, Crohn's disease.
[a] Simple fistulas are characterized by a superficial or low origin in relation to the sphincter complex, single external opening, and absence of perianal abscess, rectovaginal fistula, or anorectal stricture.
[b] Complex fistulas are characterized by a high origin in relation to the sphincter complex, multiple external openings, and/or association with a perianal abscess, rectovaginal fistula, or anorectal stricture.

of clinical symptoms, and those with a penetrating phenotype at initial diagnosis.[33] The indications for usage, advantages, and disadvantages of CTE and MRE are discussed in **Table 7**.

Numerous MR scoring systems have been developed to determine disease activity in CD, including the Magnetic Resonance Index of Activity (MaRIA) score, London score, Nancy score, and Clermont score, as shown in **Table 8**.[41] There is no standardization regarding which score to use. Of these scoring systems, the MaRIA score is best characterized and accurately predicts response to therapy in CD.[47] Perhaps the primary drawback of the MaRIA score is that it can underestimate disease severity in patients who have SB CD proximal to the terminal ileum. In addition, it is complex and cumbersome to calculate. Consequently, a simplified MaRIA (MaRIAs) has been recently developed and validated.[48] It consists of 3 parameters from the MaRIA (mural thickening, mural edema, and mucosal ulcerations), and fat stranding, a new

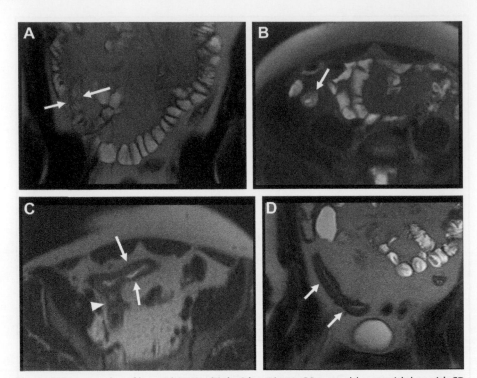

Fig. 2. MRE examples of low-risk versus high-risk patients. 30-year-old man with low-risk CD. Coronal T2-weighted image (*A*) and axial T2-weighted image with fat suppression (*B*) show a short segment of active inflammation involving the TI (*arrows*), without stricture, penetrating dx, or abscess. 26-year-old man with high-risk CD. Axial and T2-weighted image ((*C*) and (*D*), respectively) show a long segment of active inflammation involving the terminal and distal ileum (*arrows*), with perienteric soft tissue and tethering of the adjacent sigmoid suspicious for fistulization (*arrowhead*). (*From* Deepak P, Ludwig DR, Fidler JL, Guglielmo FF, Bruining DH. Medical and Endoscopic Management of Crohn's Disease. Top Magn Reson Imaging. 2021 Feb 1;30(1):43-61; with permission)

parameter. MaRIAs has been shown to accurately identify segments of disease activity using SES-CD as standard of reference.[49] In addition, a strong correlation was found between MaRIAs and CDEIS (r = 0.83) and between MaRIAs and the original MaRIA (r = 0.93).[49]

Perianal Fistula Protocol MRI of the Pelvis

Perianal fistulas can be seen in up to one-third of patients with CD, with most patients requiring medical or surgical management in their disease course.[50] A dedicated perianal fistula protocol MRI of the pelvis is important in initial treatment planning in perianal fistulizing CD (CD-PAF) and subsequently to assess treatment response of the fistulas in the perianal region.[51] It has a high sensitivity and specificity for detecting fistula tracts and abscesses, and allows for detailed assessment of the relationship between the fistula tract and pelvic floor structures.[52] MR may help to image a fistula that may be missed at a physical examination or even during an examination under anesthesia, including in the low rectum and above the sphincter complex (**Fig. 3**). The MRI pelvis protocol can be performed alone or paired with an MRE (as additional dedicated sequences) at a single visit. Studies have shown that preoperative pelvic MR changes

Table 7
Imaging modalities, indications, advantages, and disadvantages in Crohn's disease

Imaging Modality	Indications	Advantages	Disadvantages
Plain film radiography	Useful to assess obstruction and perforation as clinical presentations	- Universal availability - Very short examination time - Low cost	- Lacks sensitivity for defining disease severity - Does not provide information about mural changes or extramural complications
CT CT abdomen/pelvis CTE	• Assessment of severity and length of active CD in small bowel • Assessment of stricturing CD in small bowel and colon • Assessment of extraluminal complications including internal penetrating disease, inflammatory collections, and abscesses and to guide abscess drainage • Evaluate response to medical therapy in comparison to pretreatment images	• Generally, universal availability • Short examination time • Assess luminal and extraluminal complications • Detailed cross-sectional images	• Radiation exposure is of concern particularly in children. • Requires intravenous contrast (may not be appropriate in those with allergic reactions or renal insufficiency) • IV contrast limitation in renal disease
Magnetic Resonance MRE DWI MRI pelvis fistula protocol	• Assessment of severity and length of active CD in small bowel • Assessment of coexisting stricturing disease CD in small bowel and colon • Assessment of extraluminal complications including internal penetrating disease, inflammatory collections, and abscesses	• No radiation exposure, preferred over CTE for serial monitoring of disease activity and response to therapy • Detailed imaging with qualitative and quantitative analysis	• Limited prospective data demonstrating utility in this indication • Variable availability and insurance coverage in the community • IV contrast limitation in renal disease and pregnancy, maybe overcome with DWI sequences with T2-weighted sequences.

(continued on next page)

Table 7 (continued)			
Imaging Modality	**Indications**	**Advantages**	**Disadvantages**
	• Evaluate response to medical therapy in comparison to pretreatment images, preferred over CTE for serial monitoring of small bowel CD • Initial evaluation of perianal CD, guide management and follow-up after initial management		• DWI sequences can be heterogenous between scanners and examinations, not recommended as sole sequence. • Contraindicated with metal implants
Ultrasound Elastography CEUS SICUS	• Useful in centers with appropriate expertise in bowel ultrasound • Primarily useful to evaluate disease activity in terminal ileum and colonic CD as point of care testing. • Potential role for serial monitoring of response to therapy in select patients	• Low cost • Radiation-free	• Degree of correlation with inflammation not well defined • Highly operator-dependent • Limited by body habitus and bowel gas content

Abbreviations: CD, Crohn's disease; CEUS, contrast-enhanced ultrasound; CT, computed tomography; CTE, computed tomography enterography; DWI, diffusion-weighted imaging; IV, intravenous; MRE, magnetic resonance enterography; SICUS, small intestine contrast ultrasonography.

surgical management in up to 15% of patients.[52] MR findings consistent with CD-PAF include disruption of the normal T2 intermediate signal of the internal sphincter, with fluid-filled patent tracts demonstrating T2 hyperintensity, enhancement, and diffusion restriction (**Fig. 4**).[43]

Van Assche and colleagues developed an MR-based index in 2003 to evaluate the clinical behavior of perianal fistulizing CD before and after treatment with infliximab.[53] The Van Assche Index (VAI) consists of criteria for both local extension of fistulas and active inflammation (**Table 9**), and has been shown to correlate well with the degree of clinical severity in perianal CD.[54] Subsequently, T1 hyperintensity was shown to be a better indicator of fistula activity than T2 hyperintensity and was added to create the modified Van Assche index (mVAI) in 2011, which was shown to provide accurate assessment of the internal details of fistula tracts.[55] In addition, the MR novel index for fistula imaging in CD (MAGNIFI-CD) was recently developed, which has improved inter-rater reliability and responsiveness compared with the VAI and mVAI.[56] In

Table 8
Scoring systems using MRI for assessment of disease activity in Crohn's disease

	MaRIA[1-3]	Simplified MaRIA	CDMI[4]	MEGS[5,6]	Nancy[7,8]	Clermont[9-11]
Reference standard	Ileocolonoscopy (CDEIS)	Ileocolonoscopy (CDEIS)	Surgical specimen (AIS)	Extension of London score and correlated to clinical indices (HBI, fecal calprotectin, CRP, and CD activity score)	Ileocolonoscopy (SES-CD)	MaRIA
Validated	Yes	Yes	Yes	Yes	Yes	Yes
Responsive to treatment	Yes	Yes	No	Yes	Yes	Yes
Wall thickening	Yes	Yes	Yes	Yes	Yes	Yes
Enhancement	Yes (quantification of relative contrast enhancement)	Yes (qualitative evaluation)	Qualitative (4 different categories)	Qualitative (4 different categories)	Yes (qualitative evaluation)	Yes (qualitative evaluation)
High signal on T2	Yes (qualitative evaluation)	Yes (qualitative evaluation)	Yes (4 different categories)	Yes (4 different categories)	Yes (qualitative evaluation)	Yes (qualitative evaluation)
Ulcerations	Yes	Yes	–	–	Yes	Yes
T2 perimural signal	–	Yes	Yes (4 different categories)	Yes (4 different categories)	–	–
Mural stratification	–	–	–	–	Yes	–
Length of disease segment	–	–	–	Yes	–	–
Proximal small bowel disease assessed	–	–	–	–	–	Yes
Diffusion weighting imaging hyperintensity	–	–	–	–	Yes	Yes

Abbreviations: AIS, acute inflammation score; CD, Crohn's disease; CDEIS, Crohn's Disease Endoscopic Index of Severity; CDMI, Crohn's disease MRI index; CRP, C-reactive protein; HBI, Harvey-Bradshaw Index; MaRIA, magnetic resonance index of activity; MEGS, magnetic resonance enterography global score; SES-CD, simple endoscopic score for Crohn's disease.

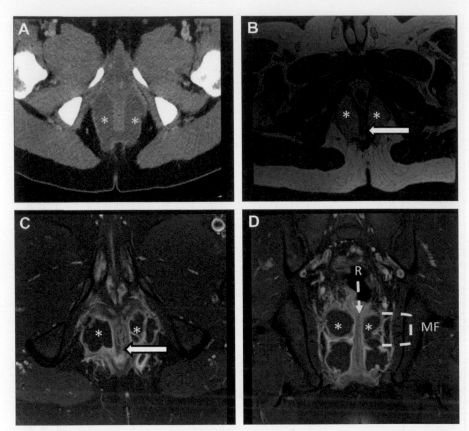

Fig. 3. Transsphincteric fistula tracts with horseshoe abscess and extensive involvement above the levator ani complex into the mesorectal fascia. 25-year-old man with perianal Crohn's disease, who initially presented to an outside hospital with a contrast-enhanced CT (*A*) demonstrating a large perirectal abscess (*). The delineations of its relationship, if any, to the sphincter complex were not well delineated on that CT examination. MR examination with turbo spin-echo T2 axial image (*B*) demonstrates a transsphincteric fistula feeding this large perirectal abscess (*arrow* in *B*). Identification of the fistulous tract (*arrow* in *C*) is more conspicuous with views of fat-saturated T1-weighted postcontrast axial image (*C*). Coronal T1-weighted postcontrast image (*D*) demonstrates the abscess extension into the mesorectal fascia ("MF" with bracket in D) to abut the rectum ("R" with dashed *arrow* in *D*). (*From* Abushamma S, Ballard DH, Smith RK, Deepak P. Multidisciplinary management of perianal Crohn's disease. Curr Opin Gastroenterol. 2021 Jul 1;37(4):295-305; with permission)

contrast with other indexes, MAGNIFI-CD includes the number and length of fistulas and omits proctitis, which is not directly associated with disease severity but may predict eventual nonhealing of fistulas. External validation of this novel index is still needed.

Bowel Ultrasound

Bowel ultrasound has become increasingly used to assess CD activity. Its strengths include that it is nonionizing, noninvasive, widely available, and relatively inexpensive

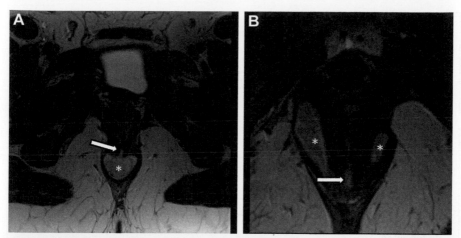

Fig. 4. Transsphincteric fistula tracts with horseshoe abscess. 18-year-old woman with peri-anal Crohn's disease. (*A, B*) Turbo spin-echo axial T2 axial images demonstrate a transsphinc-teric fistula (*arrows*) with horseshoe abscess (yellow *) interdigitating about the puborectalis muscle. A demonstrates the most confluent portion of the horseshoe abscess, whereas B demonstrates the violation of the internal sphincter. (*From* Abushamma S, Ballard DH, Smith RK, Deepak P. Multidisciplinary management of perianal Crohn's disease. Curr Opin Gastroenterol. 2021 Jul 1;37(4):295-305; with permission)

(see **Table 7**).[41] In addition, it can be used in real-time and is much more readily accepted and tolerated by patients than MRE or colonoscopy.[57] Point-of-care bowel ultrasound (POCBUS) has been incorporated into routine IBD assessment in many European centers, and has been shown to be accurate in defining disease activity and extent compared with ileocolonoscopy.[58] POCBUS consists of scanning the entire abdomen systematically with various frequency probes. A panoramic view is provided by convex probes at low frequency, whereas more detailed images are supplied by linear or microconvex probes at higher frequencies, displaying the 5 layers of the bowel wall.[59] Numerous parameters are used to evaluate disease activity, including the presence of bowel wall thickening, abnormal bowel wall pattern, increased bowel wall flow, ulcers, fistulas, abscesses, enlarged lymph nodes, and so forth.[59]

A recent prospective study of 225 CD patients used a bowel ultrasound score composed of wall thickness and wall flow to accurately predict a negative clinical course throughout a 12-month period.[60] Calabrese and colleagues also recently showed that bowel ultrasound can be used effectively in the tight control and monitoring of CD activity during different biologic therapies.[61] In addition, the sensitivity and specificity of bowel ultrasound can be increased with contrast agents administered orally (small intestine contrast US [SICUS]) or IV (contrast-enhanced US [CEUS]).[62] CEUS assesses the bowel wall microvasculature and adjacent perienteric tissues with greater precision than conventional ultrasound.[63] However, the use of contrast also limits its everyday use by increasing procedure duration and invasiveness. Several studies have shown a strong correlation between CEUS and clinical activity (using scores such as CDAI) and between CEUS and endoscopic activity.[63,64] In a prospective study, Laterza and colleagues recently showed CEUS to reliably predict endoscopic response and relapse within 1 year of anti-TNF therapy.[64]

Table 9
Scoring systems using MRI for the assessment of perianal fistulizing Crohn's disease

	Van Assche Index	Modified Van Assche Index	MAGNIFI-CD
Validated	Yes	Yes	Yes
Responsive to treatment	Yes	Yes	Unknown
Number of fistula tracts	Yes (qualitative, 4 different categories)	Yes (qualitative, 4 different categories)	Yes (quantitative evaluation)
Location	Yes (qualitative, 3 different categories)	Yes (qualitative, 3 different categories)	–
Extension	Yes	Yes	Yes
Hyperintensity on T1-weighted images	–	Yes	Yes
Hyperintensity on T2-weighted images	Yes	Yes	–
Inflammatory mass	Yes (qualitative, 3 different categories)	Yes (qualitative, 3 different categories)	Yes (qualitative, 6 different categories)
Proctitis	Yes (qualitative evaluation)	Yes (qualitative evaluation)	–
Dominant feature	–	–	Yes (qualitative, 3 different categories)

Abbreviations: CD, Crohn's disease; MAGNIFI-CD, magnetic resonance novel index for fistula imaging in CD.

BIOMARKERS
C-Reactive Protein

CRP is one the most widely used serum markers of inflammation in IBD. The utility of CRP is limited in that it may be elevated in other inflammatory disorders as well.[65] ESR is additionally affected by hematocrit, age, and pregnancy, reducing its accuracy and specificity in IBD.[66] A clear correlation exists between CRP levels and the degree of CD activity.[65] CRP has a short half-life of approximately 19 hours, making it more reliable at indicating acute inflammation than other acute phase reactants.[67] However, in 20% to 25% of patients with CD, CRP levels are normal because of the presence of a single nucleotide polymorphism in the CRP gene.[67] Assays for CRP can differ in their sensitivity, with normal cutoff values ranging from 0.8 mg/L for highly sensitive assays to 5 mg/L for standard assays.[66] A recent meta-analysis showed that patients with a CRP ≤0.5 mg/dL had a ≤1% probability of having IBD, whereas ESR did not have an adequate sensitivity to rule out IBD.[68] Normalization of CRP at 8 to 14 weeks into treatment has been associated with remission at 1 year.[69] CRP levels have also been shown to predict response and loss of response to anti-TNF treatment.[70] Decrease in CRP was also found to correlate with sustained response to infliximab in a post-hoc analysis of the ACCENT trial.[71]

Fecal Calprotectin

Fecal calprotectin (FC) is a sensitive and specific marker of inflammation, which is useful as a surrogate marker of disease activity. It is a cytosolic protein derived mainly from neutrophils and can be found in concentrations proportional to the degree of inflammation.[72] It has been shown to accurately differentiate between active and inactive IBD, though it has greater accuracy in UC than CD.[73] There have previously been concerns regarding its efficacy in detecting SB CD but a recent meta-analysis showed that an FC cutoff of 100 μg/g is effective at screening for SB CD.[74] Although cutoffs of 50 or 100 μg/g are often used by different assays, 100 to 250 is considered a "gray zone" given the low reliability of FC.[12] The STRIDE-II initiative recommends using normalization of FC (to 100–250 μg/g) and CRP as intermediate treatment targets in IBD, and to consider changing treatments if these targets have not been reached.[12] The CALM trial demonstrated that using FC and CRP in combination with clinical symptoms to guide escalation of treatment was associated with greater endoscopic healing than using clinical symptoms alone.[75] Although FC generally outperforms CRP, both a post-hoc analysis of the CALM trial and the MINI index demonstrated that using a combination of the two is superior to either one alone.[76,77] One study from 2015 showed that FC increases and remains elevated before clinical or endoscopic relapse.[78] Plevris and colleagues recently showed that normalization of FC within the first year of CD diagnosis is associated with a significantly lower risk of disease progression.[79]

There is also evidence that FC can predict the likelihood of relapse when considering withdrawal of treatment in certain patients. Indeed, the STORI study demonstrated that in patients with documented mucosal healing, discontinuing an anti-TFN in the setting of an elevated FC ($\geq$300 μg/g) was associated with a higher relapse rate (30%) when compared with patients who had lower FC levels.[80] It has also been found to be useful when monitoring for postoperative recurrence. In the POCER study, FC was significantly higher among patients who had endoscopic recurrence (Rutgeerts score $\geq$ i2), with a negative predictive value of 91% and area under the curve (AUROC) of 0.763.[15] By contrast, CRP and CDAI did not perform as well at predicting endoscopic recurrence (AUROC of 0.568 and 0.541, respectively).[15] The limitations of FC include variability between different assays and stool samples, interpatient variability, and lack of stability of samples at room temperature. It is therefore recommended to be collected as the first stool of the day and to be stored for no longer than 3 days at room temperature.[19]

Serologic Markers: ASCA, ANCA, Anti-CBir-1, and Anti-Omp-C

Serologic biomarkers have been studied extensively in IBD. Anti-Saccharomyces cerevisiae antibodies (ASCA) and perinuclear antineutrophilic cytoplasmic antibodies (pANCA) were found to have high sensitivity but low specificity for distinguishing the 2 diseases, wherein ASCA positivity is seen in 59.7% of those with CD and 13.6% with UC, whereas pANCA is positive in 49.7% of those with UC and 5.7% with CD.[81] Although there may be some utility in ordering these antibodies in undifferentiated IBD (IBD-U), their role as biomarkers for disease activity remains unclear and have no current role in diagnosing or ruling out IBD.[82] Still, ASCA positivity has been associated with a more aggressive CD phenotype[83] and higher likelihood of complications in pediatric CD patients.[84] Positivity for pANCA and antibodies to the bacterial flagellin C-Bir1 (anti-CBir-1) have been associated with a risk of pouchitis in patients undergoing ileoanal pouch surgery for UC.[85] Van Schaik and colleagues were able to predict the development of CD and UC in low-risk individuals using a

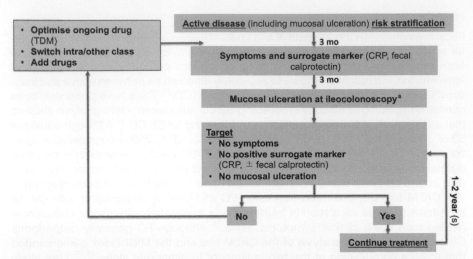

Fig. 5. Schematic representation of a treat-to-target strategy involving the assessment of intermediate and longer-term targets using biomarkers, endoscopy, and imaging per STRIDE II guidelines for Crohn's disease. [a]Or resolution of findings of inflammation on cross-sectional imaging in patients who cannot be adequately assessed with ileocolonoscopy. CRP, C-reactive protein; TDM, therapeutic drug monitoring.

combination of pANCA, ASCA, anti-CBir1, and the antibody to outer membrane porin C (OmpC).[86]

INTEGRATED USE IN CLINICAL PRACTICE

The STRIDE-II initiative recommends incorporating these various diagnostic tools into the management of patients with CD (**Fig. 5**). Although clinical response is considered an immediate treatment target, biomarkers, endoscopy, and imaging can serve important functions in the intermediate and long-term management of these patients.[12] Indeed, normalization of CRP to values under the upper limit of normal and FC to 100 to 250 µg/g is recommended as an intermediate treatment target, and changing therapy by dose/frequency escalation (partial response) or to a new mechanism-of-action (primary nonresponse) is recommended if these endpoints have not been reached. Some studies suggest that normalization of FC to 82 to 168 µg/g at weeks 12 to 14 after anti-TNF initiation is predictive of clinical remission and endoscopic healing.[87,88] Mucosal healing visualized by endoscopic examination is considered an important long-term target in CD and can be measured by an SES-CD less than 3 points or absence of ulcerations.[12] Treat-to-target approach requires an iterative approach using biomarkers every 3 months and endoscopy every 6 months until the target of mucosal healing is achieved. Following that, reassessment of the target is recommended every 1 to 2 years to maintain a "tight control," given the findings of the CALM study.

The STRIDE II initiative recommends assessing transmural healing (assessed by CTE, MRE, or bowel ultrasound) as an adjunct to mucosal healing confirmed by endoscopic remission in CD, to assess the depth of remission.[12] These imaging modalities, particularly MRE and POCBUS, allow for more frequent assessments than endoscopy and can visualize SB CD beyond the reach of a colonoscope, which is skipping the terminal ileum or is intramural.[23,89] Furthermore, improvement in radiologic

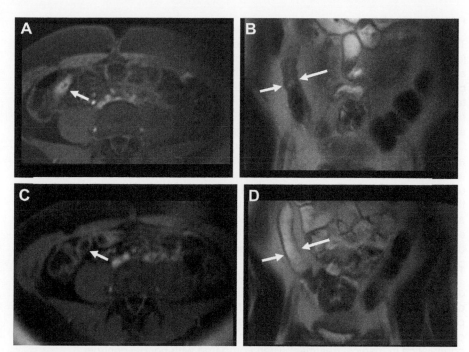

Fig. 6. Radiological response to therapy in small bowel Crohn's disease. 18-year-old woman with ileal CD with resolution of active inflammation on MRE after initiation of Humira and azathioprine. Pretreatment postcontrast T1-weighted (*A*) and coronal T2-weighted images (*B*) show hyperenhancement and mild to moderate wall thickening involving the terminal ileum (*arrows*). Following treatment, resolution of wall thickening (*C, D*). (*From* Deepak P, Ludwig DR, Fidler JL, Guglielmo FF, Bruining DH. Medical and Endoscopic Management of Crohn's Disease. Top Magn Reson Imaging. 2021;30(1):43-61. https://doi.org/10.1097/RMR. 0000000000000267; with permission)

parameters with CTE or MRE (**Fig. 6**) has been associated with improved clinical outcomes relating to hospitalizations, surgery, and steroid use.[90] In contrast, histologic healing has not been recommended as a treatment target because of a lack of well-validated and reliable scoring systems, current treatments having limited efficacy at reaching this endpoint, and lack of evidence suggesting that treatment intensification to this goal results in improved outcomes.[12]

The combined use of these targets is recommended to improve patient outcomes. Supporting evidence is provided by a post-hoc analysis of the CALM trial showing that combining CRP with FC is superior to either biomarker alone in predicting endoscopic healing at 48 weeks of treatment with adalimumab.[76] The MINI (Mucosal-Inflammation-Non-Invasively) Index also predicted endoscopic inflammation at higher rates when both FC and CRP were included, particularly when values of FC were between 100 and 600 mg/g.[77] Using the two in combination also improved the performance of the Utrecht Activity Index.[91] Numerous other studies suggest that the use of multiple targets together improves patient outcomes.[12] In a pediatric cohort, the use of a weighted pediatric CDAI in combination with FC was found to be superior than either alone in predicting deep healing in patients on infliximab.[92] Indeed, the tools available in the diagnosis and management of IBD should be considered complimentary rather than mutually exclusive.

FUTURE DIRECTIONS

There has been increasing interest in the utilization of smartphones applications (apps), activity wearable biosensors as tools to help monitor CD activity. The use of apps to monitor health has been shown to improve patient participation, increase security in their medical conditions, and improve perception regarding how well they are taken care of outside of the clinic.[93] Zhen and colleagues recently implemented an IBD health monitoring platform, HealthPROMISE, through which patients can track their symptoms, medications, quality of life scores (assessed by Short Inflammatory IBD Questionnaire [SIBDQ]), quality of care scores, clinic visits, emergency room visits, and hospitalizations.[94] The app also allows for patients to track longitudinal trends and for physicians to easily identify patients with suboptimal disease control. Patients using this app had significantly reduced ER visits and hospitalizations compared with the prior year and reported an increase in understanding of their condition.[94] There is also evidence that the use of wearable biosensors can help predict disease activity and hospital length of stay.[95,96] Patients with active disease were found to have fewer daily steps in the week before disease assessment, and daily steps were found to be predictive of disease activity.[96]

During the coronavirus disease 2019 (COVID-19) pandemic, there has been an increase in home-based point of care testing (eg, FC) and dried blood samples for drug monitoring, which have offered patients convenience and safety during the pandemic.[97] Östlund and colleagues recently found that home-based FC testing in conjunction with a digital app for symptom monitoring was associated with increased compliance in medical treatment when compared with normal controls.[98]

The PREDICTS trial found that it is possible to predict CD up to 5 years before diagnosis using a panel of 51 protein biomarkers.[99] The study was unable to replicate a predictive panel in UC. Recently, the first validated prognostic blood test was created from a gene-expression signature of CD8+ T cells in newly diagnosed patients with IBD.[100] It is currently being studied in the PROFILE trial, in which patients are assigned to different therapies based on their biomarker status.[100]

SUMMARY

Although endoscopic healing has been identified as a long-term treatment target in CD,[12] ileocolonoscopy is invasive, often poorly tolerated by patients, and often requires anesthesia. Consequently, various imaging studies, biomarkers, and scoring systems have been developed and are increasingly used in the diagnosis and management of CD. Each of these tools has its individual advantages and pitfalls. As such, these instruments are most effectively used in combination with one another, and there is increasing evidence that their integration results in improved outcomes. Several of them, including FC, CRP, SES-CD, enterography, and bowel ultrasound have been incorporated into the STRIDE II initiative as either formal treatment targets or adjunctive endpoints.[12] Tools in CD continue to become more sophisticated, with many new developments on the horizon including prognostic blood tests to guide individualized treatment, smartphone apps to track disease activity, wearable biosensors, home biomarker assays, and more.

DISCLOSURE

M. Gergely has nothing to disclose. P. Deepak has served as a consultant or on an advisory board for Janssen, Pfizer, Prometheus Biosciences, Boehringer Ingelheim, AbbVie, Arena Pharmaceuticals, and Scipher Medicine Corporation; he has also received funding under a sponsored research agreement unrelated to the data in the paper from Takeda Pharmaceutical, Arena Pharmaceuticals, Bristol-Myers Squibb, and Boehringer Ingelheim.

CLINICS CARE POINTS

- Endoscopic scoring systems such as the simple endoscopic score in Crohn's Disease (SES-CD) should be used regularly to assess disease activity and treatment response, and can be easily calculated using endoscopy documentation software.

- EGD is not routinely recommended for the evaluation of suspected Crohn's disease unless patients have specific upper GI symptoms but is useful for the dilation of short-segment fibrostenotic strictures.

- Cross-sectional imaging with CT or MR enterography or bowel ultrasound (depending on local expertise) is recommended at diagnosis in all patients with Crohn's disease to detect extent of disease activity and the presence of stricturing or penetrating complications. Serial monitoring with imaging should be utilized to assess complications of Crohn's disease or track small bowel disease activity.

- Fecal calprotectin is a useful surrogate marker of inflammation and is superior when used in combination with CRP.

- There is currently a very limited role for the use of serological markers in undifferentiated IBD.

REFERENCES

1. American Society for Gastrointestinal Endoscopy Standards of Practice C, Shergill AK, Lightdale JR, et al. The role of endoscopy in inflammatory bowel disease. Gastrointest Endosc 2015;81(5):1101–21.e1-3.
2. Terheggen G, Lanyi B, Schanz S, et al. Safety, feasibility, and tolerability of ileo-colonoscopy in inflammatory bowel disease. Endoscopy 2008;40(8):656–63.
3. Lawrance IC, Willert RP, Murray K. Bowel cleansing for colonoscopy: prospective randomized assessment of efficacy and of induced mucosal abnormality with three preparation agents. Endoscopy 2011;43(5):412–8.
4. Rejchrt S, Bures J, Siroky M, et al. A prospective, observational study of colonic mucosal abnormalities associated with orally administered sodium phosphate for colon cleansing before colonoscopy. Gastrointest Endosc 2004;59(6):651–4.
5. Mowat C, Cole A, Windsor A, et al. Guidelines for the management of inflammatory bowel disease in adults. Gut 2011;60(5):571–607.
6. Pera A, Bellando P, Caldera D, et al. Colonoscopy in inflammatory bowel disease. Diagnostic accuracy and proposal of an endoscopic score. Gastroenterology 1987;92(1):181–5.
7. Goldstein N, Dulai M. Contemporary morphologic definition of backwash ileitis in ulcerative colitis and features that distinguish it from Crohn disease. Am J Clin Pathol 2006;126(3):365–76.
8. Neurath MF, Travis SP. Mucosal healing in inflammatory bowel diseases: a systematic review. Gut 2012;61(11):1619–35.
9. Ungaro RC, Yzet C, Bossuyt P, et al. Deep Remission at 1 Year Prevents Progression of Early Crohn's Disease. Gastroenterology 2020;159(1):139–47.
10. Daperno M, D'Haens G, Van Assche G, et al. Development and validation of a new, simplified endoscopic activity score for Crohn's disease: the SES-CD. Gastrointest Endosc 2004;60(4):505–12.

11. Mary JY, Modigliani R. Development and validation of an endoscopic index of the severity for Crohn's disease: a prospective multicentre study. Groupe d'Etudes Therapeutiques des Affections Inflammatoires du Tube Digestif (GE-TAID). Gut 1989;30(7):983–9.

12. Turner D, Ricciuto A, Lewis A, et al. STRIDE-II: An Update on the Selecting Therapeutic Targets in Inflammatory Bowel Disease (STRIDE) Initiative of the International Organization for the Study of IBD (IOIBD): Determining Therapeutic Goals for Treat-to-Target strategies in IBD. Gastroenterology 2021;160(5):1570–83.

13. Nguyen GC, Loftus EV Jr, Hirano I, et al. American Gastroenterological Association Institute Guideline on the Management of Crohn's Disease After Surgical Resection. Gastroenterology 2017;152(1):271–5.

14. Rutgeerts P, Geboes K, Vantrappen G, et al. Natural history of recurrent Crohn's disease at the ileocolonic anastomosis after curative surgery. Gut 1984;25(6):665–72.

15. De Cruz P, Kamm MA, Hamilton AL, et al. Crohn's disease management after intestinal resection: a randomised trial. Lancet 2015;385(9976):1406–17.

16. Rutgeerts P, Geboes K, Vantrappen G, et al. Predictability of the postoperative course of Crohn's disease. Gastroenterology 1990;99(4):956–63.

17. Murthy SK, Feuerstein JD, Nguyen GC, et al. AGA clinical practice update on endoscopic surveillance and management of colorectal dysplasia in inflammatory bowel diseases: expert review. Gastroenterology 2021;161(3):1043–51.e4.

18. Annunziata ML, Caviglia R, Papparella LG, et al. Upper gastrointestinal involvement of Crohn's disease: a prospective study on the role of upper endoscopy in the diagnostic work-up. Dig Dis Sci 2012;57(6):1618–23.

19. Lamb CA, Kennedy NA, Raine T, et al. British Society of Gastroenterology consensus guidelines on the management of inflammatory bowel disease in adults. Gut 2019;68(Suppl 3):s1–106.

20. Paerregaard A. What does the IBD patient hide in the upper gastrointestinal tract? Inflamm Bowel Dis 2009;15(7):1101–4.

21. Chen M, Shen B. Endoscopic therapy in Crohn's disease: principle, preparation, and technique. Inflamm Bowel Dis 2015;21(9):2222–40.

22. Bessissow T, Reinglas J, Aruljothy A, et al. Endoscopic management of Crohn's strictures. World J Gastroenterol 2018;24(17):1859–67.

23. Samuel S, Bruining DH, Loftus EV Jr, et al. Endoscopic skipping of the distal terminal ileum in Crohn's disease can lead to negative results from ileocolonoscopy. Clin Gastroenterol Hepatol 2012;10(11):1253–9.

24. Kopylov U, Yung DE, Engel T, et al. Diagnostic yield of capsule endoscopy versus magnetic resonance enterography and small bowel contrast ultrasound in the evaluation of small bowel Crohn's disease: Systematic review and meta-analysis. Dig Liver Dis 2017;49(8):854–63.

25. Dionisio PM, Gurudu SR, Leighton JA, et al. Capsule endoscopy has a significantly higher diagnostic yield in patients with suspected and established small-bowel Crohn's disease: a meta-analysis. Am J Gastroenterol 2010;105(6):1240–8 [quiz: 1249].

26. Bourreille A, Ignjatovic A, Aabakken L, et al. Role of small-bowel endoscopy in the management of patients with inflammatory bowel disease: an international OMED-ECCO consensus. Endoscopy 2009;41(7):618–37.

27. Annese V, Daperno M, Rutter MD, et al. European evidence based consensus for endoscopy in inflammatory bowel disease. J Crohns Colitis 2013;7(12):982–1018.

28. Pasha SF, Pennazio M, Rondonotti E, et al. Capsule Retention in Crohn's Disease: A Meta-analysis. Inflamm Bowel Dis 2020;26(1):33–42.
29. Cotter J, Dias de Castro F, Magalhaes J, et al. Validation of the Lewis score for the evaluation of small-bowel Crohn's disease activity. Endoscopy 2015;47(4): 330–5.
30. Gralnek IM, Defranchis R, Seidman E, et al. Development of a capsule endoscopy scoring index for small bowel mucosal inflammatory change. Aliment Pharmacol Ther 2008;27(2):146–54.
31. Niv Y, Ilani S, Levi Z, et al. Validation of the Capsule Endoscopy Crohn's Disease Activity Index (CECDAI or Niv score): a multicenter prospective study. Endoscopy 2012;44(1):21–6.
32. Gal E, Geller A, Fraser G, et al. Assessment and validation of the new capsule endoscopy Crohn's disease activity index (CECDAI). Dig Dis Sci 2008;53(7): 1933–7.
33. Lichtenstein GR, Loftus EV, Isaacs KL, et al. ACG Clinical Guideline: Management of Crohn's Disease in Adults. Am J Gastroenterol 2018;113(4):481–517.
34. Takabayashi K, Hosoe N, Kato M, et al. Significance of endoscopic deep small bowel evaluation using balloon-assisted enteroscopy for Crohn's disease in clinical remission. J Gastroenterol 2021;56(1):25–33.
35. Takenaka K, Ohtsuka K, Kitazume Y, et al. Utility of Magnetic Resonance Enterography For Small Bowel Endoscopic Healing in Patients With Crohn's Disease. Am J Gastroenterol 2018;113(2):283–94.
36. Feakins RM, British Society of G. Inflammatory bowel disease biopsies: updated British Society of Gastroenterology reporting guidelines. J Clin Pathol 2013; 66(12):1005–26.
37. Rubio CA, Orrego A, Nesi G, et al. Frequency of epithelioid granulomas in colonoscopic biopsy specimens from paediatric and adult patients with Crohn's colitis. J Clin Pathol 2007;60(11):1268–72.
38. Chachu KA, Osterman MT. How to Diagnose and Treat IBD Mimics in the Refractory IBD Patient Who Does Not Have IBD. Inflamm Bowel Dis 2016;22(5): 1262–74.
39. Christensen B, Erlich J, Gibson PR, et al. Histologic healing is more strongly associated with clinical outcomes in ileal crohn's disease than endoscopic healing. Clin Gastroenterol Hepatol 2020;18(11):2518–25.e1.
40. Hu AB, Tan W, Deshpande V, et al. Ileal or colonic histologic activity is not associated with clinical relapse in patients with crohn's disease in endoscopic remission. Clin Gastroenterol Hepatol 2021;19(6):1226–33.e1.
41. Deepak P, Axelrad JE, Ananthakrishnan AN. The role of the radiologist in determining disease severity in inflammatory bowel diseases. Gastrointest Endosc Clin N Am 2019;29(3):447–70.
42. Biernacka KB, Baranska D, Grzelak P, et al. Up-to-date overview of imaging techniques in the diagnosis and management of inflammatory bowel diseases. Prz Gastroenterol 2019;14(1):19–25.
43. Deepak P, Sheedy SP, Lightner AL, et al. Chapter 7 - Role of Abdominal Imaging in the Diagnosis of IBD Strictures, Fistulas, and Postoperative Complications. In: Shen B, editor. Interventional inflammatory bowel disease: endoscopic management and treatment of complications. Cambridge, Massachusetts, USA: Academic Press; 2018. p. 79–95.
44. Guglielmo FF, Anupindi SA, Fletcher JG, et al. Small Bowel Crohn Disease at CT and MR enterography: imaging atlas and glossary of terms. Radiographics 2020;40(2):354–75.

45. Sandborn WJ, Fazio VW, Feagan BG, et al, American Gastroenterological Association Clinical Practice Committee. AGA technical review on perianal Crohn's disease. Gastroenterology 2003;125(5):1508–30.
46. Church PC, Turner D, Feldman BM, et al. Systematic review with meta-analysis: magnetic resonance enterography signs for the detection of inflammation and intestinal damage in Crohn's disease. Aliment Pharmacol Ther 2015;41(2):153–66.
47. Rimola J, Ordas I, Rodriguez S, et al. Magnetic resonance imaging for evaluation of Crohn's disease: validation of parameters of severity and quantitative index of activity. Inflamm Bowel Dis 2011;17(8):1759–68.
48. Ordas I, Rimola J, Alfaro I, et al. Development and Validation of a Simplified Magnetic Resonance Index of Activity for Crohn's Disease. Gastroenterology 2019;157(2):432–9.e1.
49. Roseira J, Ventosa AR, de Sousa HT, et al. The new simplified MARIA score applies beyond clinical trials: A suitable clinical practice tool for Crohn's disease that parallels a simple endoscopic index and fecal calprotectin. United Eur Gastroenterol J 2020;8(10):1208–16.
50. Adegbola SO, Dibley L, Sahnan K, et al. Burden of disease and adaptation to life in patients with Crohn's perianal fistula: a qualitative exploration. Health Qual Life Outcomes 2020;18(1):370.
51. Lee MJ, Parker CE, Taylor SR, et al. Efficacy of medical therapies for fistulizing crohn's disease: systematic review and meta-analysis. Clin Gastroenterol Hepatol 2018;16(12):1879–92.
52. Schwartz DA, Wiersema MJ, Dudiak KM, et al. A comparison of endoscopic ultrasound, magnetic resonance imaging, and exam under anesthesia for evaluation of Crohn's perianal fistulas. Gastroenterology 2001;121(5):1064–72.
53. Van Assche G, Vanbeckevoort D, Bielen D, et al. Magnetic resonance imaging of the effects of infliximab on perianal fistulizing Crohn's disease. Am J Gastroenterol 2003;98(2):332–9.
54. Kulkarni S, Gomara R, Reeves-Garcia J, et al. MRI-based score helps in assessing the severity and in follow-up of pediatric patients with perianal Crohn disease. J Pediatr Gastroenterol Nutr 2014;58(2):252–7.
55. Horsthuis K, Ziech ML, Bipat S, et al. Evaluation of an MRI-based score of disease activity in perianal fistulizing Crohn's disease. Clin Imaging 2011;35(5):360–5.
56. Hindryckx P, Jairath V, Zou G, et al. Development and Validation of a Magnetic Resonance Index for Assessing Fistulas in Patients With Crohn's Disease. Gastroenterology 2019;157(5):1233–44.e5.
57. Buisson A, Gonzalez F, Poullenot F, et al. Comparative acceptability and perceived clinical utility of monitoring tools: a nationwide survey of patients with inflammatory bowel disease. Inflamm Bowel Dis 2017;23(8):1425–33.
58. Sathananthan D, Rajagopalan A, Van De Ven L, et al. Point-of-care gastrointestinal ultrasound in inflammatory bowel disease: An accurate alternative for disease monitoring. JGH Open 2020;4(2):273–9.
59. Allocca M, Furfaro F, Fiorino G, et al. Point-of-care ultrasound in inflammatory bowel disease. J Crohns Colitis 2021;15(1):143–51.
60. Allocca M, Craviotto V, Bonovas S, et al. Predictive value of bowel ultrasound in crohn's disease: a 12-month prospective study. Clin Gastroenterol Hepatol 2021. https://doi.org/10.1016/j.cgh.2021.04.029.
61. Calabrese E, Rispo A, Zorzi F, et al. Ultrasonography tight control and monitoring in crohn's disease during different biological therapies: a multicenter

study. Clin Gastroenterol Hepatol 2021. https://doi.org/10.1016/j.cgh.2021.03.030.

62. Servais L, Boschetti G, Meunier C, et al. Intestinal conventional ultrasonography, contrast-enhanced ultrasonography and magnetic resonance enterography in assessment of crohn's disease activity: a comparison with surgical histopathology analysis. Dig Dis Sci 2021. https://doi.org/10.1007/s10620-021-07074-3.

63. Wong DD, Forbes GM, Zelesco M, et al. Crohn's disease activity: quantitative contrast-enhanced ultrasound assessment. Abdom Imaging 2012;37(3):369–76.

64. Laterza L, Ainora ME, Garcovich M, et al. Bowel contrast-enhanced ultrasound perfusion imaging in the evaluation of Crohn's disease patients undergoing anti-TNFalpha therapy. Dig Liver Dis 2021;53(6):729–37.

65. Sands BE. Biomarkers of Inflammation in Inflammatory Bowel Disease. Gastroenterology 2015;149(5):1275–85, e1272.

66. Mendoza JL, Abreu MT. Biological markers in inflammatory bowel disease: practical consideration for clinicians. Gastroenterol Clin Biol 2009;33(Suppl 3):S158–73.

67. Jones J, Loftus EV Jr, Panaccione R, et al. Relationships between disease activity and serum and fecal biomarkers in patients with Crohn's disease. Clin Gastroenterol Hepatol 2008;6(11):1218–24.

68. Menees SB, Powell C, Kurlander J, et al. A meta-analysis of the utility of C-reactive protein, erythrocyte sedimentation rate, fecal calprotectin, and fecal lactoferrin to exclude inflammatory bowel disease in adults with IBS. Am J Gastroenterol 2015;110(3):444–54.

69. Sollelis E, Quinard RM, Bouguen G, et al. Combined evaluation of biomarkers as predictor of maintained remission in Crohn's disease. World J Gastroenterol 2019;25(19):2354–64.

70. Echarri A, Ollero V, Barreiro-de Acosta M, et al. Clinical, biological, and endoscopic responses to adalimumab in antitumor necrosis factor-naive Crohn's disease: predictors of efficacy in clinical practice. Eur J Gastroenterol Hepatol 2015;27(4):430–5.

71. Cornillie F, Hanauer SB, Diamond RH, et al. Postinduction serum infliximab trough level and decrease of C-reactive protein level are associated with durable sustained response to infliximab: a retrospective analysis of the ACCENT I trial. Gut 2014;63(11):1721–7.

72. Ricciuto A, Griffiths AM. Clinical value of fecal calprotectin. Crit Rev Clin Lab Sci 2019;56(5):307–20.

73. Lin JF, Chen JM, Zuo JH, et al. Meta-analysis: fecal calprotectin for assessment of inflammatory bowel disease activity. Inflamm Bowel Dis 2014;20(8):1407–15.

74. Jung ES, Lee SP, Kae SH, et al. Diagnostic accuracy of fecal calprotectin for the detection of small bowel crohn's disease through capsule endoscopy: an updated meta-analysis and systematic review. Gut Liver 2020;15(5):732–41.

75. Colombel JF, Panaccione R, Bossuyt P, et al. Effect of tight control management on Crohn's disease (CALM): a multicentre, randomised, controlled phase 3 trial. Lancet 2017;390(10114):2779–89.

76. Reinisch W, Panaccione R, Bossuyt P, et al. Association of biomarker cutoffs and endoscopic outcomes in crohn's disease: a post hoc analysis from the CALM Study. Inflamm Bowel Dis 2020;26(10):1562–71.

77. Cozijnsen MA, Ben Shoham A, Kang B, et al. Development and validation of the mucosal inflammation noninvasive index for pediatric crohn's disease. Clin Gastroenterol Hepatol 2020;18(1):133–40.e1.

78. Molander P, Farkkila M, Ristimaki A, et al. Does fecal calprotectin predict short-term relapse after stopping TNFalpha-blocking agents in inflammatory bowel disease patients in deep remission? J Crohns Colitis 2015;9(1):33–40.

79. Plevris N, Fulforth J, Lyons M, et al. Normalization of Fecal Calprotectin Within 12 Months of Diagnosis Is Associated With Reduced Risk of Disease Progression in Patients With Crohn's Disease. Clin Gastroenterol Hepatol 2021;19(9): 1835–44.e6.

80. Louis E, Mary JY, Vernier-Massouille G, et al. Maintenance of remission among patients with Crohn's disease on antimetabolite therapy after infliximab therapy is stopped. Gastroenterology 2012;142(1):63–70.e5 [quiz: e31].

81. Peeters M, Joossens S, Vermeire S, et al. Diagnostic value of anti-Saccharomyces cerevisiae and antineutrophil cytoplasmic autoantibodies in inflammatory bowel disease. Am J Gastroenterol 2001;96(3):730–4.

82. Joossens S, Reinisch W, Vermeire S, et al. The value of serologic markers in indeterminate colitis: a prospective follow-up study. Gastroenterology 2002; 122(5):1242–7.

83. Walker LJ, Aldhous MC, Drummond HE, et al. Anti-Saccharomyces cerevisiae antibodies (ASCA) in Crohn's disease are associated with disease severity but not NOD2/CARD15 mutations. Clin Exp Immunol 2004;135(3):490–6.

84. Forcione DG, Rosen MJ, Kisiel JB, et al. Anti-Saccharomyces cerevisiae antibody (ASCA) positivity is associated with increased risk for early surgery in Crohn's disease. Gut 2004;53(8):1117–22.

85. Fleshner P, Ippoliti A, Dubinsky M, et al. Both preoperative perinuclear antineutrophil cytoplasmic antibody and anti-CBir1 expression in ulcerative colitis patients influence pouchitis development after ileal pouch-anal anastomosis. Clin Gastroenterol Hepatol 2008;6(5):561–8.

86. van Schaik FD, Oldenburg B, Hart AR, et al. Serological markers predict inflammatory bowel disease years before the diagnosis. Gut 2013;62(5):683–8.

87. Boschetti G, Garnero P, Moussata D, et al. Accuracies of serum and fecal S100 proteins (calprotectin and calgranulin C) to predict the response to TNF antagonists in patients with Crohn's disease. Inflamm Bowel Dis 2015;21(2):331–6.

88. Guidi L, Marzo M, Andrisani G, et al. Faecal calprotectin assay after induction with anti-Tumour Necrosis Factor alpha agents in inflammatory bowel disease: Prediction of clinical response and mucosal healing at one year. Dig Liver Dis 2014;46(11):974–9.

89. Nehra AK, Sheedy SP, Wells ML, et al. Imaging findings of ileal inflammation at computed tomography and magnetic resonance enterography: what do they mean when ileoscopy and biopsy are negative? J Crohns Colitis 2020;14(4): 455–64.

90. Deepak P, Fletcher JG, Fidler JL, et al. Radiological response is associated with better long-term outcomes and is a potential treatment target in patients with small bowel crohn's disease. Am J Gastroenterol 2016;111(7):997–1006.

91. Minderhoud IM, Steyerberg EW, van Bodegraven AA, et al. Predicting endoscopic disease activity in crohn's disease: a new and validated noninvasive disease activity index (the utrecht activity index). Inflamm Bowel Dis 2015;21(10): 2453–9.

92. D'Arcangelo G, Oliva S, Dilillo A, et al. Predictors of long-term clinical and endoscopic remission in children with crohn disease treated with infliximab. J Pediatr Gastroenterol Nutr 2019;68(6):841–6.

93. Wang J, Wang Y, Wei C, et al. Smartphone interventions for long-term health management of chronic diseases: an integrative review. Telemed J E Health 2014;20(6):570–83.
94. Zhen J, Marshall JK, Nguyen GC, et al. Impact of Digital Health Monitoring in the Management of Inflammatory Bowel Disease. J Med Syst 2021;45(2):23.
95. Yi Y, Sossenheimer PH, Erondu AI, et al. Using Wearable Biosensors to Predict Length of Stay for Patients with IBD After Bowel Surgery. Dig Dis Sci 2021. https://doi.org/10.1007/s10620-021-06910-w.
96. Sossenheimer PH. Abstract 539, Digestive Disease Week, May 18-21, 2019.
97. Solitano V, Alfarone L, D'Amico F, et al. IBD goes home: from telemedicine to self-administered advanced therapies. Expert Opin Biol Ther 2021;1–13. https://doi.org/10.1080/14712598.2021.1942833.
98. Ostlund I, Werner M, Karling P. Self-monitoring with home based fecal calprotectin is associated with increased medical treatment. A randomized controlled trial on patients with inflammatory bowel disease. Scand J Gastroenterol 2021; 56(1):38–45.
99. Torres J, Petralia F, Sato T, et al. Serum biomarkers identify patients who will develop inflammatory bowel diseases up to 5 years before diagnosis. Gastroenterology 2020;159(1):96–104.
100. Biasci D, Lee JC, Noor NM, et al. A blood-based prognostic biomarker in IBD. Gut 2019;68(8):1386–95.

Mimics of Crohn's Disease

Sanchit Gupta, MD, MS[a,b], Jessica R. Allegretti, MD, MPH[a,b],*

KEYWORDS

• Crohn's disease • Inflammatory bowel disease • Mimics • Differential diagnosis

KEY POINTS

• Crohn's disease can manifest with a variety of symptoms.
• Mimics of Crohn's disease include alternate gastrointestinal diseases, vascular causes, autoimmune processes, infections, malignancies and complications, drug- or treatment-induced conditions, and genetic diseases.
• A broad differential diagnosis is important when assessing presenting symptoms and evaluating the patient with symptomatic or refractory inflammatory bowel disease.

INTRODUCTION

Crohn's disease (CD) is a chronic inflammatory bowel disease (IBD) of the gastrointestinal tract of unknown cause.[1] Presenting symptoms can include abdominal pain, diarrhea, hematochezia, weight loss, nausea, or vomiting. Classic features of CD include transmural inflammation, skip lesions, and ulcers, with involvement of any part of the gastrointestinal tract from mouth to anus.[2] Noncaseating granulomas on histopathology are a key feature of CD if present. Complications of CD include abscesses, strictures, and fistulas, and extraintestinal manifestations can affect multiple organs.[3,4] CD is a clinical diagnosis, established based on a combination of clinical, endoscopic, histologic, and radiologic findings, and there is no single component diagnostic of CD.[4] Diagnostic confusion exists even within IBD, where ulcerative colitis with rectal sparing or cecal patch can suggest CD. Multiple diseases, including luminal, vascular, autoimmune, infectious, malignant, drug-induced, and radiation-induced conditions, can mimic CD by causing luminal inflammation, or complications such as bowel stricture, fistula formation, or abdominal abscess (**Tables 1–3**).

DISCUSSION
Gastrointestinal Conditions

Diverticular disease can present with multiple symptoms that suggest CD. Acute diverticulitis may present with abdominal pain, typically left lower quadrant, and

---

[a] Division of Gastroenterology, Hepatology, and Endoscopy, Brigham and Women's Hospital, 850 Boyslton Street, Suite 201, Chestnut Hill, MA 02467, USA; [b] Harvard Medical School, 25 Shattuck Street, Boston, MA 02115, USA
* Corresponding author. 850 Boylston Street, Suite 201, Chestnut Hill, MA 02467.
E-mail address: jallegretti@bwh.harvard.edu

Gastroenterol Clin N Am 51 (2022) 241–269
https://doi.org/10.1016/j.gtc.2021.12.006
0889-8553/22/© 2021 Elsevier Inc. All rights reserved.

Table 1
Locations of involvement by noninfectious mimics of Crohn's disease

Location	Cause	Potential Distinguishing Features from Crohn's Disease
Small intestine	Meckel diverticulum	Imaging: Meckel scan (99m technetium pertechnetate scan)
		Histology: submucosal fibrosis
	Chronic mesenteric ischemia	Imaging: atherosclerotic/thrombotic disease, pneumatosis, portal venous gas
	Fibromuscular dysplasia	Epigastric or flank bruit
	Autoimmune enteropathy	Association with IPEX, APECED
		Laboratory: autoantibodies (antienterocyte, antigoblet cell)
Colon	Acute/complicated diverticulitis	Imaging: diverticulitis
	Segmental colitis associated with diverticulosis	Endoscopy: inflammation in area of diverticulosis
	Ischemic colitis	Imaging: thumbprinting
		Endoscopy: necrosis, colon single-stripe sign
		Histology: fibrin thrombi, ghost cells, infarction
	Mesenteric venous disease (IMHMV, MIVOD)	Imaging, endoscopy: uncommon rectal involvement
		Histology: smooth muscle proliferation, lymphocytic inflammatory infiltrate
	Cord colitis	History of umbilical cord blood for hematopoietic stem cell transplant
Any	Microscopic polyangiitis	Palpable purpura, bruits
	Granulomatosis with polyangiitis	Laboratory: ANA, ANCA, low complement/C4, cryoglobulins, viral hepatitis
	Eosinophilic granulomatosis with polyangiitis (Churg-Strauss)	
	IgA vasculitis (Henoch-Schonlein purpura)	
	Cryoglobulinemic vasculitis	
	Polyarteritis nodosa	
	Behcet disease	Laboratory: pathergy test
		Histology: neutrophilic infiltration of vasculature
	Sarcoidosis	Systemic/pulmonary disease involvement
		Laboratory: serum ACE, calcium levels
	Eosinophilic gastrointestinal disorders	Laboratory: peripheral eosinophilia
		Histology: infiltration with eosinophils
	Common variable immunodeficiency	Laboratory: reduced IgG and low IgA and/or IgM
	Primary gastrointestinal/colorectal lymphomas	Histology: definitive diagnosis of neoplasm
	Neuroendocrine tumors/carcinoid syndrome	Laboratory: urine/serum 5-HIAA, serum chromogranin
		Imaging: masses, hepatic metastases, somatostatin receptor scintigraphy/PET
		Histology: definitive diagnosis of neoplasm

(continued on next page)

Table 1 (continued)		
Location	Cause	Potential Distinguishing Features from Crohn's Disease
	Radiation-induced	Endoscopy: telangiectasias Histology: collagen deposition, vascular sclerosis
	NSAID-induced	History of chronic or excess NSAID use Endoscopy: diaphragm-like stricture Histology: submucosal fibrosis, normal epithelium
	ICI gastritis, enterocolitis	History of ICI therapy, rapid response to treatment initiation Histology: intraepithelial lymphocytes
	Chronic granulomatous disease	Laboratory: neutrophil function testing, phagocyte oxidase genetic testing

Abbreviations: ACE, angiotensin-converting enzyme; ANA, antinuclear antibody; ANCA, antineutrophil cytoplasmic antibody; HIAA, hydroxyindoleacetic acid; ICI, immune checkpoint inhibitors; Ig, immunoglobulin; IMHMV, idiopathic myointimal hyperplasia of the mesenteric veins; MIVOD, mesenteric inflammatory venoocclusive disease; NSAID, nonsteroidal antiinflammatory drug.

include symptoms such as changes in bowel habits, nausea, and fever.[5] Rectal bleeding or diarrhea may not be present. Diagnosis can be made expediently with imaging, and colonoscopy should be avoided in the acute setting for risk of perforation. Complicated diverticulitis including perforated diverticulitis can lead to stricture, fistula, or phlegmon/abscess formation, and smoldering diverticulitis may lead to abdominal pain and ongoing inflammation on imaging.[5]

Patients with diverticular disease may develop segmental colitis associated with diverticulosis (SCAD). Presenting symptoms include abdominal pain, diarrhea, and rectal bleeding.[6] Histologic features include acute or chronic inflammatory infiltrate, crypt abscesses or distortion, and Paneth cell metaplasia, which can be potentially indistinguishable from CD. SCAD is characterized by localization of inflammation in colonic areas with diverticulosis and usually excludes the rectum. The clinical course can range from acute inflammation that resolves to chronic recurrent symptoms, which can add to diagnostic uncertainty in distinguishing SCAD from CD.[7,8]

Meckel diverticula typically present in childhood but may cause varied symptoms in adults, including melena or hematochezia with anemia, abominable pain, and intestinal obstruction.[9] Pain can arise from diverticular inflammation, foreign body impaction, or perforation.[10–12] Terminal ileal inflammation may develop due to acid secretion from ectopic gastric mucosa contained in the Meckel diverticulum, and histopathologic features can include ulceration and submucosal fibrosis.[13,14]

Vascular Diseases

Ischemic colitis develops after a vascular insult to watershed areas of the colon supplied by mesenteric and iliac arteries with limited collateral flow.[15] Classically, systemic hypotension or decreased cardiac output precipitates injury. Segmental damage can occur based on vascular anatomy to the right colon, splenic flexure, and rectosigmoid colon.[16] Those with comorbid hypertension, atherosclerotic disease, diabetes, chronic kidney disease, and older patients are at increased risk.[15] Symptoms include acute abdominal pain, tenesmus, diarrhea, and rectal bleeding.[15,16] Imaging can show circumferential and segmental colonic wall thickening and thumbprinting indicating pneumatosis, and

Table 2
Locations of involvement by infectious mimics of Crohn's disease

Location	Cause	Potential Distinguishing Features from Crohn's Disease
Stomach/Small intestine	Norovirus Rotavirus Sapovirus Adenovirus Astrovirus Enterovirus Coxsackievirus	Laboratory: stool PCR; may represent asymptomatic carriage
	Anisakidosis	Endoscopy: larvae
	Nontyphoidal salmonella	Laboratory: stool culture
	Aeromonas gastroenteritis	Laboratory: stool culture (may require special request)
Small intestine	Coccidioidomycosis	Laboratory: serum IgM, IgG, biopsy fungal culture
	Giardiasis	Laboratory: stool microscopy, stool antigen/PCR Endoscopy: scalloping of duodenum/ileum Histology: villous blunting, trophozoites
	Strongyloidiasis	Cutaneous larva currens rash Laboratory: stool microscopy, stool PCR, serum IgG Endoscopy: discoloration, xanthoma-like lesions Histology: parasites in crypts, eosinophilic infiltration
	Whipple disease	Endoscopy: dilated villi, ectatic lymph, yellow color Histology: PAS staining, immunohistochemistry, PCR
Ileocolonic/ Terminal ileitis	Schistosomiasis	Laboratory: peripheral eosinophilia, stool microscopy, stool/urine/serum antigen, serum antibody Histology: ova deposition
	Campylobacter	Laboratory: stool culture/PCR; blood culture
	Typhoid fever (Salmonella)	Rose spots Laboratory: stool culture, blood culture
	Yersiniosis	Laboratory: stool/blood culture Histology: suppurative granuloma
	Hereditary angioedema	Endoscopy: normal mucosa Laboratory: C1-INH level/function, C4/complement levels, coagulation factor XII genetic testing
Colon	Amebiasis	Laboratory: stool microscopy, stool/serum antigen Endoscopy: flasklike erosions Histology: cysts or trophozoites
	C difficile infection	Laboratory: stool immunoassays for GDH or A/B, stool toxigenic PCR Endoscopy: pseudomembranes
	EHEC, STEC, EPEC, ETEC, EIEC, EAEC (E coli)	Laboratory: stool culture, PCR
	Shigellosis	Laboratory: stool culture, PCR
	Infectious proctitis	Laboratory: N gonorrhoeae culture/PCR, C trachomatis PCR, HSV-2 viral culture/PCR, syphilis serum RPR/VDRL

(continued on next page)

Table 2 (continued)		
Location	Cause	Potential Distinguishing Features from Crohn's Disease
Any	Cytomegalovirus	Laboratory: anti-CMV IgM, serum/stool PCR Histopathology: viral inclusion bodies, immunohistochemical staining
	Histoplasmosis	Laboratory: urine/serum antigen, biopsy fungal culture Histology: macrophage clusters, immunohistochemistry
	Abdominal tuberculosis	Laboratory: ascites ADA, protein, AFB smear, mycobacterial culture/PCR; stool mycobacterial culture/PCR Endoscopy: patulous IC valve, fish-mouth opening Histology: submucosal granulomas, AFB staining
	Actinomycosis	Imaging: contrast-enhancing, multicystic lesion Laboratory: pus culture Histology: sulfur granules

Abbreviations: AFB, acid-fact bacteria; *C difficile, Clostridiodes difficile*; IC, ileocecal; PAS, Periodic acid–Schiff; PCR, polymerase chain reaction; RPR, rapid plasma reagin; VDRL, venereal disease research laboratory.

angiography findings do not typically correlate with ischemic colitis.[15,16] Colonoscopy findings include edema, erythema, and necrosis, and the colon single-stripe sign is specific for colonic ischemia.[16] Histology can be variable and show edema, capillary fibrin thrombi, and neutrophilic infiltration, and pathognomonic features include ghost cells and infarction.[15]

Chronic mesenteric ischemia can be caused by both arterial and venous disease, such as embolism, atherosclerosis, impaired venous outflow including median arcuate ligament syndrome, thrombosis, and vasoconstriction.[17,18] Risk factors include low-flow states such as congestive heart failure or chronic kidney disease.[19] Symptoms include abdominal or postprandial pain, nausea, vomiting, early satiety, diarrhea, constipation, and weight loss.[17] Imaging can reveal small bowel wall thickening and mesenteric stranding, along with pneumatosis and portal venous gas.[17] Endoscopy is often of limited utility, as only small portions of the small intestine can be assessed, but can demonstrate edema, erythema, atrophy, and ulcers.[19]

Small vessel inflammatory vasculitides affect arteries, arterioles, capillaries, and venules, leading to ischemic injury in the gastrointestinal tract that can resemble CD.[20] These injuries include the antineutrophil cytoplasmic antibody-associated vasculitides microscopic polyangiitis, granulomatosis with polyangiitis, and eosinophilic granulomatosis with polyangiitis (Churg-Strauss), along with immunoglobulin A (IgA) vasculitis (Henoch-Schonlein purpura), and more rarely, cryoglobulinemic vasculitis.[20] Patients may present with abdominal pain, nausea, vomiting, fever, diarrhea, rectal bleeding, bowel infarct, and perforation. Endoscopy can show inflammation, erosions, petechiae, nodularity, hemorrhage, strictures, and ulcers, and histology may be nonspecific.[21] In particular, granulomas may be present in patients with granulomatosis with polyangiitis, and terminal ileitis has been reported in IgA vasculitis.[22,23]

Polyarteritis nodosa, a necrotizing vasculitis of medium-sized vessels, can be associated with hepatitis B. Gastrointestinal involvement is common, usually affecting the

Table 3
Rare causes to consider as possible mimics of Crohn's disease

Location	Cause	Typical Features
Small intestine	Median arcuate ligament syndrome/ celiac artery compression syndrome[235,236]	Symptoms: postprandial abdominal pain, nausea, vomiting, weight loss, diarrhea Imaging: bowel thickening, celiac trunk stenosis, increased celiac artery velocity Endoscopy: erythema, altered vascular pattern, granularity
	Superior mesenteric artery syndrome (Wilkie syndrome)[237–240]	Symptoms: abdominal pain, nausea, vomiting, distension, weight loss Imaging: compression of third portion of duodenum between aorta and superior mesenteric artery Endoscopy: extrinsic duodenal stenosis
	ARB-associated sprue-like enteropathy[241–243]	Symptoms: abdominal pain, nausea, vomiting, diarrhea, malabsorption Laboratory: possible positive HLA-DQ2/DQ8 serology, negative TTG Endoscopy: scalloping of duodenum Histology: villous atrophy, crypt distortion, intraepithelial lymphocytes
Ileocolonic	Postappendectomy fistula, abscess, mucocele[244–246]	Symptoms: abdominal pain, drainage, wound Imaging: fistula, abscess, postappendectomy state, stump appendicitis
Colon	Solitary rectal ulcer syndrome[247,248]	Symptoms: pain, hematochezia, mucous discharge, constipation, straining Endoscopy: ulcer, hyperemia, nodularity, polypoid lesion, yellow slough Histology: fibromuscular obliteration of lamina propria, smooth muscle hyperplasia, surface ulceration, crypt distortion, chronic inflammatory infiltrate
	Diversion colitis[249–251]	Symptoms: pain, rectal bleeding Endoscopy: ulceration, friability Histology: lymphoid follicle hyperplasia, mucin granuloma
Any	Gastrointestinal amyloidosis	Symptoms: dysphagia, reflux, nausea, vomiting, constipation, diarrhea, malabsorption, weight loss, bleeding Endoscopy: erythema, ulcerations, granularity, polypoid protrusion Histology: ulceration, crypt hyperplasia, lamina propria hyalinization, vascular deposits, apple-green birefringence with Congo red staining

(continued on next page)

Table 3 (continued)		
Location	Cause	Typical Features
	Cronkhite-Canada syndrome[252,253]	Symptoms: pain, diarrhea, hematochezia, hypogeusia, alopecia, skin pigmentation, malabsorption, weight loss Endoscopy: sessile/pedunculated polyps (classically sparing the esophagus), nodularity, edema, erythema, villous atrophy/irregularity Histology: polyps (inflammatory, hyperplastic, hamartomatous, adenomatous), chronic inflammatory infiltrate, crypt changes viral inclusion bodies, immunohistochemical staining
	Acute intermittent porphyria[254,255]	Symptoms: abdominal pain, vomiting, obstruction, constipation Laboratory: liver enzyme elevations, urine/plasma porphobilinogen
	Mitochondrial neurogastrointestinal encephalopathy[256,257]	Symptoms: abdominal pain, vomiting, bloating, diarrhea, cachexia, extraocular muscle weakness, neuropathy, leukoencephalopathy Laboratory: TYMP mutation Imaging: terminal ileal thickening Endoscopy: dilated small intestine, ulceration Histology: chronic inflammation, cryptitis, megalomitochondria
	Endometriosis[258–261]	Symptoms: diarrhea, constipation, rectal bleeding, chronic pain, pain during menstruation, bloating, obstruction, abscess, fistulae Imaging: nodules, thickening, infiltrative lesions, endometrioma (transvaginal ultrasound, rectal endoscopic ultrasound, cross-sectional CT/MRI) Endoscopy: normal mucosa, infiltrative implants, lumen stenosis
	Kaposi sarcoma[262–265]	Symptoms: violaceous skin plaques, abdominal pain, diarrhea, weight loss, obstruction Laboratory: HHV-8, HIV Imaging: bowel thickening, mass, obstruction Endoscopy: mucosal inflammation, polypoid mass, nodules, submucosal infiltration Histology: vascular slits, HHV-8 staining

Abbreviations: CT, computed tomography; HHV, human herpesvirus; HIV, human immunodeficiency virus.

small bowel and gallbladder.[24] The most common gastrointestinal symptom is abdominal pain, particularly after meals. Other symptoms include nausea, vomiting, diarrhea, and bleeding. Polyarteritis nodosa can lead to transmural ischemia of the intestine, leading to necrosis, stenosis, and perforation.[24]

Behcet disease is a variable-vessel vasculitis classically diagnosed with the triad of oral aphthous ulcers, uveitis, and genital ulcers. Gastrointestinal symptoms include abdominal pain, fever, diarrhea, and rectal bleeding. Oval or round, deep ulcers can be present anywhere in the gastrointestinal tract, although ileocolonic involvement is most common and segmental regions can be affected.[25] Histology reveals neutrophilic infiltration of the vessel walls, and venules may be more frequently affected than arteries. Behcet disease and CD may be difficult to distinguish, although the pathergy test can be positive in Behcet disease.[26–28]

Fibromuscular dysplasia (FMD) is a noninflammatory and nonatherosclerotic arterial disease that can lead to vascular stenosis, dissection, occlusion, and aneurysm.[29] Although FMD is mainly associated with renal, carotid, and vertebral arteries, it can affect any arterial system, including the mesenteric vasculature. Epigastric or flank bruit may suggest FMD.[30] Reported cases include symptoms consistent with chronic mesenteric ischemia, and a patient who underwent bowel resection for refractory CD was ultimately found to have mesenteric FMD on histopathology.[31,32]

Mesenteric venous disease, including idiopathic myointimal hyperplasia of the mesenteric veins (IMHMV) and mesenteric inflammatory venoocclusive disease (MIVOD), is rare and primarily affects the colon.[33] Symptoms include abdominal pain, cramping, diarrhea, rectal bleeding, and weight loss. Endoscopy can show edema, friability, and ulcerations in the colon, and histology can demonstrate ischemic injury.[33,34] Histologic findings include smooth muscle proliferation in IMHMV and lymphocytic inflammatory infiltrate in MIVOD.[33,35–37] Ischemia of the rectum is uncommon and can help distinguish IMHMV from ischemic colitis.[34,38]

Immune-mediated Diseases

Sarcoidosis is a systemic disease with the hallmark feature of noncaseating granulomas.[39] Gastrointestinal manifestations are uncommon but can include abdominal pain, weight loss, dysphagia, and anemia. Endoscopy may show esophagitis, erosion, nodularity, ulcers, polypoid lesions, and stenosis.[39] Dysphagia may be secondary to extrinsic esophageal compression from mediastinal lymphadenopathy. Mucosal and muscular infiltration may contribute to symptoms and lead to complications including stricture development.[39] Histology shows noncaseating granulomas, and clinical evidence for systemic sarcoid can help in differentiating sarcoidosis from CD.[40]

Eosinophilic gastrointestinal disorders include eosinophilic esophagitis, eosinophilic gastroenteritis, eosinophilic enteritis, and eosinophilic colitis and may suggest CD, given the multiple areas of the gastrointestinal tract that can be affected.[41–45] The gastrointestinal mucosa is infiltrated with eosinophils, and peripheral eosinophilia may or may not be present.[46] Symptoms include dysphagia, food impaction, abdominal pain, nausea, vomiting, diarrhea, weight loss, malabsorption, and protein-losing enteropathy.[46,47] Depth of infiltration can affect severity of illness: mucosal infiltration causes milder symptoms; muscular layer disease can lead to esophageal stricture, pseudoachalasia, gastric outlet obstruction, bowel obstruction, and rarely perforation; and subserosal disease may lead to eosinophilic ascites or pleural effusion with or without other associated symptoms.[41] Eosinophilia in the esophagus may be increased in patients with IBD with higher prevalence of eosinophilic esophagitis and may be more common in younger and male patients.[48,49] The differential diagnosis for eosinophilic gastrointestinal disorders includes CD, and careful assessment including, but not limited to, histology should be conducted for the diagnosis.[50]

Autoimmune enteropathy is an autoimmune disease of the small intestine, characterized by villous atrophy, autoantibodies, and chronic diarrhea.[51,52] Symptoms include severe diarrhea, malabsorption, and weight loss and can be associated with systemic diseases including immunodysregulation polyendocrinopathy enteropathy X-linked syndrome and autoimmune phenomena, polyendocrinopathy, candidiasis, and ectodermal dystrophy.[51] Autoimmune enteropathy is distinct from celiac disease, and histology can show villous blunting, intraepithelial or crypt lymphocytosis, and crypt apoptotic bodies.[52] The presence of autoantibodies, including antienterocyte and antigoblet cell antibodies, can support the diagnosis of autoimmune enteropathy.[51]

Common variable immunodeficiency (CVID) is a disorder of B-cell differentiation leading to impaired immunoglobulin production.[53] Gastrointestinal manifestations include diarrhea, malabsorption, anemia, and weight loss, and CVID may be associated with primary gastrointestinal lymphoma and gastric cancer.[54] CVID is diagnosed based on reductions in total IgG, IgA, and/or IgM and poor antibody response to vaccination.[54–56] Laboratory findings may include elevated fecal calprotectin, and bile acid malabsorption may be present.[56] Endoscopic findings include candida esophagitis, ulceration, polyps, and nodularity. Histology may show atrophic gastritis, villous blunting, increased intraepithelial lymphocytes, follicular lymphatic hyperplasia, ileitis, cryptitis, and crypt distortion, which may be seen more commonly in the colon than upper gastrointestinal tract.[56]

INFECTIONS
Viral

Many viral infections cause gastroenteritis and may lead to diarrhea in patients with CD. Notable viruses include norovirus, rotavirus, sapovirus, adenovirus, astrovirus, enterovirus, coxsackievirus, and cytomegalovirus.[57,58] Moreover, viral gastroenteritis may be associated with CD flare, although the relationship between carriage and infection is uncertain.[59,60] Norovirus has been associated with CD flare, but norovirus carriage has also been detected at higher rates in patients with active CD.[57,61,62] Viral infections should remain on the differential for diarrheal disease and can be distinguished from CD by absence of additional characteristic clinical features. Conversely, patients may initially present with a history that suggests recent viral infection but ultimately have CD.

Although uncommon, cytomegalovirus (CMV) can lead to gastrointestinal symptoms with tissue-invasive disease in the absence of viremia, and stool and tissue testing should be considered.[63,64] Both primary infections and reactivation of latent CMV can occur, potentially in the setting of critical illness, immunosuppression, or malignancy.[63] Presenting symptoms include odynophagia, dysphagia, abdominal pain, nausea, vomiting, diarrhea, and rectal bleeding.[63] Endoscopic findings include erythema, edema, erosions, pseudotumors, and severe ulceration.[64] Patients with CMV colitis following hematopoietic stem cell transplantation have been found to have granulomatous inflammation on histology.[65] Refractory IBD, immunosuppression, and age greater than 30 years may be associated with CMV disease in patients with IBD, although local CMV reactivation may be a consequence of severe CD without active infection.[64,66,67] CMV in the patient without IBD may be difficult to distinguish from CD, and in the patient with IBD, careful consideration is required for diagnostic certainty and potential treatment benefit.[64,68]

Fungal

Coccidioidomycosis, known as Valley fever, typically causes pulmonary disease after inhalation of *Coccidioides* spores and is endemic to the southwestern United States.[69]

Extrapulmonary disease is rare, but risk factors include immunocompromised hosts and pregnant women.[70] Gastrointestinal or peritoneal coccidiomycosis can present with symptoms including abdominal pain, fevers, ascites, fatigue, obstruction, and perforation.[71–74] Endoscopic features are not well described, although biopsies may show caseating granulomas with giant cells and thick-walled spherules with endospores.[70]

Histoplasmosis, endemic to the Mississippi and Ohio river valleys in the United States, results from inhalation of *Histoplasma capsulatum* spores.[75] Histoplasmosis typically affects the lungs, liver, bone marrow, and spleen.[76,77] Gastrointestinal disease is present in almost all cases of disseminated disease, particularly in immunocompromised patients.[78] Symptoms include abdominal pain, fever, diarrhea, weight loss, bowel obstruction, and rectal bleeding.[76,79] Gastrointestinal involvement usually occurs in the ileocecal region but can also involve the upper gastrointestinal tract, small intestine, and colon.[76] On endoscopy, polypoid masses including apple core lesions, focal erosions, and skip lesions can be seen.[80] Pathology can show macrophage clusters with both caseating and noncaseating granulomas.[70] Diagnosis can be made by culture and antigen detection.[75,81]

Parasitic

Amebiasis due to infection by *Entamoeba histolytica* is an important cause of diarrhea globally.[82,83] Disease transmission via fecal-oral spread usually occurs after ingestion of contaminated water but can be via sexual transmission.[84,85] Invasive disease may cause intestinal lesions including necrotizing colitis and liver abscesses.[83] Symptoms include abdominal pain or cramping, fever, diarrhea, mucus in stool, and rectal bleeding.[86] Endoscopy can show left- and right-sided colitis with edema, masses, and characteristic "flask-like" erosions or ulcerations, with the cecum most commonly affected.[83,87] Biopsies from ulcer edges can show cryptitis and crypt abscesses suggesting CD, but may not detect cysts or trophozoites, and additional stool/serologic tests should be considered for diagnosis.[82,83] A patient thought to have CD died of fulminant colitis with perforation ultimately diagnosed as amebiasis on autopsy, highlighting the importance of including amebiasis on the differential diagnosis.[88]

Giardiasis, caused by *Giardia duodenalis*, is a worldwide cause of diarrheal disease. Giardia cysts are transmitted by the fecal-oral route through contaminated food products or water supply, including areas inhabited by infected wild animals such as rivers and springs.[89] Patients may have asymptomatic infection but can shed cysts for several months.[90] Symptoms include nausea, bloating, fever, malaise, steatorrhea, diarrhea, malabsorption, and weight loss.[91,92] Chronic giardiasis can lead to persistent symptoms including arthritis lasting months and can suggest a diagnosis of CD.[93,94] Endoscopy may be normal but can show scalloping in the duodenum or ileum, and some patients with dyspepsia may have gastric giardiasis.[95,96] Histologic features include villous blunting and trophozoites in the mucosa and inflammatory cells in the lamina propria.[97] Stool microscopy may not be sufficiently sensitive for diagnosis, and immunoassay or nucleic acid amplification testing can be used.[98,99]

Schistosomiasis is caused by blood flukes of *Schistosoma spp.*, and many people may be asymptomatic or experience a self-limited acute illness.[100,101] Chronic disease is due to a granulomatous inflammatory response to Schistosoma eggs deposited in the bowel wall.[102] Presenting symptoms include abdominal pain, diarrhea, tenesmus, and eosinophilia.[103] Complications include intestinal fibrosis, stricture, appendicitis, obstruction, and polyp formation, which may suggest CD.[101,104–106] Fecal occult blood and elevated calprotectin may be detected.[107] Endoscopic findings include erythema, edema, ulceration, and segmental colitis, and histology may show ova deposition, inflammatory infiltrate, submucosal fibrosis, and dysplasia including carcinoma.[108]

Strongyloidiasis, caused by *Strongyloides stercoralis,* can lead to gastrointestinal symptoms during both acute and chronic infection. Initial symptoms follow migration of larva from the skin, where irritation, rash, and urticaria may develop.[109] After the small intestine is infected, symptoms can include abdominal pain, anorexia, diarrhea, constipation, rectal bleeding, malnutrition, and ascites.[109,110] Production of new larvae causes a cycle of autoinfection from the perianal skin or intestinal mucosa with larvae migrating through subcutaneous tissues, leading to the pathognomonic larva currens urticarial rash and chronic symptoms, which are typically mild.[109] Severe manifestations in hyperinfection syndrome and disseminated strongyloidiasis are more common in immunocompromised patients.[109,111] Endoscopic findings in the duodenum and colon include edema, erythema, erosions, discoloration, nodular xanthoma-like lesions, skip lesions, and aphthous or serpiginous ulcers.[110,112–115] Histologic features include visible parasites in crypts and eosinophilic infiltration of lamina propria.[112–114] Diagnosis can be made by stool and serologic testing but may be delayed due to nonspecific symptoms or suspicion for other conditions.[109,116]

Anisakidosis is caused by the nematode *Anisakis*, found in raw fish. Infection occurs primarily in Japan and coastal areas of Europe, although increased consumption of raw or undercooked fish may contribute to increasing incidence elsewhere.[117] Ingested larvae penetrate gastric and intestinal mucosa and die in the incidental human host, leading to an inflammatory reaction. Gastric anisakidosis occurs within hours after ingestion and can resolve with nonspecific persistent symptoms afterward.[118] Intestinal anisakiasis can present with intermittent abdominal pain, due to inflammation primarily in the terminal ileum. Additional features can include ascites, stenosis, appendicitis, bowel obstruction, and perforation.[117] Endoscopy may demonstrate larvae, erosions, edema, erythema, nodules, and ulcerations.[119] Histology may show an inflammatory infiltrate, abscess, and granuloma formation, and larvae may be detected but may have degenerated or passed by time of examination.[117] Gastric anisakidosis can be treated by endoscopic removal of the culprit larva, and intestinal anisakidosis can usually be treated with conservative therapy.[117]

Bacterial

Clostridiodes difficile, a spore-forming bacteria, is an important cause of nosocomial and community-acquired diarrheal disease.[120] *C difficile* infection (CDI) presents with diarrhea and abdominal pain, and severe or fulminant disease can include fever, ileus, and toxic megacolon.[121] Risk factors for CDI include antibiotic use, hospitalization, age greater than 65 years, immunosuppression use, and female sex.[122] Patients with IBD are at increased risk of both CDI and asymptomatic *C difficile* carriage, and the patient with symptomatic IBD may have CDI, IBD flare, or both.[123] Endoscopic features include characteristic pseudomembranes, inflammation, and normal mucosa.[124]

Enterotoxigenic, enteropathogenic, enteroinvasive, and enteroaggregative strains of *Escherichia coli*, including Shiga toxin-producing strains, can cause watery diarrhea, abdominal pain, nausea, and vomiting.[125,126] Enterohemorrhagic *E coli* (EHEC) invades the intestinal mucosa, and serotype 0157:H7 is responsive for virulent disease, often found in undercooked beef.[127,128] EHEC is associated with bloody diarrhea and hemolytic uremic syndrome.[129] Histologic findings can include pseudomembranes, ischemia, or chronic inflammation that may be difficult to distinguish from IBD.[130,131]

Shigella species frequently cause diarrhea, and a low inoculum can be sufficient, as these organisms are less susceptible to gastric acid degradation.[132] Waterborne and foodborne transmission with person-to-person spread can contribute to disease.[132-134] Shigellosis presents with abdominal pain, vomiting, fever, malaise, diarrhea, and rectal bleeding.[135] Complications include toxic megacolon and perforation, bowel obstruction, and rectal prolapse.[136] Extraintestinal manifestations can include reactive arthritis and hemolytic uremic syndrome.[135]

Campylobacter infection leads to acute diarrhea, caused by *Campylobacter jejuni* or *Campylobacter coli*. Poultry is the main host for foodborne or waterborne transmission.[137-139] Presenting symptoms include nausea, vomiting, abdominal pain, cramping, diarrhea, and rectal bleeding.[137] Infection starts in the ileum and jejunum, extending distally to the colon. Endoscopic features include segmental edema, loss of vascular pattern, and ulceration, and histology typically shows acute plasma cell infiltrate without chronicity and cryptitis or crypt abscess.[140,141] Patients with ileocolic infection may be misdiagnosed with appendicitis, particularly in the absence of diarrhea; however, campylobacter may also cause acute appendicitis.[142-144] Extraintestinal manifestations include rash, soft tissue infections, cholecystitis, small intestinal immunoproliferative disease, and peritonitis.[145-148] Delayed complications include reactive arthritis, more often among patients with HLA-B27 phenotype, and Guillain-Barre syndrome.[149,150]

Salmonella species cause nontyphoid acute diarrheal gastroenteritis and are considered a foodborne pathogen. Contaminated products include eggs, poultry, and dairy, and severity of illness is linked to inoculum dose.[139] Symptoms include abdominal pain, fever, diarrhea, and rectal bleeding. Nontyphoidal salmonellosis can be mild, although postinfectious complications include reactive arthritis, bacteremia, abscess, and osteomyelitis.[151-153] Typhoid and paratyphoid fever, linked to *Salmonella enterica* serotypes, present with fever, terminal ileitis, and rose spots.[154-156] *Salmonella typhi* can also lead to bowel perforation, septic or reactive arthritis, and bacteremia and has been linked to gallbladder carcinoma.[151,157-159] Chronic carriers of salmonella may contribute to disease spread and require eradication with antibiotics.[151,160]

Yersiniosis, mainly caused by *Yersinia enterocolitia,* can also be caused by *Yersinia pseudotuberculosis.*[161,162] These foodborne or waterborne pathogens are primarily transmitted by undercooked or raw pork and reservoirs include wildlife and domesticated animals.[163] Presenting symptoms include abdominal pain, fever, and diarrhea.[162] Imaging may show mesenteric lymphadenopathy, appendicitis, or pseudotumor, and endoscopic findings include terminal ileitis with ileal and cecal ulcers.[70,164,165] Histology can suggest CD with transmural inflammation, cryptitis, and epithelioid or suppurative granulomas.[70] Complications can include peritonitis, intussusception, toxic megacolon, bowel necrosis, and perforation.[162]

Aeromonas is a gram-negative anaerobe in soil and aquatic environments and may be associated with foodborne illness, gastroenteritis, and traveler's diarrhea.[166,167] Illness is typically self-limiting, and asymptomatic carriage may be present.[168] Symptoms include abdominal pain, diarrhea, and rectal bleeding, with findings of segmental colitis with ulceration and architectural distortion on histology.[169,170]

Mycobacterium tuberculosis is an acid-fast bacillus that causes tuberculosis. Gastrointestinal tuberculosis can represent a primary infection in the absence of pulmonary findings, consequence of reactivation, or spread from primary pulmonary tuberculosis.[171] Involved organs include the gastrointestinal tract, lymph nodes, peritoneum, and liver. Symptoms include weight loss, fever, dyspepsia, pain, ascites, diarrhea, rectal bleeding, bowel wall thickening, and obstruction.[171-173] Esophageal manifestations are uncommon, but odynophagia or dysphagia may occur due to mucosal disease or extrinsic compression from lymphadenopathy.[173,174] Imaging can show lymphadenitis, bowel wall thickening, fistula tracts, fat stranding, abscess, and calcification.[174] Endoscopic findings include ulcerations in the ileum and small intestine, and histology reveals chronic changes with caseating granulomas. Diagnosis can be limited by low yield of acid-fast staining or culture, and fecal mycobacterial culture may be helpful.[172,175]

Actinomycosis is caused by the gram-positive anaerobe *Actinomyces israelii* and can cause a rare chronic granulomatous disease. Invasive disease leads to granulomatous reactions with necrosis, fistulas, and abscesses.[176] Ileocecal or appendiceal involvement is most common in abdominal actinomycosis.[177] Symptoms can be vague, with abdominal pain, fever, malaise, weight loss, or palpable mass.[178] Imaging may show a contrast-enhancing multicystic lesion.[178,179] Dysphagia or odynophagia may result from esophageal ulceration.[180] Colonoscopy can reveal nodularity, ulcers, mucosal thickening, and inflamed mucosa or seem normal.[181–183] Histology can demonstrate sulfur granules, which can be scarce and can limit diagnostic yield of mucosal biopsies.[184] Diagnosis is sometimes made after laparotomy for suspected malignancy.[185]

Whipple disease is a rare chronic infection caused by *Tropheryma whipplei*, which resides within intestinal macrophages. The classic tetrad of Whipple disease includes fever, abdominal pain, arthralgias, and diarrhea, and Caucasian males are thought to be most affected.[186] A variety of symptoms may be present for multiple years before diagnosis. Gastrointestinal manifestations include steatorrhea, hematochezia, malabsorption, malaise, and weight loss. The small intestine is the main source of infection, and endoscopy may show normal duodenal mucosa or dilated villi with ectatic lymph and yellow color, with histology identifying the bacterium.[187]

Infectious proctitis can be caused by gonorrhea, chlamydia including lymphogranuloma venereum, herpes simplex virus-2, and syphilis.[188] Lymphogranuloma venereum, in particular, can lead to development of strictures and fistulae with granulomas that suggest CD or masses suspicious for malignancy.[189–191] Symptoms include rectal pain, diarrhea, bleeding, mucus, and constipation. Endoscopy may show ulcers, erythema, and skip lesions, and histology may demonstrate inflammatory colitis and granulomas but can lack chronic crypt damage that may be seen in CD.[188,192] Laboratory testing for these pathogens should be considered.

Primary Malignancy and Oncologic Complications

Primary gastrointestinal/colorectal lymphomas are among the most common extranodal lymphomas and include non-Hodgkin lymphomas such as Burkitt lymphoma, follicular lymphoma, diffuse large B-cell lymphoma, mantle cell lymphoma, and marginal zone lymphoma and also include mucosa-associated lymphoid tissue lymphoma and enteropathy-associated T-cell lymphoma.[193,194] Ileocecal involvement is common, potentially related to lymphoid tissue in Peyer patches of the terminal ileum.[193] Risk of lymphoma attributable to immunosuppressants should be considered in patients with IBD, including hepatosplenic T-cell lymphoma associated with thiopurines. Presenting symptoms can include abdominal pain, bloating, dyspepsia, nausea, vomiting, diarrhea, rectal bleeding, weight loss, and obstruction. Endoscopic features include mass, polyps, large ulcers, and inflamed mucosa with erythema, edema, and nodularity, and histology can reveal the diagnosis.[194]

Neuroendocrine tumors can develop in the entire gastrointestinal tract.[195] Serotonin, histamine, tachykinins, and other substances released by these tumors into the portal circulation are inactivated by the liver. In the presence of hepatic metastases, these products are released into systemic circulation and can cause carcinoid syndrome.[196] Symptoms include flushing, frequent watery diarrhea, and abdominal cramping.[196,197] Jejunal, ileal, and cecal tumors are most commonly associated with carcinoid syndrome.[195] Imaging may detect tumors and hepatic metastases, but location and size can vary. Polypoid lesions can seem smooth and subepithelial on endoscopy, and endoscopic ultrasound is often helpful for further evaluation.[195] Imaging, endoscopy, and biochemical testing should be considered to identify possible metastases and the primary tumor site.

Cord colitis syndrome has been associated with umbilical cord blood for hematopoietic stem cell transplantation (HSCT). After HSCT, culprits of abdominal symptoms and diarrhea include infections, neutropenic enterocolitis or typhlitis, posttransplantation lymphoproliferative disease, and graft-versus host disease. Symptoms of cord colitis syndrome include fever, weight loss, diarrhea, and rectal bleeding, and imaging can show focal or diffuse bowel wall thickening. Endoscopy reveals erythema, edema, and ulceration with histology demonstrating chronic active colitis, neutrophilic infiltration with Paneth-cell metaplasia, crypt apoptosis, and granulomas in both upper and lower gastrointestinal tract.[198,199]

Radiation therapy is used for a range of malignancies and can affect the gastrointestinal tract. Intestinal mucosa and tissue stem cells can be injured by radiation, leading to submucosal fibrosis and endothelial damage in chronic injury.[200,201] Acute toxicity is often mild or self-limiting, in up to 75% of patients within 90 days of treatment. Chronic toxicity can occur 3 months to years after therapy.[202] Patients with IBD may be at higher risk for radiation toxicity.[203] Clinical symptoms include dyspepsia, nausea, vomiting, abdominal pain, diarrhea, rectal bleeding, and perianal skin lesions.[200,204] Endoscopic features include ulceration, erythema, friability, telangiectasias, and stricture, which can also lead to bowel obstruction.[204]

Drug-induced Conditions

Nonsteroidal antiinflammatory drugs (NSAIDs) can cause injury in multiple areas of the gastrointestinal tract.[205] Although commonly linked to peptic ulcer disease, NSAIDs can also cause ulcers and strictures in the small intestine and less often, the colon, and complications include perforation.[206–210] NSAID-induced enteropathy may be mediated by localized mucosal injury.[211] Ulcers may be identified on video capsule endoscopy, balloon-assisted enteroscopy, or colonoscopy.[212,213] Strictures related to NSAIDs can have a characteristic concentric shape with a small lumen, termed a diaphragm-like stricture, with submucosal fibrosis and normal epithelium on histology; focal granuloma can also develop.[214–216]

Immune checkpoint inhibitors (ICI) target regulatory pathways that can lead to immune-related adverse events, and gastrointestinal toxicity is common.[217] Patients can develop ICI gastritis, enteritis, enterocolitis, or segmental colitis that can mimic CD, and colitis is most common.[218] Symptoms include abdominal pain, reflux, nausea, vomiting, diarrhea, and hematochezia that can be graded on severity.[218] Imaging may be of low sensitivity, and fecal calprotectin and lactoferrin may be elevated.[219–221] Endoscopy may show erythema, cobblestoning and ulceration, and segmental colitis.[222] Histology may show noncaseating granulomas, cryptitis, and intraepithelial lymphocytes.[222,223] Patients with IBD may be at higher risk of enterocolitis or relapse.[224,225] Treatment response to immunosuppressants is often rapid, in contrast to CD.[218]

Genetic Conditions

Hereditary angioedema (HAE) leads to recurrent angioedema from increased production of bradykinin and can affect the skin, respiratory tract, and gastrointestinal tract. Symptoms include acute episodic abdominal pain, nausea, vomiting, and diarrhea, and complications include intussusception.[226,227] Imaging can demonstrate bowel wall thickening.[226] HAE may develop due to deficiency (type I) or low levels (type II) of complement component 1 inhibitor (C1-INH) protein or can occur in patients with normal levels associated with mutations in coagulation factor XII (type III).[228] HAE with normal C1-INH may more commonly affect women, be diagnosed in adulthood, and present with fewer episodes of abdominal pain.[229] Diagnosis can be made by testing for complement levels, C1-INH level and function, and mutations in coagulation factor XII.[228]

Chronic granulomatous disease (CGD) is a primary immunodeficiency in which reactive oxygen species production is impaired due to a defect in NADPH oxidase, precluding phagocytic antimicrobial activity. Patients suffer from frequent infections and complications of abnormal inflammatory responses; gastrointestinal manifestations are common.[230] Symptoms include abdominal pain, diarrhea, constipation, and rectal bleeding. Anorectal fissures, fistulae, and stenoses may develop. Endoscopy may show inflammation, erosions, ulcers, discolored mucosa, strictures, and skip lesions. Histologic features include crypt distortion, basal cell plasmacytosis, cryptitis and crypt abscesses, granulomas, and pigmented macrophages.[231] CGD-related IBD is a distinct entity from CD and may have limited current treatment options.[232–234]

SUMMARY

CD can present similarly to a wide variety of diseases. These range from noninfectious causes, where a range of diagnostic tools can help evaluate for these conditions (see **Table 1**), to infectious causes, where acuity of symptoms and exposure/travel history along with organism identification can be critical to differentiate infection from CD (see **Table 2**). In addition, many diseases typically affecting other organ systems may present with gastrointestinal manifestations. Potential additional rare causes to consider are listed in **Table 3**. Infectious, luminal, vascular, immune-mediated, malignant, and genetic processes and treatment complications should be considered in patients presenting with symptoms suspicious for CD. Social, travel, and sexual history may provide additional clues to guide evaluation, and specific laboratory testing or imaging may be warranted to evaluate for mimics of CD. Identifying the correct diagnosis has major implications for patient management and treatment outcomes.

CLINICS CARE POINTS

- Symptoms of Crohn's disease are not specific and may overlap with many disease states
- Patients with so-called refractory Crohn's disease may in fact carry an alternate diagnosis
- The differential diagnosis of Crohn's disease is broad

DISCLOSURE

S. Gupta: supported by NIH Training Grant NIDDK T32DK007533-35, J.R. Allegretti: consultant for Janssen, Pfizer, Pandion, Servatus, Finch Therapeutics, Iterative Scopes, BMS, Baccain, Morphic and Artugen, and has grant support from Merck.

REFERENCES

1. Chang JT. Pathophysiology of inflammatory bowel diseases. N Engl J Med 2020;383(27):2652–64.
2. Abraham C, Cho JH. Inflammatory bowel disease. N Engl J Med 2009;361(21):2066–78.

3. Peyrin-Biroulet L, Loftus EV, Colombel J-F, et al. Long-term complications, extra-intestinal manifestations, and mortality in adult Crohn's disease in population-based cohorts. Inflamm Bowel Dis 2011;17(1):471–8.

4. Lichtenstein GR, Loftus EV, Isaacs KL, et al. ACG clinical guideline: management of crohn's disease in adults. Am J Gastroenterol 2018;113(4):481–517.

5. Peery AF, Shaukat A, Strate LL. AGA clinical practice update on medical management of colonic diverticulitis: expert review. Gastroenterology 2021;160(3):906–11.e1.

6. Lamps LW, Knapple WL. Diverticular disease-associated segmental colitis. Clin Gastroenterol Hepatol 2007;5(1):27–31.

7. Freeman H-J. Segmental colitis associated with diverticulosis syndrome. World J Gastroenterol 2008;14(42):6442–3.

8. Schembri J, Bonello J, Christodoulou DK, et al. Segmental colitis associated with diverticulosis: is it the coexistence of colonic diverticulosis and inflammatory bowel disease? Ann Gastroenterol 2017;30(3):257–61.

9. Hansen C-C, Søreide K. Systematic review of epidemiology, presentation, and management of Meckel's diverticulum in the 21st century. Medicine 2018;97(35):e12154.

10. Dumper J, Mackenzie S, Mitchell P, et al. Complications of Meckel's diverticula in adults. Can J Surg 2006;49(5):353–7.

11. Nikolopoulos I, Ntakomyti E, El-Gaddal A, et al. Extracorporeal laparoscopically assisted resection of a perforated Meckel's diverticulum due to a chicken bone. BMJ Case Rep 2015;2015. https://doi.org/10.1136/bcr-2014-209051.

12. Modi S, Kanapathy Pillai S, DeClercq S. Perforated Meckel's diverticulum in an adult due to faecolith: A case report and review of literature. Int J Surg Case Rep 2015;15:143–5.

13. Hamilton CM, Arnason T. Ileitis associated with Meckel's diverticulum. Histopathology 2015;67(6):783–91.

14. Andreyev HJ, Owen RA, Thomas PA, et al. Acid secretion from a Meckel's diverticulum: the unsuspected mimic of Crohn's disease? Am J Gastroenterol 1994;89(9):1552–4.

15. Brandt LJ, Feuerstadt P, Longstreth GF, et al. ACG clinical guideline: epidemiology, risk factors, patterns of presentation, diagnosis, and management of colon ischemia (CI). Am J Gastroenterol 2015;110(1):18–44.

16. Misiakos EP, Tsapralis D, Karatzas T, et al. Advents in the diagnosis and management of ischemic colitis. Front Surg 2017;4:47.

17. Clair DG, Beach JM. Mesenteric Ischemia. N Engl J Med 2016;374(10):959–68.

18. Al-Diery H, Phillips A, Evennett N, et al. The pathogenesis of nonocclusive mesenteric ischemia: implications for research and clinical practice. J Intensive Care Med 2019;34(10):771–81.

19. Terlouw LG, Moelker A, Abrahamsen J, et al. European guidelines on chronic mesenteric ischaemia - joint United European Gastroenterology, European Association for Gastroenterology, Endoscopy and Nutrition, European Society of Gastrointestinal and Abdominal Radiology, Netherlands Association of Hepato-gastroenterologists, Hellenic Society of Gastroenterology, Cardiovascular and Interventional Radiological Society of Europe, and Dutch Mesenteric Ischemia Study group clinical guidelines on the diagnosis and treatment of patients with chronic mesenteric ischaemia. United Eur Gastroenterol J 2020;8(4):371–95.

20. Jennette JC, Falk RJ, Bacon PA, et al. 2012 revised International Chapel Hill Consensus Conference Nomenclature of Vasculitides. Arthritis Rheum 2013; 65(1):1–11.
21. Hatemi I, Hatemi G, Çelik AF. Systemic vasculitis and the gut. Curr Opin Rheumatol 2017;29(1):33–8.
22. Sampat HN, McAllister BP, Gaines DD, et al. Terminal Ileitis as a Feature of Henoch-Schönlein Purpura Masquerading as Crohn's Disease in Adults. J Clin Rheumatol 2016;22(2):82–5.
23. Deniz K, Ozşeker HS, Balas S, et al. Intestinal involvement in Wegener's granulomatosis. J Gastrointestin Liver Dis 2007;16(3):329–31.
24. Ebert EC, Hagspiel KD, Nagar M, et al. Gastrointestinal involvement in polyarteritis nodosa. Clin Gastroenterol Hepatol 2008;6(9):960–6.
25. Kobayashi K, Ueno F, Bito S, et al. Development of consensus statements for the diagnosis and management of intestinal Behçet's disease using a modified Delphi approach. J Gastroenterol 2007;42(9):737–45.
26. Rodrigues-Pinto E, Magro F, Pimenta S, et al. Mimicry between intestinal Behçet's disease and inflammatory bowel disease. J Crohn's Colitis 2014;8(7): 714–5.
27. Hatemi I, Hatemi G, Celik AF, et al. Frequency of pathergy phenomenon and other features of Behçet's syndrome among patients with inflammatory bowel disease. Clin Exp Rheumatol 2008;26(4 Suppl 50):S91–5.
28. International Team for the Revision of the International Criteria for Behçet's Disease (ITR-ICBD). The International Criteria for Behçet's Disease (ICBD): a collaborative study of 27 countries on the sensitivity and specificity of the new criteria. J Eur Acad Dermatol Venereol 2014;28(3):338–47.
29. Gornik HL, Persu A, Adlam D, et al. First International Consensus on the diagnosis and management of fibromuscular dysplasia. Vasc Med 2019;24(2): 164–89.
30. Olin JW, Froehlich J, Gu X, et al. The United States Registry for Fibromuscular Dysplasia: results in the first 447 patients. Circulation 2012;125(25):3182–90.
31. Chaturvedi R, Vaideeswar P, Joshi A, et al. Unusual mesenteric fibromuscular dysplasia a rare cause for chronic intestinal ischaemia. J Clin Pathol 2008; 61(2):237.
32. Du S, Yang S, Jia K, et al. Fibromuscular dysplasia of mesenteric arteries: a rare cause of multiple bowel resections-a case report and literature review. BMC Gastroenterol 2021;21(1):133.
33. Al Ansari A, Ahmed S, Mansour E, et al. Idiopathic myointimal hyperplasia of the mesenteric veins. J Surg Case Rep 2021;2021(1). https://doi.org/10.1093/jscr/rjaa453.
34. Wangensteen KJ, Fogt F, Kann BR, et al. Idiopathic myointimal hyperplasia of the mesenteric veins diagnosed preoperatively. J Clin Gastroenterol 2015; 49(6):491–4.
35. Miracle AC, Behr SC, Benhamida J, et al. Mesenteric inflammatory veno-occlusive disease: radiographic and histopathologic evaluation of 2 cases. Abdom Imaging 2014;39(1):18–24.
36. Flaherty MJ, Lie JT, Haggitt RC. Mesenteric inflammatory veno-occlusive disease. A seldom recognized cause of intestinal ischemia. Am J Surg Pathol 1994;18(8):779–84.
37. Hu JCC, Forshaw MJ, Thebe P, et al. Mesenteric inflammatory veno-occlusive disease as a cause of acute abdomen: report of five cases. Surg Today 2005; 35(11):961–4.

38. Martin FC, Yang LS, Fehily SR, et al. Idiopathic myointimal hyperplasia of the mesenteric veins: Case report and review of the literature. JGH Open 2020; 4(3):345–50.
39. Brito-Zerón P, Bari K, Baughman RP, et al. Sarcoidosis involving the gastrointestinal tract: diagnostic and therapeutic management. Am J Gastroenterol 2019; 114(8):1238–47.
40. Govender P, Berman JS. The diagnosis of sarcoidosis. Clin Chest Med 2015; 36(4):585–602.
41. Talley NJ, Shorter RG, Phillips SF, et al. Eosinophilic gastroenteritis: a clinicopathological study of patients with disease of the mucosa, muscle layer, and subserosal tissues. Gut 1990;31(1):54–8.
42. Schoonbroodt D, Horsmans Y, Laka A, et al. Eosinophilic gastroenteritis presenting with colitis and cholangitis. Dig Dis Sci 1995;40(2):308–14.
43. Haberkern CM, Christie DL, Haas JE. Eosinophilic gastroenteritis presenting as ileocolitis. Gastroenterology 1978;74(5 Pt 1):896–9.
44. Matsushita M, Hajiro K, Morita Y, et al. Eosinophilic gastroenteritis involving the entire digestive tract. Am J Gastroenterol 1995;90(10):1868–70.
45. Cianferoni A, Spergel J. Eosinophilic esophagitis: A comprehensive review. Clin Rev Allergy Immunol 2016;50(2):159–74.
46. Gonsalves N. Eosinophilic Gastrointestinal Disorders. Clin Rev Allergy Immunol 2019;57(2):272–85.
47. Chehade M, Magid MS, Mofidi S, et al. Allergic eosinophilic gastroenteritis with protein-losing enteropathy: intestinal pathology, clinical course, and long-term follow-up. J Pediatr Gastroenterol Nutr 2006;42(5):516–21.
48. Fan YC, Steele D, Kochar B, et al. Increased Prevalence of Esophageal Eosinophilia in Patients with Inflammatory Bowel Disease. Inflamm Intest Dis 2019; 3(4):180–6.
49. Mintz MJ, Ananthakrishnan AN. Phenotype and natural history of inflammatory bowel disease in patients with concomitant eosinophilic esophagitis. Inflamm Bowel Dis 2021;27(4):469–75.
50. Katsanos KH, Zinovieva E, Lambri E, et al. Eosinophilic-Crohn's overlap colitis and review of the literature. J Crohns Colitis 2011;5(3):256–61.
51. Gentile NM, Murray JA, Pardi DS. Autoimmune enteropathy: a review and update of clinical management. Curr Gastroenterol Rep 2012;14(5):380–5.
52. Chen CB, Tahboub F, Plesec T, et al. A review of autoimmune enteropathy and its associated syndromes. Dig Dis Sci 2020;65(11):3079–90.
53. Gereige JD, Maglione PJ. Current understanding and recent developments in common variable immunodeficiency associated autoimmunity. Front Immunol 2019;10:2753.
54. Ghafoor A, Joseph SM. Making a diagnosis of common variable immunodeficiency: A review. Cureus 2020;12(1):e6711.
55. Cunningham-Rundles C, Maglione PJ. Common variable immunodeficiency. J Allergy Clin Immunol 2012;129(5):1425–6.e3.
56. Pikkarainen S, Martelius T, Ristimäki A, et al. A high prevalence of gastrointestinal manifestations in common variable immunodeficiency. Am J Gastroenterol 2019;114(4):648–55.
57. Axelrad JE, Joelson A, Green PHR, et al. Enteric Infections Are Common in Patients with Flares of Inflammatory Bowel Disease. Am J Gastroenterol 2018; 113(10):1530–9.
58. Norman JM, Handley SA, Baldridge MT, et al. Disease-specific alterations in the enteric virome in inflammatory bowel disease. Cell 2015;160(3):447–60.

59. García Rodríguez LA, Ruigómez A, Panés J. Acute gastroenteritis is followed by an increased risk of inflammatory bowel disease. Gastroenterology 2006;130(6): 1588–94.

60. Masclee GMC, Penders J, Pierik M, et al. Enteropathogenic viruses: triggers for exacerbation in IBD? A prospective cohort study using real-time quantitative polymerase chain reaction. Inflamm Bowel Dis 2013;19(1):124–31.

61. Khan RR, Lawson AD, Minnich LL, et al. Gastrointestinal norovirus infection associated with exacerbation of inflammatory bowel disease. J Pediatr Gastroenterol Nutr 2009;48(3):328–33.

62. Limsrivilai J, Saleh ZM, Johnson LA, et al. Prevalence and Effect of Intestinal Infections Detected by a PCR-Based Stool Test in Patients with Inflammatory Bowel Disease. Dig Dis Sci 2020;65(11):3287–96.

63. Fakhreddine AY, Frenette CT, Konijeti GG. A practical review of cytomegalovirus in gastroenterology and hepatology. Gastroenterol Res Pract 2019;2019: 6156581.

64. Beswick L, Ye B, van Langenberg DR. Toward an Algorithm for the Diagnosis and Management of CMV in Patients with Colitis. Inflamm Bowel Dis 2016; 22(12):2966–76.

65. Shimoji S, Kato K, Eriguchi Y, et al. Evaluating the association between histological manifestations of cord colitis syndrome with GVHD. Bone Marrow Transplant 2013;48(9):1249–52.

66. Lawlor G, Moss AC. Cytomegalovirus in inflammatory bowel disease: pathogen or innocent bystander? Inflamm Bowel Dis 2010;16(9):1620–7.

67. quiz e7 McCurdy JD, Jones A, Enders FT, et al. A model for identifying cytomegalovirus in patients with inflammatory bowel disease. Clin Gastroenterol Hepatol 2015;13(1):131–7.

68. Yerushalmy-Feler A, Padlipsky J, Cohen S. Diagnosis and management of CMV colitis. Curr Infect Dis Rep 2019;21(2):5.

69. Johnson RH, Sharma R, Kuran R, et al. Coccidioidomycosis: a review. J Investig Med 2021;69(2):316–23.

70. Amarnath S, Deeb L, Philipose J, et al. A comprehensive review of infectious granulomatous diseases of the gastrointestinal tract. Gastroenterol Res Pract 2021;2021:8167149.

71. Storage TR, Segal J, Brown J. Peritoneal coccidioidomycosis: a rare case report and review of the literature. J Gastrointestin Liver Dis 2015;24(4):527–30.

72. Zhou S, Ma Y, Chandrasoma P. Small bowel dissemination of coccidioidomycosis. Case Rep Pathol 2015;2015:403671.

73. Weatherhead JE, Barrows BD, Stager CE, et al. Gastrointestinal Coccidioidomycosis. J Clin Gastroenterol 2015;49(7):628–9.

74. Weisman IM, Moreno AJ, Parker AL, et al. Gastrointestinal dissemination of coccidioidomycosis. Am J Gastroenterol 1986;81(7):589–93.

75. Kauffman CA. Histoplasmosis: a clinical and laboratory update. Clin Microbiol Rev 2007;20(1):115–32.

76. Patel NM, Schwartz DJ. Lower GI bleeding from ileocolonic histoplasmosis. Gastrointest Endosc 2011;74(6):1404–5.

77. Assi M, McKinsey DS, Driks MR, et al. Gastrointestinal histoplasmosis in the acquired immunodeficiency syndrome: report of 18 cases and literature review. Diagn Microbiol Infect Dis 2006;55(3):195–201.

78. Lamps LW, Molina CP, West AB, et al. The pathologic spectrum of gastrointestinal and hepatic histoplasmosis. Am J Clin Pathol 2000;113(1):64–72.

79. Panchabhai TS, Bais RK, Pyle RC, et al. An Apple-core Lesion in the Colon: An Infectious Etiology. J Glob Infect Dis 2011;3(2):195–8.
80. Zhu L-L, Wang J, Wang Z-J, et al. Intestinal histoplasmosis in immunocompetent adults. World J Gastroenterol 2016;22(15):4027–33.
81. Toscanini MA, Nusblat AD, Cuestas ML. Diagnosis of histoplasmosis: current status and perspectives. Appl Microbiol Biotechnol 2021;105(5):1837–59.
82. Shirley D-AT, Farr L, Watanabe K, et al. A review of the global burden, new diagnostics, and current therapeutics for amebiasis. Open Forum Infect Dis 2018;5(7):ofy161.
83. Kantor M, Abrantes A, Estevez A, et al. Entamoeba histolytica: updates in clinical manifestation, pathogenesis, and vaccine development. Can J Gastroenterol Hepatol 2018;2018:4601420.
84. Billet AC, Salmon Rousseau A, Piroth L, et al. An underestimated sexually transmitted infection: amoebiasis. BMJ Case Rep 2019;12(5). https://doi.org/10.1136/bcr-2018-228942.
85. Salit IE, Khairnar K, Gough K, et al. A possible cluster of sexually transmitted Entamoeba histolytica: genetic analysis of a highly virulent strain. Clin Infect Dis 2009;49(3):346–53.
86. Van Den Broucke S, Verschueren J, Van Esbroeck M, et al. Clinical and microscopic predictors of Entamoeba histolytica intestinal infection in travelers and migrants diagnosed with Entamoeba histolytica/dispar infection. Plos Negl Trop Dis 2018;12(10):e0006892.
87. Lee K-C, Lu C-C, Hu W-H, et al. Colonoscopic diagnosis of amebiasis: a case series and systematic review. Int J Colorectal Dis 2015;30(1):31–41.
88. Wang H, Kanthan R. Multiple colonic and ileal perforations due to unsuspected intestinal amoebiasis-Case report and review. Pathol Res Pract 2020;216(1):152608.
89. McClung RP, Roth DM, Vigar M, et al. Waterborne disease outbreaks associated with environmental and undetermined exposures to water - United States, 2013-2014. Am J Transplant 2018;18(1):262–7.
90. Pickering LK, Woodward WE, DuPont HL, et al. Occurrence of Giardia lamblia in children in day care centers. J Pediatr 1984;104(4):522–6.
91. Allain T, Buret AG. Pathogenesis and post-infectious complications in giardiasis. Adv Parasitol 2020;107:173–99.
92. Ryan U, Hijjawi N, Feng Y, et al. Giardia: an under-reported foodborne parasite. Int J Parasitol 2019;49(1):1–11.
93. Gunasekaran TS, Hassall E. Giardiasis mimicking inflammatory bowel disease. J Pediatr 1992;120(3):424–6.
94. Halliez MCM, Buret AG. Extra-intestinal and long term consequences of Giardia duodenalis infections. World J Gastroenterol 2013;19(47):8974–85.
95. Lebwohl B, Deckelbaum RJ, Green PHR. Giardiasis. Gastrointest Endosc 2003;57(7):906–13.
96. Doglioni C, De Boni M, Cielo R, et al. Gastric giardiasis. J Clin Pathol 1992;45(11):964–7.
97. Oberhuber G, Stolte M. Giardiasis: analysis of histological changes in biopsy specimens of 80 patients. J Clin Pathol 1990;43(8):641–3.
98. Aziz H, Beck CE, Lux MF, et al. A comparison study of different methods used in the detection of Giardia lamblia. Clin Lab Sci 2001;14(3):150–4.
99. Heyworth MF. Diagnostic testing for Giardia infections. Trans R Soc Trop Med Hyg 2014;108(3):123–5.

100. Gryseels B, De Vlas SJ. Worm burdens in schistosome infections. Parasitol Today 1996;12(3):115–9.

101. Shuja A, Guan J, Harris C, et al. Intestinal Schistosomiasis: A Rare Cause of Abdominal Pain and Weight loss. Cureus 2018;10(1):e2086.

102. Schwartz C, Fallon PG. Schistosoma "Eggs-Iting" the Host: Granuloma Formation and Egg Excretion. Front Immunol 2018;9:2492.

103. Elbaz T, Esmat G. Hepatic and intestinal schistosomiasis: review. J Advanc Res 2013;4(5):445–52.

104. Mu A, Fernandes I, Phillips D. A 57-Year-Old Woman With a Cecal Mass. Clin Infect Dis 2016;63(5):703–5.

105. Lamyman MJ, Noble DJ, Narang S, et al. Small bowel obstruction secondary to intestinal schistosomiasis. Trans R Soc Trop Med Hyg 2006;100(9):885–7.

106. Gabbi C, Bertolotti M, Iori R, et al. Acute abdomen associated with schistosomiasis of the appendix. Dig Dis Sci 2006;51(1):215–7.

107. Bustinduy AL, Sousa-Figueiredo JC, Adriko M, et al. Fecal occult blood and fecal calprotectin as point-of-care markers of intestinal morbidity in Ugandan children with Schistosoma mansoni infection. Plos Negl Trop Dis 2013;7(11): e2542.

108. Cao J, Liu W-J, Xu X-Y, et al. Endoscopic findings and clinicopathologic characteristics of colonic schistosomiasis: a report of 46 cases. World J Gastroenterol 2010;16(6):723–7.

109. Krolewiecki A, Nutman TB. Strongyloidiasis: A neglected tropical disease. Infect Dis Clin North Am 2019;33(1):135–51.

110. Sreenivas DV, Kumar A, Kumar YR, et al. Intestinal strongyloidiasis–a rare opportunistic infection. Indian J Gastroenterol 1997;16(3):105–6.

111. Karanam LSK, Basavraj GK, Papireddy CKR. Strongyloides stercoralis Hyper infection Syndrome. Indian J Surg 2020;1–5.

112. Rivasi F, Pampiglione S, Boldorini R, et al. Histopathology of gastric and duodenal Strongyloides stercoralis locations in fifteen immunocompromised subjects. Arch Pathol Lab Med 2006;130(12):1792–8.

113. Overstreet K, Chen J, Rodriguez JW, et al. Endoscopic and histopathologic findings of Strongyloides stercoralis infection in a patient with AIDS. Gastrointest Endosc 2003;58(6):928–31.

114. Thompson BF, Fry LC, Wells CD, et al. The spectrum of GI strongyloidiasis: an endoscopic-pathologic study. Gastrointest Endosc 2004;59(7):906–10.

115. Qu Z, Kundu UR, Abadeer RA, et al. Strongyloides colitis is a lethal mimic of ulcerative colitis: the key morphologic differential diagnosis. Hum Pathol 2009; 40(4):572–7.

116. Paul M, Meena S, Gupta P, et al. Clinico-epidemiological spectrum of strongyloidiasis in India: Review of 166 cases. J Fam Med Prim Care 2020;9(2):485–91.

117. Hochberg NS, Hamer DH. Anisakidosis: Perils of the deep. Clin Infect Dis 2010; 51(7):806–12.

118. Kakizoe S, Kakizoe H, Kakizoe K, et al. Endoscopic findings and clinical manifestation of gastric anisakiasis. Am J Gastroenterol 1995;90(5):761–3.

119. Muraoka A, Suehiro I, Fujii M, et al. Acute gastric anisakiasis: 28 cases during the last 10 years. Dig Dis Sci 1996;41(12):2362–5.

120. Guh AY, Mu Y, Winston LG, et al. Trends in U.S. Burden of Clostridioides difficile Infection and Outcomes. N Engl J Med 2020;382(14):1320–30.

121. McDonald LC, Gerding DN, Johnson S, et al. Clinical Practice Guidelines for Clostridium difficile Infection in Adults and Children: 2017 Update by the

Infectious Diseases Society of America (IDSA) and Society for Healthcare Epidemiology of America (SHEA). Clin Infect Dis 2018;66(7):e1–48.

122. Lessa FC, Mu Y, Bamberg WM, et al. Burden of Clostridium difficile infection in the United States. N Engl J Med 2015;372(9):825–34.

123. Dalal RS, Allegretti JR. Diagnosis and management of Clostridioides difficile infection in patients with inflammatory bowel disease. Curr Opin Gastroenterol 2021. https://doi.org/10.1097/MOG.0000000000000739.

124. Burkart NE, Kwaan MR, Shepela C, et al. Indications and Relative Utility of Lower Endoscopy in the Management of Clostridium difficile Infection. Gastroenterol Res Pract 2011;2011:626582.

125. Nataro JP, Kaper JB. Diarrheagenic Escherichia coli. Clin Microbiol Rev 1998; 11(1):142–201.

126. Vila J, Sáez-López E, Johnson JR, et al. Escherichia coli: an old friend with new tidings. FEMS Microbiol Rev 2016;40(4):437–63.

127. Lim JY, Yoon J, Hovde CJ. A brief overview of Escherichia coli O157:H7 and its plasmid O157. J Microbiol Biotechnol 2010;20(1):5–14.

128. Johnson KE, Thorpe CM, Sears CL. The emerging clinical importance of non-O157 Shiga toxin-producing Escherichia coli. Clin Infect Dis 2006;43(12): 1587–95.

129. Goldwater PN, Bettelheim KA. Treatment of enterohemorrhagic Escherichia coli (EHEC) infection and hemolytic uremic syndrome (HUS). BMC Med 2012;10:12.

130. Lamps LW. Infective disorders of the gastrointestinal tract. Histopathology 2007; 50(1):55–63.

131. Bhaijee F, Arnold C, Lam-Himlin D, et al. Infectious mimics of inflammatory bowel disease. Diagn Histopathol 2015;21(7):267–75.

132. DuPont HL, Levine MM, Hornick RB, et al. Inoculum size in shigellosis and implications for expected mode of transmission. J Infect Dis 1989;159(6):1126–8.

133. Baker S, The HC. Recent insights into Shigella. Curr Opin Infect Dis 2018;31(5): 449–54.

134. Williams PCM, Berkley JA. Guidelines for the treatment of dysentery (shigellosis): a systematic review of the evidence. Paediatr Int Child Health 2018; 38(sup1):S50–65.

135. Dekker JP, Frank KM. Salmonella, Shigella, and yersinia. Clin Lab Med 2015; 35(2):225–46.

136. Kotloff KL, Riddle MS, Platts-Mills JA, et al. Shigellosis. Lancet 2018;391(10122): 801–12.

137. Burnham PM, Hendrixson DR. Campylobacter jejuni: collective components promoting a successful enteric lifestyle. Nat Rev Microbiol 2018;16(9):551–65.

138. Silva J, Leite D, Fernandes M, et al. Campylobacter spp. as a Foodborne Pathogen: A Review. Front Microbiol 2011;2:200.

139. Tack DM, Ray L, Griffin PM, et al. Preliminary Incidence and Trends of Infections with Pathogens Transmitted Commonly Through Food - Foodborne Diseases Active Surveillance Network, 10 U.S. Sites, 2016-2019. MMWR Morb Mortal Wkly Rep 2020;69(17):509–14.

140. Loss RW, Mangla JC, Pereira M. Campylobacter colitis presentin as inflammatory bowel disease with segmental colonic ulcerations. Gastroenterology 1980;79(1):138–40.

141. van Spreeuwel JP, Duursma GC, Meijer CJ, et al. Campylobacter colitis: histological immunohistochemical and ultrastructural findings. Gut 1985;26(9): 945–51.

142. van Spreeuwel JP, Lindeman J, Bax R, et al. Campylobacter-associated appendicitis: prevalence and clinicopathologic features. Pathol Annu 1987;22(Pt 1): 55–65.

143. Puylaert JB, Vermeijden RJ, van der Werf SD, et al. Incidence and sonographic diagnosis of bacterial ileocaecitis masquerading as appendicitis. Lancet 1989; 2(8654):84–6.

144. Oh SJ, Pimentel M, Leite GGS, et al. Acute appendicitis is associated with appendiceal microbiome changes including elevated Campylobacter jejuni levels. BMJ Open Gastroenterol 2020;7(1). https://doi.org/10.1136/bmjgast-2020-000412.

145. Lecuit M, Abachin E, Martin A, et al. Immunoproliferative small intestinal disease associated with Campylobacter jejuni. N Engl J Med 2004;350(3):239–48.

146. Monselise A, Blickstein D, Ostfeld I, et al. A case of cellulitis complicating Campylobacter jejuni subspecies jejuni bacteremia and review of the literature. Eur J Clin Microbiol Infect Dis 2004;23(9):718–21.

147. Lang CL, Chiang CK, Hung KY, et al. Campylobacter jejuni peritonitis and bacteremia in a patient undergoing continuous ambulatory peritoneal dialysis. Clin Nephrol 2009;71(1):96–8.

148. Wang C-H, Tai T-H, Weng S-Y, et al. Spontaneous bacterial peritonitis caused by Campylobacter Coli in cirrhotic patient: A rare case report (CARE-compliant). Medicine 2020;99(21):e19887.

149. Kaakoush NO, Castaño-Rodríguez N, Mitchell HM, et al. Global Epidemiology of Campylobacter Infection. Clin Microbiol Rev 2015;28(3):687–720.

150. Schaad UB. Reactive arthritis associated with Campylobacter enteritis. Pediatr Infect Dis 1982;1(5):328–32.

151. Gal-Mor O. Persistent Infection and Long-Term Carriage of Typhoidal and Non-typhoidal Salmonellae. Clin Microbiol Rev 2019;32(1). https://doi.org/10.1128/CMR.00088-18.

152. Cohen JI, Bartlett JA, Corey GR. Extra-intestinal manifestations of salmonella infections. Medicine 1987;66(5):349–88.

153. Keithlin J, Sargeant JM, Thomas MK, et al. Systematic review and meta-analysis of the proportion of non-typhoidal Salmonella cases that develop chronic sequelae. Epidemiol Infect 2015;143(7):1333–51.

154. Crump JA, Sjölund-Karlsson M, Gordon MA, et al. Epidemiology, clinical presentation, laboratory diagnosis, antimicrobial resistance, and antimicrobial management of invasive salmonella infections. Clin Microbiol Rev 2015;28(4): 901–37.

155. Balthazar EJ, Charles HW, Megibow AJ. Salmonella- and Shigella-induced ileitis: CT findings in four patients. J Comput Assist Tomogr 1996;20(3):375–8.

156. Dionisio D, Esperti F, Vivarelli A, et al. Acute terminal ileitis mimicking Crohn's disease caused by Salmonella veneziana. Int J Infect Dis 2001;5(4):225–7.

157. Eng S-K, Pusparajah P, Ab Mutalib N-S, et al. Salmonella : A review on pathogenesis, epidemiology and antibiotic resistance. Front Life Sci 2015;8(3): 284–93.

158. Nagaraja V, Eslick GD. Systematic review with meta-analysis: the relationship between chronic Salmonella typhi carrier status and gall-bladder cancer. Aliment Pharmacol Ther 2014;39(8):745–50.

159. Mogasale V, Desai SN, Mogasale VV, et al. Case fatality rate and length of hospital stay among patients with typhoid intestinal perforation in developing countries: a systematic literature review. PLoS One 2014;9(4):e93784.

160. Gunn JS, Marshall JM, Baker S, et al. Salmonella chronic carriage: epidemiology, diagnosis, and gallbladder persistence. Trends Microbiol 2014;22(11): 648–55.
161. McNally A, Thomson NR, Reuter S, et al. Add, stir and reduce ': Yersinia spp. as model bacteria for pathogen evolution. Nat Rev Microbiol 2016;14(3):177–90.
162. Triantafillidis JK, Thomaidis T, Papalois A. Terminal ileitis due to yersinia infection: an underdiagnosed situation. Biomed Res Int 2020;2020:1240626.
163. Sabina Y, Rahman A, Ray RC, et al. Yersinia enterocolitica: Mode of Transmission, Molecular Insights of Virulence, and Pathogenesis of Infection. J Pathog 2011;2011:429069.
164. Matsumoto T, Iida M, Matsui T, et al. Endoscopic findings in Yersinia enterocolitica enterocolitis. Gastrointest Endosc 1990;36(6):583–7.
165. Ijichi S, Kusaka T, Okada H, et al. Terminal ileitis caused by Yersinia pseudotuberculosis mimicking Crohn's disease in childhood. J Pediatr Gastroenterol Nutr 2012;55(4):e125.
166. Zhou Y, Yu L, Nan Z, et al. Taxonomy, virulence genes and antimicrobial resistance of Aeromonas isolated from extra-intestinal and intestinal infections. BMC Infect Dis 2019;19(1):158.
167. Chopra AK, Houston CW. Enterotoxins in Aeromonas-associated gastroenteritis. Microbes Infect 1999;1(13):1129–37.
168. Batra P, Mathur P, Misra MC. Aeromonas spp.: An Emerging Nosocomial Pathogen. J Lab Physicians 2016;8(1):1–4.
169. Farraye FA, Peppercorn MA, Ciano PS, et al. Segmental colitis associated with Aeromonas hydrophila. Am J Gastroenterol 1989;84(4):436–8.
170. Deutsch SF, Wedzina W. Aeromonas sobria-associated left-sided segmental colitis. Am J Gastroenterol 1997;92(11):2104–6.
171. Evans RPT, Mourad MM, Dvorkin L, et al. Hepatic and Intra-abdominal Tuberculosis: 2016 Update. Curr Infect Dis Rep 2016;18(12):45.
172. Mamo JP, Brij SO, Enoch DA. Abdominal tuberculosis: a retrospective review of cases presenting to a UK district hospital. QJM 2013;106(4):347–54.
173. Rathi P, Gambhire P. Abdominal Tuberculosis. J Assoc Physicians India 2016; 64(2):38–47.
174. Ladumor H, Al-Mohannadi S, Ameerudeen FS, et al. TB or not TB: A comprehensive review of imaging manifestations of abdominal tuberculosis and its mimics. Clin Imaging 2021;76:130–43.
175. Kurnick A, Bar N, Maharshak N. Intestinal tuberculosis and crohn's disease is always a diagnostic challenge: A case report and review of the literature on the importance of fecal mycobacterial cultures and the limitations of latent infection testing. Cureus 2019;11(9):e5689.
176. Klaaborg KE, Kronborg O, Olsen H. Enterocutaneous fistulization due to Actinomyces odontolyticus. Report of a case. Dis Colon Rectum 1985;28(7):526–7.
177. Horvath BA, Maryamchik E, Miller GC, et al. Actinomyces in Crohn's-like appendicitis. Histopathology 2019;75(4):486–95.
178. Valour F, Sénéchal A, Dupieux C, et al. Actinomycosis: etiology, clinical features, diagnosis, treatment, and management. Infect Drug Resist 2014;7:183–97.
179. Cintron JR, Del Pino A, Duarte B, et al. Abdominal actinomycosis. Dis Colon Rectum 1996;39(1):105–8.
180. Abdalla J, Myers J, Moorman J. Actinomycotic infection of the oesophagus. J Infect 2005;51(2):E39–43.
181. Piper MH, Schaberg DR, Ross JM, et al. Endoscopic detection and therapy of colonic actinomycosis. Am J Gastroenterol 1992;87(8):1040–2.

182. Yang SH, Li AF, Lin JK. Colonoscopy in abdominal actinomycosis. Gastrointest Endosc 2000;51(2):236–8.
183. Kim JB, Han DS, Lee HL, et al. Diagnosis and partial treatment of actinomycosis by colonoscopic biopsy. Gastrointest Endosc 2004;60(1):162–4.
184. Wong VK, Turmezei TD, Weston VC. Actinomycosis. BMJ 2011;343:d6099.
185. Dayan K, Neufeld D, Zissin R, et al. Actinomycosis of the large bowel: unusual presentations and their surgical treatment. Eur J Surg 1996;162(8):657–60.
186. Elfanagely Y, Jamot S, Dapaah-Afriyie K, et al. Whipple's disease mimicking common digestive disorders. R Med J (2013) 2021;104(4):43–5.
187. Dolmans RA, Boel CH, Lacle MM, et al. Clinical manifestations, treatment, and diagnosis of Tropheryma whipplei infections. Clin Microbiol Rev 2017;30(2): 529–55.
188. Hoentjen F, Rubin DT. Infectious proctitis: when to suspect it is not inflammatory bowel disease. Dig Dis Sci 2012;57(2):269–73.
189. Di Altobrando A, Tartari F, Filippini A, et al. Lymphogranuloma venereum proctitis mimicking inflammatory bowel diseases in 11 patients: a 4-year single-center experience. Crohns Colitis 360 2019;1(1).
190. Neri B, Stingone C, Romeo S, et al. Inflammatory bowel disease versus Chlamydia trachomatis infection: a case report and revision of the literature. Eur J Gastroenterol Hepatol 2020;32(3):454–7.
191. Bancil AS, Alexakis C, Pollok R. Delayed diagnosis of lymphogranuloma venereum-associated colitis in a man first suspected to have rectal cancer. JRSM Open 2016;8(1). 2054270416660933.
192. Arnold CA, Roth R, Arsenescu R, et al. Sexually transmitted infectious colitis vs inflammatory bowel disease: distinguishing features from a case-controlled study. Am J Clin Pathol 2015;144(5):771–81.
193. Hangge PT, Calderon E, Habermann EB, et al. Primary colorectal lymphoma: institutional experience and review of a national database. Dis Colon Rectum 2019;62(10):1167–76.
194. Shirwaikar Thomas A, Schwartz M, Quigley E. Gastrointestinal lymphoma: the new mimic. BMJ Open Gastroenterol 2019;6(1):e000320.
195. Ahmed M. Gastrointestinal neuroendocrine tumors in 2020. World J Gastrointest Oncol 2020;12(8):791–807.
196. Modlin IM, Kidd M, Latich I, et al. Current status of gastrointestinal carcinoids. Gastroenterology 2005;128(6):1717–51.
197. von der Ohe MR, Camilleri M, Kvols LK, et al. Motor dysfunction of the small bowel and colon in patients with the carcinoid syndrome and diarrhea. N Engl J Med 1993;329(15):1073–8.
198. Gupta NK, Masia R. Cord colitis syndrome: a cause of granulomatous inflammation in the upper and lower gastrointestinal tract. Am J Surg Pathol 2013;37(7): 1109–13.
199. Herrera AF, Soriano G, Bellizzi AM, et al. Cord colitis syndrome in cord-blood stem-cell transplantation. N Engl J Med 2011;365(9):815–24.
200. Araujo IK, Muñoz-Guglielmetti D, Mollà M. Radiation-induced damage in the lower gastrointestinal tract: Clinical presentation, diagnostic tests and treatment options. Best Pract Res Clin Gastroenterol 2020;48-49:101707.
201. Hasleton PS, Carr N, Schofield PF. Vascular changes in radiation bowel disease. Histopathology 1985;9(5):517–34.
202. Lawrie TA, Green JT, Beresford M, et al. Interventions to reduce acute and late adverse gastrointestinal effects of pelvic radiotherapy for primary pelvic cancers. Cochrane Database Syst Rev 2018;1:CD012529.

203. Tromp D, Christie DRH. Acute and Late Bowel Toxicity in Radiotherapy Patients with Inflammatory Bowel Disease: A Systematic Review. Clin Oncol (R Coll Radiol) 2015;27(9):536–41.
204. Shadad AK, Sullivan FJ, Martin JD, et al. Gastrointestinal radiation injury: prevention and treatment. World J Gastroenterol 2013;19(2):199–208.
205. Allison MC, Howatson AG, Torrance CJ, et al. Gastrointestinal damage associated with the use of nonsteroidal antiinflammatory drugs. N Engl J Med 1992; 327(11):749–54.
206. Bjarnason I, Hayllar J, MacPherson AJ, et al. Side effects of nonsteroidal antiinflammatory drugs on the small and large intestine in humans. Gastroenterology 1993;104(6):1832–47.
207. Day TK. Intestinal perforation associated with osmotic slow release indomethacin capsules. Br Med J (Clin Res Ed) 1983;287(6406):1671–2.
208. Kaufman HL, Fischer AH, Carroll M, et al. Colonic ulceration associated with nonsteroidal anti-inflammatory drugs. Report of three cases. Dis Colon Rectum 1996;39(6):705–10.
209. Klein M, Linnemann D, Rosenberg J. Non-steroidal anti-inflammatory drug-induced colopathy. BMJ Case Rep 2011;2011.
210. Kessler WF, Shires GT, Fahey TJ. Surgical complications of nonsteroidal antiinflammatory drug-induced small bowel ulceration. J Am Coll Surg 1997;185(3): 250–4.
211. Bjarnason I, Fehilly B, Smethurst P, et al. Importance of local versus systemic effects of non-steroidal anti-inflammatory drugs in increasing small intestinal permeability in man. Gut 1991;32(3):275–7.
212. Graham DY, Opekun AR, Willingham FF, et al. Visible small-intestinal mucosal injury in chronic NSAID users. Clin Gastroenterol Hepatol 2005;3(1):55–9.
213. Hayashi Y, Yamamoto H, Kita H, et al. Non-steroidal anti-inflammatory drug-induced small bowel injuries identified by double-balloon endoscopy. World J Gastroenterol 2005;11(31):4861–4.
214. Lang J, Price AB, Levi AJ, et al. Diaphragm disease: pathology of disease of the small intestine induced by non-steroidal anti-inflammatory drugs. J Clin Pathol 1988;41(5):516–26.
215. Woodman I, Schofield JB, Haboubi N. The histopathological mimics of inflammatory bowel disease: a critical appraisal. Tech Coloproctol 2015;19(12): 717–27.
216. Baert F, Hart J, Blackstone MO. A case of diclofenac-induced colitis with focal granulomatous change. Am J Gastroenterol 1995;90(10):1871–3.
217. Pauken KE, Dougan M, Rose NR, et al. Adverse events following cancer immunotherapy: obstacles and opportunities. Trends Immunol 2019;40(6):511–23.
218. Dougan M, Wang Y, Rubio-Tapia A, et al. AGA clinical practice update on diagnosis and management of immune checkpoint inhibitor colitis and hepatitis: expert review. Gastroenterology 2021;160(4):1384–93.
219. Gong Z, Wang Y. Immune Checkpoint Inhibitor-Mediated Diarrhea and Colitis: A Clinical Review. JCO Oncol Pract 2020;16(8):453–61.
220. Durbin SM, Mooradian MJ, Fintelmann FJ, et al. Diagnostic utility of CT for suspected immune checkpoint inhibitor enterocolitis. J Immunother Cancer 2020; 8(2). https://doi.org/10.1136/jitc-2020-001329.
221. Garcia-Neuer M, Marmarelis ME, Jangi SR, et al. Diagnostic Comparison of CT Scans and Colonoscopy for Immune-Related Colitis in Ipilimumab-Treated Advanced Melanoma Patients. Cancer Immunol Res 2017;5(4):286–91.

222. Wang Y, Abu-Sbeih H, Mao E, et al. Endoscopic and Histologic Features of Immune Checkpoint Inhibitor-Related Colitis. Inflamm Bowel Dis 2018;24(8): 1695–705.

223. Isidro RA, Ruan AB, Gannarapu S, et al. Medication-specific variations in morphological patterns of injury in immune check-point inhibitor-associated colitis. Histopathology 2021;78(4):532–41.

224. Grover S, Ruan AB, Srivoleti P, et al. Safety of Immune Checkpoint Inhibitors in Patients With Pre-Existing Inflammatory Bowel Disease and Microscopic Colitis. JCO Oncol Pract 2020;16(9):e933–42.

225. Meserve J, Facciorusso A, Holmer AK, et al. Systematic review with meta-analysis: safety and tolerability of immune checkpoint inhibitors in patients with pre-existing inflammatory bowel diseases. Aliment Pharmacol Ther. 2021;53(3): 374–82.

226. Mumneh N, Tick M, Borum M. Angioedema with severe acute abdominal pain: Think of hereditary angioedema. Clin Res Hepatol Gastroenterol 2021;101702. https://doi.org/10.1016/j.clinre.2021.101702.

227. Roy J, Vunnam R, Gorrepati VS, et al. Colonic intussusception secondary to hereditary angioedema. ACG Case Rep J 2021;8(1):e00498.

228. Busse PJ, Christiansen SC, Riedl MA, et al. US HAEA medical advisory board 2020 guidelines for the management of hereditary angioedema. J Allergy Clin Immunol Pract 2021;9(1):132–50.e3.

229. Bork K, Gül D, Hardt J, et al. Hereditary angioedema with normal C1 inhibitor: clinical symptoms and course. Am J Med 2007;120(11):987–92.

230. Marciano BE, Rosenzweig SD, Kleiner DE, et al. Gastrointestinal involvement in chronic granulomatous disease. Pediatrics 2004;114(2):462–8.

231. Khangura SK, Kamal N, Ho N, et al. Gastrointestinal features of chronic granulomatous disease found during endoscopy. Clin Gastroenterol Hepatol 2016; 14(3):395–402.e5.

232. Uzel G, Orange JS, Poliak N, et al. Complications of tumor necrosis factor-α blockade in chronic granulomatous disease-related colitis. Clin Infect Dis 2010;51(12):1429–34.

233. Kamal N, Marciano B, Curtin B, et al. The response to vedolizumab in chronic granulomatous disease-related inflammatory bowel disease. Gastroenterol Rep (Oxf) 2020;8(5):404–6.

234. Bhattacharya S, Marciano BE, Malech HL, et al. Safety and efficacy of ustekinumab in the inflammatory bowel disease of chronic granulomatous disease. Clin Gastroenterol Hepatol 2021. https://doi.org/10.1016/j.cgh.2021.03.039.

235. Goodall R, Langridge B, Onida S, et al. Median arcuate ligament syndrome. J Vasc Surg 2020;71(6):2170–6.

236. Chaum M, Shouhed D, Kim S, et al. Clinico-pathologic findings in patients with median arcuate ligament syndrome (celiac artery compression syndrome). Ann Diagn Pathol 2021;52:151732.

237. Warncke ES, Gursahaney DL, Mascolo M, et al. Superior mesenteric artery syndrome: a radiographic review. Abdom Radiol (Ny) 2019;44(9):3188–94.

238. Wang T, Wang Z-X, Wang H-J. Clinical Insights into Superior Mesenteric Artery Syndrome with Multiple Diseases: A Case Report. Dig Dis Sci 2019;64(6): 1711–4.

239. Zhang ZA. Superior mesenteric artery syndrome: a vicious cycle. BMJ Case Rep 2018;2018. https://doi.org/10.1136/bcr-2018-226002.

240. Ganss A, Rampado S, Savarino E, et al. Superior mesenteric artery syndrome: a prospective study in a single institution. J Gastrointest Surg 2019;23(5): 997–1005.

241. Malfertheiner P, Formigoni C. Severe cases of sprue-like enteropathy associated with angiotensin receptor blockers other than olmesartan. GastroHep - The Int J Gastroenterol Hepatol Endosc 2021;3(2):88–99.

242. Kamal A, Fain C, Park A, et al. Angiotensin II receptor blockers and gastrointestinal adverse events of resembling sprue-like enteropathy: a systematic review. Gastroenterol Rep (Oxf) 2019;7(3):162–7.

243. Soldera J, Gastrointerestinal Salgado K. Valsartan induced sprue-like enteropathy. J Gastroenterol Hepatol 2020;35(8):1262.

244. Agostinho N, Bains HK, Sardelic F. Enterocutaneous fistula secondary to stump appendicitis. Case Rep Surg 2017;2017:1–3.

245. Dobremez E, Lavrand F, Lefevre Y, et al. Treatment of post-appendectomy intra-abdominal deep abscesses. Eur J Pediatr Surg 2003;13(6):393–7.

246. Ali SM, Al-Tarakji M, Shahid F, et al. From diagnosis to management; mucocele of stump appendicitis, extremely rare finding in an uncommon surgical disease: literature review. Int J Surg Oncol 2021;2021:8816643.

247. Zhu Q-C, Shen R-R, Qin H-L, et al. Solitary rectal ulcer syndrome: clinical features, pathophysiology, diagnosis and treatment strategies. World J Gastroenterol 2014;20(3):738–44.

248. Forootan M, Darvishi M. Solitary rectal ulcer syndrome: A systematic review. Medicine 2018;97(18):e0565.

249. Glotzer DJ, Glick ME, Goldman H. Proctitis and colitis following diversion of the fecal stream. Gastroenterology 1981;80(3):438–41.

250. Edwards CM, George B, Warren B. Diversion colitis–new light through old windows. Histopathology 1999;34(1):1–5.

251. Guillemot F, Colombel JF, Neut C, et al. Treatment of diversion colitis by short-chain fatty acids. Prospective and double-blind study. Dis Colon Rectum 1991;34(10):861–4.

252. Wu Z-Y, Sang L-X, Chang B. Cronkhite-Canada syndrome: from clinical features to treatment. Gastroenterol Rep (Oxf) 2020;8(5):333–42.

253. Liu S, You Y, Ruan G, et al. The Long-Term Clinical and Endoscopic Outcomes of Cronkhite-Canada Syndrome. Clin Transl Gastroenterol 2020;11(4):e00167.

254. Bissell DM, Anderson KE, Bonkovsky HL. Porphyria. N Engl J Med 2017;377(9): 862–72.

255. Ma Y, Teng Q, Zhang Y, et al. Acute intermittent porphyria: focus on possible mechanisms of acute and chronic manifestations. Intractable Rare Dis Res 2020;9(4):187–95.

256. Patel R, Coulter LL, Rimmer J, et al. Mitochondrial neurogastrointestinal encephalopathy: a clinicopathological mimic of Crohn's disease. BMC Gastroenterol 2019;19(1):11.

257. Habibzadeh P, Silawi M, Dastsooz H, et al. Clinical and molecular characterization of a patient with mitochondrial Neurogastrointestinal Encephalomyopathy. BMC Gastroenterol 2020;20(1):142.

258. Zondervan KT, Becker CM, Koga K, et al. Endometriosis. Nat Rev Dis Primers 2018;4(1):9.

259. Nezhat C, Li A, Falik R, et al. Bowel endometriosis: diagnosis and management. Am J Obstet Gynecol 2018;218(6):549–62.

260. Chiaffarino F, Cipriani S, Ricci E, et al. Endometriosis and inflammatory bowel disease: A systematic review of the literature. Eur J Obstet Gynecol Reprod Biol 2020;252:246–51.
261. Foulon A, Pichois R, Sabbagh C, et al. Bowel endometriosis mimicking crohn disease. Inflamm Bowel Dis 2021;27(3):e26–7.
262. Claytor J, Viramontes O, Conner S, et al. Kaposi sarcoma in an immunosuppressed patient with presumed crohn's disease: iatrogenic or epidemic? Gastroenterology 2021;160(3):S1.
263. Stasi E, De Santis S, Cavalcanti E, et al. Iatrogenic Kaposi sarcoma of the terminal ileum following short-term treatment with immunomodulators for Crohn's disease: A case report. Medicine 2019;98(20):e15714.
264. Kilincalp S, Akıncı H, Hamamci M, et al. Kaposi's sarcoma developing in a HIV-negative Crohn's disease patient shortly after azathioprine and corticosteroid treatment. J Crohns Colitis 2014;8(6):558–9.
265. Windon AL, Shroff SG. Iatrogenic Kaposi's Sarcoma in an HIV-Negative Young Male With Crohn's Disease and IgA Nephropathy: A Case Report and Brief Review of the Literature. Int J Surg Pathol 2018;26(3):276–82.

Conventional Therapies for Crohn's Disease

Stacey Rolak, MD, MPH[a],*, Sunanda V. Kane, MD, MSPH[b]

KEYWORDS

- Crohn's disease • Treatments • Aminosalicylates • Immunomodulators • Biologics
- Anti-TNF • Anti-Integrins • Anti-interleukins

KEY POINTS

- Mesalamine is used frequently in ulcerative colitis but has a limited role in the treatment of Crohn's disease. Sulfasalazine can be used in colonic Crohn's disease.
- Corticosteroids are effective in disease flares and in inducing remission of disease. Steroids cannot be used long-term because of their significant adverse effect profile.
- Immunomodulators including methotrexate, 6-mercaptopurine, and azathioprine are effective maintenance treatments.
- Anti-TNF agents are effective in the induction of remission of disease and as maintenance treatments.
- The anti-integrins are effective in the induction and maintenance of remission of disease.

5-AMINOSALICYLIC ACIDS

Although aminosalicylates are established and effective therapies in the treatment of ulcerative colitis, their use in Crohn's disease is more limited. Several organizations including the American College of Gastroenterology (ACG), the American Gastroenterological Association, and the European Crohn's and Colitis Organization recommend against the use of 5-aminosalicylates for the maintenance of medically induced remission in patients with Crohn's disease.[1–3]

Sulfasalazine and mesalamine contain the active ingredient 5-aminosalicylate (5-ASA), which works as a topical anti-inflammatory agent in the gut. Sulfasalazine is a prodrug composed of 5-ASA linked to sulfapyridine. Sulfapyridine is rapidly absorbed in the colon. This combination allows enhanced delivery and absorption of the anti-inflammatory properties of 5-ASA to the colon. Mesalamine does not contain the sulfa group and is generally better tolerated than sulfasalazine. There are multiple formulations and delivery systems of mesalamine; however, none are FDA approved to treat Crohn's disease. They are approved in the treatment of ulcerative colitis.

[a] Department of Internal Medicine, Mayo Clinic College of Medicine and Science, 200 First Street, Southwest, Rochester, MN 55905, USA; [b] Division of Gastroenterology and Hepatology, Mayo Clinic Rochester, 200 First Street, Southwest, Rochester, MN 55905, USA
* Corresponding author.
E-mail address: Rolak.stacey@mayo.edu

Gastroenterol Clin N Am 51 (2022) 271–282
https://doi.org/10.1016/j.gtc.2021.12.004
0889-8553/22/© 2022 Elsevier Inc. All rights reserved.

Oral mesalamine is generally not more effective than placebo in the induction of remission or achievement of mucosal healing in patients with Crohn's disease. ACG guidelines recommend that mesalamine not be used to treat patients with active Crohn's disease.[1] In one meta-analysis, high doses of moisture-dependent mesalamine (>2.4 g/d) were associated with greater rates of remission when compared with placebo.[4] However, other studies have shown there is no benefit to olsalazine, low-dose mesalamine, or high-dose mesalamine in inducing remission over placebo.[5–7]

Sulfasalazine at 3g to 6 g daily can be effective in treating the symptoms of mild to moderately severe colonic Crohn's disease.[1,5] It should not be used in patients with isolated small bowel disease. One systematic review of 20 randomized controlled trials evaluating the efficacy of sulfasalazine or mesalamine in the treatment of mild to moderate Crohn's disease compared with placebo, corticosteroids, and other aminosalicylates demonstrated a nonsignificant trend supporting the use of sulfasalazine over placebo.[8] However, this study also found that sulfasalazine is inferior to corticosteroids and corticosteroids plus combination therapy in the treatment of mild to moderate Crohn's disease.[8] Another meta-analysis revealed a nonsignificant trend favoring sulfasalazine over placebo for achieving remission in active Crohn's disease.[7] Other studies have shown that sulfasalazine is not more effective than placebo for achieving mucosal healing in patients with Crohn's disease.[1,9,10] The primary adverse effects of sulfasalazine include dose-dependent nausea, dyspepsia, photosensitivity, and headaches. More rarely, pancreatitis, hepatotoxicity, bone marrow toxicity, and hypersensitivity reactions can occur.

CORTICOSTEROIDS

There are several steroid preparations that can be used in the treatment of Crohn's disease. Steroids are efficacious in inducing remission of disease.[1] However, they are not preferred for the maintenance of remission because of their significant adverse effects and limited effectiveness long-term.[11]

Oral budesonide is a gut-selective steroid that can be useful in the induction of remission in mild to moderate cases of ileocecal Crohn's disease.[1,3,12] Budesonide undergoes significant first-pass metabolism in the liver, leading to reduced systemic absorption. One meta-analysis of 3 randomized controlled trials comparing budesonide 9 mg/d with placebo demonstrated the superiority of budesonide in inducing clinical remission at 8 weeks.[13–16] However, budesonide is significantly less effective than conventional steroids (such as prednisone, dexamethasone, and methylprednisolone), especially in severe Crohn's disease.[13] Although effective in Crohn's disease flares, budesonide should not be used to maintain remission of Crohn's disease beyond 4 months.[1] Several randomized controlled studies evaluating the maintenance of remission with 3 mg or 6 mg of budesonide showed that it has no significant benefit over placebo long-term.[17–19] Budesonide is safer than conventional corticosteroids, which can lead to infections, osteoporosis, Cushing syndrome, hypertension, and diabetes mellitus.[12,20] Budesonide has more adverse effects than placebo.[21,22]

Conventional oral steroids with increased systemic bioavailability are very effective in inducing remission in moderate to severe Crohn's disease, and are significantly more effective than placebo.[9,10,23] However, they should not be used for the maintenance of remission of disease. A meta-analysis of 3 randomized controlled trials demonstrated that conventional systemic corticosteroids do not reduce the risk of disease relapse at 6, 12, and 24 months.[24]

Severe Crohn's disease flares often require intravenous steroids. If a patient requires 2 or more steroid courses per year for disease flares, this indicates that they would likely benefit from optimization of their maintenance therapy. It may also indicate the need for surgical consideration.[12] Ideally, corticosteroid tapers should not exceed 3 months without attempting to introduce a steroid-sparing agent.[1] Steroids are relatively contraindicated in penetrating Crohn's disease with the presence of abscess or fistulas.[11]

IMMUNOMODULATORS

The immunomodulators used in the treatment of Crohn's disease are methotrexate and the thiopurines, azathioprine, and 6-mercaptopurine. Immunomodulators should not be used for the induction of remission of disease, but are effective as maintenance treatments and are popular steroid-sparing agents.[1]

Methotrexate is a folate antimetabolite that binds to and inhibits dihydrofolate reductase, ultimately inhibiting DNA synthesis, repair, and cellular replication. The ACG recommends methotrexate at a dose of up to 25 mg once weekly, intramuscularly or subcutaneously, for steroid-dependent Crohn's disease, and for the maintenance of remission of disease.[1] In a double-blind placebo-controlled study of patients who had entered remission after treatment with 25 mg of methotrexate weekly, patients who were assigned intramuscular methotrexate 15 mg weekly for 40 weeks maintained remission significantly more often (65%) than those who received placebo (39%). Those in the methotrexate maintenance group also required fewer courses of prednisone for relapse.[25] A systematic review found intramuscular methotrexate 15 mg weekly to be safe and effective for the maintenance of remission. Low-dose oral methotrexate at 12.5 mg to 15 mg per week did not have similar effectiveness for the maintenance of remission.[26] Additional studies have supported the efficacy and safety of intramuscular methotrexate.[27] Significant adverse effects of methotrexate include alopecia, rash, stomatitis, nausea and vomiting, bone marrow suppression, hepatotoxicity, and pulmonary toxicity. Folate supplementation can reduce gastrointestinal side effects and hepatotoxicity.[28] White blood cell counts and liver function tests should be monitored while on this medication. Methotrexate is contraindicated in pregnancy.

The thiopurines include 6-mercaptopurine and azathioprine. Mercaptopurine is a purine antagonist that inhibits DNA and RNA synthesis. Azathioprine is a derivative of mercaptopurine and similarly inhibits purine synthesis. Azathioprine and mercaptopurine should not be used for the induction of remission of Crohn's disease. The ACG recommends these agents as steroid-sparing maintenance therapies.[1] Thiopurines appear to have minimal benefit over placebo in the treatment of early Crohn's disease. The Azathioprine for Treatment of Early Crohn's (AZTEC) study, a prospective double-blind trial including adult patients with a recent diagnosis of Crohn's disease within 8 weeks, found that thiopurines have minimal benefit over placebo in achieving steroid-free remission. Patients were randomized to receive either azathioprine 2.5 mg/kg per day or placebo. After 76 weeks of treatment, 44.1% of those taking azathioprine were in steroid-free remission compared with 36.5% of those in the placebo group. A post-hoc analysis demonstrated significantly lower relapse rates in the azathioprine group.[29] Another trial focusing on patients with a recent diagnosis of Crohn's disease found that consistent administration of azathioprine early on in disease had no benefit over conventional management in prolonging disease remission.[30] In a Cochrane review evaluating thiopurines in Crohn's disease, a pooled analysis failed to demonstrate a benefit of thiopurines over placebo for the induction of remission of disease.[31]

Although thiopurines may be of limited benefit early on in disease, several studies have shown a modest advantage in the use of thiopurines over placebo for the maintenance of remission of Crohn's disease.[32–34] Thiopurines also have some benefit in preventing postoperative recurrence in patients with Crohn's disease. One meta-analysis demonstrated that treatment with thiopurines was superior to placebo for the prevention of clinical and endoscopic recurrence at 1 year postoperatively.[35] However, there is an increased risk of adverse events among patients taking azathioprine, including leukopenia, nausea, allergic reactions, and pancreatitis.[34,35] It is reasonable to test for thiopurine S-methyltransferase (TPMT) and nudix hydrolase 15 (NUDT15) deficiency before initiating azathioprine or mercaptopurine, as patients with either deficiency are at increased risk for severe drug toxicity and may require decreased doses. Additional toxicities of these medications include bone marrow suppression, nonmelanoma skin cancers, and lymphoma.[36–38]

Immunomodulator monotherapy is less effective than biologic monotherapy or combination therapy of immunomodulator with a biologic in maintaining remission of disease.[1,12] The Study of Biologic and Immunomodulator Naïve Patients in Crohn's disease (SONIC) trial demonstrated this. The SONIC trial was a randomized double-blind clinical trial comparing the efficacy of infliximab monotherapy, azathioprine monotherapy, and combination therapy with infliximab and azathioprine in patients with moderate to severe Crohn's disease who were naïve to these therapies. The primary endpoint of the trial was steroid-free clinical remission at week 26. A significantly greater proportion of patients receiving combination therapy were in steroid-free clinical remission at 26 weeks (56.8%) when compared with the infliximab (44.4%) or azathioprine (30.0%) monotherapy groups. Similar results were demonstrated at 50 weeks of follow-up.[39] Immunomodulators also reduce the immunogenicity of therapeutic antibodies in Crohn's disease.[39,40]

ANTI-TNF AGENTS

TNFα is an inflammatory cytokine produced by macrophages, monocytes, and T-lymphocytes during acute inflammation. It is involved in multiple cell signaling pathways and induces proinflammatory cytokines including interleukin (IL)-1 β and IL-6, enhances leukocyte migration and activation, induces acute phase reactants, and inhibits apoptosis of inflammatory cells. Elevated TNFα levels are thought to be involved in the pathogenesis of intestinal inflammation in Crohn's disease.[41] Anti-TNF agents bind with TNFα and neutralize its activity.

The antitumor necrosis factor (TNF) agents used in the treatment of Crohn's disease are infliximab and its biosimilars (Remicade, Avsola, Inflectra, and Renflexis), adalimumab (Humira), and certolizumab pegol (Cimzia). The ACG recommends that anti-TNF agents be used to treat Crohn's disease that is resistant to treatment with corticosteroids, thiopurines, or methotrexate.[1] Combination therapy with infliximab and immunomodulators (thiopurines) is more effective than treatment with either immunomodulators alone or infliximab alone in patients who are naïve to these agents, as demonstrated in the SONIC trial.[1,39] There is less data available to support the combination of adalimumab or certolizumab pegol with immunomodulators.[1]

Infliximab is a chimeric mouse-human monoclonal antibody that binds to TNFα, and is approved for the treatment of moderate to severe Crohn's disease and fistulizing Crohn's disease that has failed to respond to conventional therapy.[1] Infliximab 5 mg/kg or 10 mg/kg given intravenously every 8 weeks is effective for the maintenance of remission in patients who responded to infliximab induction.[42] Adalimumab is a recombinant fully human IgG1 monoclonal antibody that binds to TNFα. The CLASSIC-I trial demonstrated that adalimumab 160 mg at week 0 followed by 80 mg at week 2 was superior to placebo for induction of remission in patients with moderate to severe Crohn's disease naïve to anti-TNF therapy.[43] The Crohn's Trial of the Fully Human Antibody Adalimumab for Remission Maintenance (CHARM) trial also supported the efficacy of adalimumab in maintaining remission in moderate to severe Crohn's disease among patients who initially responded to adalimumab therapy, compared with placebo.[44] It is usually given subcutaneously at a maintenance dose of 40 mg every other week. Certolizumab pegol is a pegylated humanized Fab fragment of TNFα monoclonal antibody, which binds to and selectively neutralizes TNFα activity. It is usually given at a maintenance dose of 400 mg subcutaneously every 4 weeks. A 26-week placebo-controlled trial of induction and maintenance treatment with certolizumab pegol in patients with moderate to severe Crohn's disease demonstrated modest improvement with certolizumab compared with placebo. There was no significant improvement in remission rates.[45] Another trial supported the use of certolizumab pegol in the maintenance of remission among initial responders.[46] Both adalimumab and certolizumab pegol are now approved for moderate to severe Crohn's disease that have failed to respond to conventional therapy.[1] Multiple studies have supported the efficacy of anti-TNF agents over placebo for induction, maintenance of remission, and mucosal healing in patients with Crohn's disease.[7,47–50]

There are also anti-TNF biosimilar agents for infliximab and adalimumab available, with similar indications and efficacy as their originator molecules. These biosimilars are effective treatments for patients with moderate to severe Crohn's disease and can be used as induction and maintenance treatments.[1]

In general, anti-TNF medication discontinuation is discouraged among patients who achieve disease remission. One meta-analysis demonstrated that the overall risk of relapse after discontinuation of anti-TNF therapy was 44% among those with Crohn's disease. The relapse rate was 40% at 12 months and almost 50% at more than 25 months. Retreatment with the same anti-TNF agent induced remission again in approximately 80% of cases.[51] If medication is discontinued during remission and then restarted, it is usually recommended that the first anti-TNF agent be restarted rather than switching to a different agent.[11,52,53] Patients on anti-TNF therapy who develop antibiologic antibodies require transition to a different maintenance therapy. There is insufficient evidence to support proactive monitoring of biologic drug trough levels and antibodies.[12]

There is a black box warning for the 3 anti-TNF agents used in the treatment of Crohn's disease for an increased risk of developing serious infections that may lead to hospitalization or death. There are also increased reports of lymphoma and other malignancies in children, adolescents, and young adult patients treated with anti-TNF agents. Providers must stay vigilant for signs of infection in patients on these agents. Combination therapy with anti-TNF agents and immunomodulators appears to further increase the risk for opportunistic infections such as herpes zoster, as well as for nonmelanoma skin cancers, and non-Hodgkin lymphoma.[11,54 56]

Before initiating biologic therapy, patients should be assessed for latent and active tuberculosis. Interferon-γ release assays are preferred over the tuberculin skin test in those who have previously received the Bacillus Calmette-Guerin (BCG) vaccine. Patients should be treated appropriately for latent tuberculosis, if detected. Patients should also be assessed for viral hepatitis B before starting treatment. If they are seronegative for hepatitis B, they should be vaccinated.[1]

ANTI-INTEGRINS

The anti-integrin therapies used in the treatment of Crohn's disease are vedolizumab (Entyvio) and natalizumab (Tysabri). For patients with moderate to severe Crohn's disease and objective evidence of active disease, anti-integrin therapy with vedolizumab with or without an immunomodulator can be used for induction of symptomatic remission. Natalizumab can also be used for induction of symptomatic remission in patients with active Crohn's disease.[1] Vedolizumab should be used for the maintenance of remission of vedolizumab-induced remission of disease.

Integrins are cell adhesion molecules present on the surface of circulating leukocytes, which allow leukocytes to interact with vascular endothelial cells and ultimately migrate to target tissues. Anti-integrin therapies block the action of integrins on the endothelium, decreasing immune cell recruitment to target tissues. Natalizumab is a chimeric recombinant human IgG4 antibody that targets the α_4 subunit of integrin molecules.[57] It was initially approved for the treatment of multiple sclerosis. It is typically given as a 300 mg infusion every 4 weeks. Vedolizumab is a humanized monoclonal IgG1 antibody that binds to the $\alpha_4\beta_7$ integrin receptor on T-lymphocytes. Vedolizumab is typically given as 300 mg at 0, 2, and 6 weeks and then every 8 weeks thereafter. It can be given every 4 weeks if patient response every 8 weeks is not satisfactory.[58] Although natalizumab inhibits immune trafficking in multiple organs, vedolizumab is more gut-selective.[57]

In the Efficacy of Natalizumab in Crohn's disease Response and Remission (ENCORE) trial, patients with moderate to severe Crohn's disease were randomly assigned to receive either 300 mg natalizumab or placebo. Response and remission rates were superior in the natalizumab group compared with placebo at 4, 8, and 12 weeks.[59] A systematic review of 5 randomized controlled trials also found evidence supporting the effectiveness of natalizumab in the induction of remission of disease in patients with moderate to severe Crohn's disease.[60] Although effective, the utility of natalizumab is limited by its adverse effect profile. There is a black box warning on natalizumab for an increased risk of progressive multifocal leukoencephalopathy (PML). PML is a fatal demyelinating disease of the central nervous system caused by infection from a human polyomavirus, John Cunningham (JC) virus. Risk factors for the development of PML include the presence of anti-JC virus antibodies, duration of therapy greater than 2 years, and prior use of immunosuppressants.[61] Because of this, natalizumab is only approved for patients with moderate to severe Crohn's disease not responding to, or intolerant of, conventional treatment.[62] The ACG recommends that natalizumab be considered for the maintenance of remission of natalizumab-induced remission of Crohn's disease only if patients are not seropositive for the anti-JC virus antibody.[1] Patients should be tested for the antibody every 6 months, and treatment should be discontinued if the result is positive.[1,63] Natalizumab should not be combined with immunomodulators.

Vedolizumab acts more selectively on the gut, and to date, no cases of PML have been reported with vedolizumab.[64,65] Vedolizumab is safe and effective in achieving remission and clinical response.[65] In a randomized controlled trial, patients who responded to induction therapy with vedolizumab and continued to receive vedolizumab were more likely to remain in remission at 52 weeks than those receiving maintenance with placebo.[66] Vedolizumab has increased efficacy over placebo in patients with Crohn's disease regardless of whether they are naïve to TNFα antagonist therapy.[67,68]

Data are sparse regarding the efficacy of vedolizumab monotherapy over combination therapy of vedolizumab with an immunomodulator. A recently published retrospective study demonstrated that there is no benefit to combination therapy. This study examined patients receiving maintenance therapy with vedolizumab or with ustekinumab. There was no difference in clinical response or remission between those on vedolizumab monotherapy and those on combination therapy with methotrexate or with a thiopurine. Similarly, there was no difference in clinical response or remission between the ustekinumab monotherapy and combination therapy groups. These results were evident at 14 weeks and at 1 year.[69] The ACG conditionally recommends using vedolizumab for the maintenance of remission of vedolizumab-induced remission of Crohn's disease.[1]

ANTI-INTERLEUKINS

Ustekinumab (Stelara) is an anti-interleukin used in the treatment of Crohn's disease. Ustekinumab is a monoclonal antibody that inhibits the p40 subunit of IL-12 and IL-23. The ACG recommends ustekinumab in patients with moderate to severe Crohn's disease who have failed previous treatment with steroids, thiopurines, methotrexate, or anti-TNF inhibitors, or have had no prior exposure to anti-TNF inhibitors.[1] Ustekinumab is also recommended for the maintenance of remission in ustekinumab-induced remission.[1,70]

The bowel mucosa in Crohn's disease has increased production of IL-12, a proinflammatory cytokine that induces IFN-γ production and promotes TH1 cell differentiation. IL-23 shares the p40 subunit with IL-12.[71] Ustekinumab was initially approved for the treatment of psoriatic arthritis. The UNITI trials demonstrated the efficacy of ustekinumab over placebo in the induction of remission and in the maintenance of remission in patients with moderate to severe Crohn's disease. In 2 induction trials, patients were randomly assigned to receive a single intravenous dose of ustekinumab at either 130 mg or 6 mg/kg, or a placebo. Clinical response at week 6 among patients receiving ustekinumab was significantly greater than the placebo group.[70] The IM-UNITI trial demonstrated that continued treatment with subcutaneous ustekinumab in patients who initially responded to induction with ustekinumab maintains clinical response and remission over a 3-year period. Adverse events were similar between the ustekinumab and placebo groups.[72]

Ustekinumab is usually given as a single IV infusion dose for induction, then as 90 mg subcutaneously for maintenance every 8 weeks after IV induction. A retrospective study of 110 patients demonstrated that shortening the ustekinumab 90 mg dose interval to every 4 weeks among patients not responding clinically to dosing every 8 weeks improved clinical and biological indices of disease activity. Specifically, C-reactive protein, fecal calprotectin, and endoscopic disease activity improved. This suggests that shortening the dose interval is effective and safe in those who are not responding to standard dosing.[73] Ustekinumab is well-tolerated.[74] The majority of safety data available comes from studies in patients with psoriatic arthritis.[75]

Few studies have compared the efficacy of ustekinumab, vedolizumab, and anti-TNF agents as first-line agents. The decision of which biologic treatment to start with should be determined through shared decision-making between the patient and provider.[1] A recently published observational study examined patients with Crohn's disease who failed anti-TNF treatment and started vedolizumab or ustekinumab. Patients treated with ustekinumab were more likely to achieve steroid-free clinical remission, biochemical remission with lower C-reactive protein and fecal cal-protectin, and combined steroid-free clinical and biochemical remission compared with those treated with vedolizumab. Infections and hospitalizations were comparable between the 2 groups.[76] Further studies are needed to guide the initial choice of biologic therapy.

CLINICS CARE POINTS

- There are no conclusive data that mesalamine works for anything except mild Crohns limited to the colon.
- Combination therapy is more effective at attaining remission than monotherapy.
- If using an immunomodulator for preventing antibody formation, it is only needed for the first 6 months for combination therapy.

REFERENCES

1. Lichtenstein GR, Loftus EV, Isaacs KL, et al. ACG Clinical Guideline: Management of Crohn's Disease in Adults. Am J Gastroenterol 2018;113(4):481–517.
2. Feuerstein JD, Ho EY, Shmidt E, et al. AGA Clinical Practice Guidelines on the Medical Management of Moderate to Severe Luminal and Perianal Fistulizing Crohn's Disease. Gastroenterology 2021;160(7):2496–508.
3. Torres J, Bonovas S, Doherty G, et al. ECCO Guidelines on Therapeutics in Crohn's Disease: Medical Treatment. J Crohns Colitis 2020;14(1):4–22.
4. Coward S, Kuenzig ME, Hazlewood G, et al. Comparative Effectiveness of Mesalamine, Sulfasalazine, Corticosteroids, and Budesonide for the Induction of Remission in Crohn's Disease: A Bayesian Network Meta-analysis. Inflamm Bowel Dis 2017;23(3):461–72.
5. Lim WC, Hanauer S. Aminosalicylates for induction of remission or response in Crohn's disease. Cochrane Database Syst Rev 2010;(12):CD008870.
6. Akobeng AK, Zhang D, Gordon M, et al. Oral 5-aminosalicylic acid for maintenance of medically-induced remission in Crohn's disease. Cochrane Database Syst Rev 2016;9:CD003715.
7. Ford AC, Kane SV, Khan KJ, et al. Efficacy of 5-aminosalicylates in Crohn's disease: systematic review and meta-analysis. Am J Gastroenterol 2011;106(4):617–29.
8. Lim WC, Wang Y, MacDonald JK, et al. Aminosalicylates for induction of remission or response in Crohn's disease. Cochrane Database Syst Rev 2016;7:CD008870.
9. Malchow H, Ewe K, Brandes JW, et al. European Cooperative Crohn's Disease Study (ECCDS): results of drug treatment. Gastroenterology 1984;86(2):249–66.
10. Summers RW, Switz DM, Sessions JT, et al. National Cooperative Crohn's Disease Study: results of drug treatment. Gastroenterology 1979;77(4 Pt 2):847–69.
11. Nakase H, Uchino M, Shinzaki S, et al. Evidence-based clinical practice guidelines for inflammatory bowel disease 2020. J Gastroenterol 2021;56(6):489–526.
12. Cushing K, Higgins PDR. Management of Crohn's Disease: A Review. JAMA 05 2021;325(1):69–80.
13. Rezaie A, Kuenzig ME, Benchimol EI, et al. Budesonide for induction of remission in Crohn's disease. Cochrane Database Syst Rev 2015;(6):CD000296.

14. Suzuki Y, Motoya S, Takazoe M, et al. Efficacy and tolerability of oral budesonide in Japanese patients with active Crohn's disease: a multicentre, double-blind, randomized, parallel-group Phase II study. J Crohns Colitis 2013;7(3):239–47.

15. Tremaine WJ, Hanauer SB, Katz S, et al. Budesonide CIR capsules (once or twice daily divided-dose) in active Crohn's disease: a randomized placebo-controlled study in the United States. Am J Gastroenterol 2002;97(7):1748–54.

16. Greenberg GR, Feagan BG, Martin F, et al. Oral budesonide for active Crohn's disease. Canadian Inflammatory Bowel Disease Study Group. N Engl J Med 1994;331(13):836–41.

17. Cortot A, Colombel JF, Rutgeerts P, et al. Switch from systemic steroids to budesonide in steroid dependent patients with inactive Crohn's disease. Gut 2001; 48(2):186–90.

18. Hanauer S, Sandborn WJ, Persson A, et al. Budesonide as maintenance treatment in Crohn's disease: a placebo-controlled trial. Aliment Pharmacol Ther 2005;21(4):363–71.

19. Simms L, Steinhart AH. Budesonide for maintenance of remission in Crohn's disease. Cochrane Database Syst Rev 2001;1:CD002913.

20. Singleton JW, Law DH, Kelley ML, et al. National Cooperative Crohn's Disease Study: adverse reactions to study drugs. Gastroenterology 1979;77(4 Pt 2): 870–82.

21. Papi C, Luchetti R, Gili L, et al. Budesonide in the treatment of Crohn's disease: a meta-analysis. Aliment Pharmacol Ther 2000;14(11):1419–28.

22. Benchimol EI, Seow CH, Otley AR, et al. Budesonide for maintenance of remission in Crohn's disease. Cochrane Database Syst Rev 2009;(1):CD002913.

23. Benchimol EI, Seow CH, Steinhart AH, et al. Traditional corticosteroids for induction of remission in Crohn's disease. Cochrane Database Syst Rev 2008;(2): CD006792.

24. Steinhart AH, Ewe K, Griffiths AM, et al. Corticosteroids for maintenance of remission in Crohn's disease. Cochrane Database Syst Rev 2003;4:CD000301.

25. Feagan BG, Fedorak RN, Irvine EJ, et al. A comparison of methotrexate with placebo for the maintenance of remission in Crohn's disease. North American Crohn's Study Group Investigators. N Engl J Med 2000;342(22):1627–32.

26. Patel V, Macdonald JK, McDonald JW, et al. Methotrexate for maintenance of remission in Crohn's disease. Cochrane Database Syst Rev 2009;(4):CD006884.

27. Patel V, Wang Y, MacDonald JK, et al. Methotrexate for maintenance of remission in Crohn's disease. Cochrane Database Syst Rev 2014;(8):CD006884.

28. Liu L, Liu S, Wang C, et al. Folate Supplementation for Methotrexate Therapy in Patients With Rheumatoid Arthritis: A Systematic Review. J Clin Rheumatol 2019;25(5):197–202.

29. Panés J, López-Sanromán A, Bermejo F, et al. Early azathioprine therapy is no more effective than placebo for newly diagnosed Crohn's disease. Gastroenterology 2013;145(4):766–74.e1.

30. Cosnes J, Bourrier A, Laharie D, et al. Early administration of azathioprine vs conventional management of Crohn's Disease: a randomized controlled trial. Gastroenterology 2013;145(4):758–65, e2; quiz e14-5.

31. Chande N, Townsend CM, Parker CE, et al. Azathioprine or 6-mercaptopurine for induction of remission in Crohn's disease. Cochrane Database Syst Rev 2016;10: CD000545.

32. Chande N, Patton PH, Tsoulis DJ, et al. Azathioprine or 6-mercaptopurine for maintenance of remission in Crohn's disease. Cochrane Database Syst Rev 2015;(10):CD000067.

33. Candy S, Wright J, Gerber M, et al. A controlled double blind study of azathioprine in the management of Crohn's disease. Gut 1995;37(5):674–8.
34. Prefontaine E, Macdonald JK, Sutherland LR. Azathioprine or 6-mercaptopurine for induction of remission in Crohn's disease. Cochrane Database Syst Rev 2010;(6):CD000545.
35. Peyrin-Biroulet L, Deltenre P, Ardizzone S, et al. Azathioprine and 6-mercaptopurine for the prevention of postoperative recurrence in Crohn's disease: a meta-analysis. Am J Gastroenterol 2009;104(8):2089–96.
36. de Boer NKH, Peyrin-Biroulet L, Jharap B, et al. Thiopurines in Inflammatory Bowel Disease: New Findings and Perspectives. J Crohns Colitis 2018;12(5): 610–20.
37. Kotlyar DS, Lewis JD, Beaugerie L, et al. Risk of lymphoma in patients with inflammatory bowel disease treated with azathioprine and 6-mercaptopurine: a meta-analysis. Clin Gastroenterol Hepatol 2015;13(5):847–58, e4; quiz e48-50.
38. Long MD, Herfarth HH, Pipkin CA, et al. Increased risk for non-melanoma skin cancer in patients with inflammatory bowel disease. Clin Gastroenterol Hepatol 2010;8(3):268–74.
39. Colombel JF, Sandborn WJ, Reinisch W, et al. Infliximab, azathioprine, or combination therapy for Crohn's disease. N Engl J Med 2010;362(15):1383–95.
40. Krieckaert CL, Bartelds GM, Lems WF, et al. The effect of immunomodulators on the immunogenicity of TNF-blocking therapeutic monoclonal antibodies: a review. Arthritis Res Ther 2010;12(5):217.
41. Adegbola SO, Sahnan K, Warusavitarne J, et al. Anti-TNF Therapy in Crohn's Disease. Int J Mol Sci 2018;19(8).
42. Behm BW, Bickston SJ. Tumor necrosis factor-alpha antibody for maintenance of remission in Crohn's disease. Cochrane Database Syst Rev 2008;(1):CD006893.
43. Hanauer SB, Sandborn WJ, Rutgeerts P, et al. Human anti-tumor necrosis factor monoclonal antibody (adalimumab) in Crohn's disease: the CLASSIC-I trial. Gastroenterology 2006;130(2):323–33, quiz 591.
44. Colombel JF, Sandborn WJ, Rutgeerts P, et al. Adalimumab for maintenance of clinical response and remission in patients with Crohn's disease: the CHARM trial. Gastroenterology 2007;132(1):52–65.
45. Sandborn WJ, Feagan BG, Stoinov S, et al. Certolizumab pegol for the treatment of Crohn's disease. N Engl J Med 2007;357(3):228–38.
46. Schreiber S, Khaliq-Kareemi M, Lawrance IC, et al. Maintenance therapy with certolizumab pegol for Crohn's disease. N Engl J Med 2007;357(3):239–50.
47. Kawalec P, Mikrut A, Wiśniewska N, et al. Tumor necrosis factor-α antibodies (infliximab, adalimumab and certolizumab) in Crohn's disease: systematic review and meta-analysis. Arch Med Sci 2013;9(5):765–79.
48. Sandborn WJ, Rutgeerts P, Enns R, et al. Adalimumab induction therapy for Crohn's disease previously treated with infliximab: a randomized trial. Ann Intern Med 2007;146(12):829–38.
49. Sands BE, Anderson FH, Bernstein CN, et al. Infliximab maintenance therapy for fistulizing Crohn's disease. N Engl J Med 2004;350(9):876–85.
50. Rutgeerts P, Van Assche G, Sandborn WJ, et al. Adalimumab induces and maintains mucosal healing in patients with Crohn's disease: data from the EXTEND trial. Gastroenterology 2012;142(5):1102–11.e2.
51. Gisbert JP, Marín AC, Chaparro M. The Risk of Relapse after Anti-TNF Discontinuation in Inflammatory Bowel Disease: Systematic Review and Meta-Analysis. Am J Gastroenterol 2016;111(5):632–47.

52. Van Assche G, Vermeire S, Ballet V, et al. Switch to adalimumab in patients with Crohn's disease controlled by maintenance infliximab: prospective randomised SWITCH trial. Gut 2012;61(2):229–34.
53. Casanova MJ, Chaparro M, García-Sánchez V, et al. Evolution After Anti-TNF Discontinuation in Patients With Inflammatory Bowel Disease: A Multicenter Long-Term Follow-Up Study. Am J Gastroenterol 2017;112(1):120–31.
54. Osterman MT, Haynes K, Delzell E, et al. Effectiveness and Safety of Immuno-modulators With Anti-Tumor Necrosis Factor Therapy in Crohn's Disease. Clin Gastroenterol Hepatol 2015;13(7):1293–301, e5; quiz e70, e72.
55. Lichtenstein GR, Rutgeerts P, Sandborn WJ, et al. A pooled analysis of infections, malignancy, and mortality in infliximab- and immunomodulator-treated adult patients with inflammatory bowel disease. Am J Gastroenterol 2012;107(7): 1051–63.
56. Krichgesnar J, Lemaitre M, Carrat F, et al. Risk of Serious and Opportunistic Infections Associated With Treatment of Inflammatory Bowel Diseases. Gastroenterology 2018;(2):155. https://doi.org/10.1053/j.gastro.2018.04.012.
57. Park SC, Jeen YT. Anti-integrin therapy for inflammatory bowel disease. World J Gastroenterol 2018;24(17):1868–80.
58. Rosario M, Dirks NL, Milch C, et al. A Review of the Clinical Pharmacokinetics, Pharmacodynamics, and Immunogenicity of Vedolizumab. Clin Pharmacokinet 2017;56(11):1287–301. https://doi.org/10.1007/s40262-017-0546-0.
59. Targan SR, Feagan BG, Fedorak RN, et al. Natalizumab for the treatment of active Crohn's disease: results of the ENCORE Trial. Gastroenterology 2007;132(5): 1672–83.
60. Nelson SM, Nguyen TM, McDonald JW, et al. Natalizumab for induction of remission in Crohn's disease. Cochrane Database Syst Rev 2018;8:CD006097.
61. Bloomgren G, Richman S, Hotermans C, et al. Risk of natalizumab-associated progressive multifocal leukoencephalopathy. N Engl J Med 2012;366(20): 1870–80.
62. Honey K. The comeback kid: TYSABRI now FDA approved for Crohn's disease. J Clin Invest 2008;118(3):825–6.
63. Van Assche G, Van Ranst M, Sciot R, et al. Progressive multifocal leukoencephalopathy after natalizumab therapy for Crohn's disease. N Engl J Med 2005;353(4): 362–8.
64. Card T, Xu J, Liang H, et al. What Is the Risk of Progressive Multifocal Leukoencephalopathy in Patients With Ulcerative Colitis or Crohn's Disease Treated With Vedolizumab? Inflamm Bowel Dis 2018;24(5):953–9.
65. Lin L, Liu X, Wang D, et al. Efficacy and safety of antiintegrin antibody for inflammatory bowel disease: a systematic review and meta-analysis. Medicine (Baltimore) 2015;94(10):e556.
66. Sandborn WJ, Feagan BG, Rutgeerts P, et al. Vedolizumab as induction and maintenance therapy for Crohn's disease. N Engl J Med 2013;369(8):711–21.
67. Sands BE, Sandborn WJ, Van Assche G, et al. Vedolizumab as Induction and Maintenance Therapy for Crohn's Disease in Patients Naïve to or Who Have Failed Tumor Necrosis Factor Antagonist Therapy. Inflamm Bowel Dis 2017; 23(1):97–106.
68. Chandar AK, Singh S, Murad MH, et al. Efficacy and Safety of Natalizumab and Vedolizumab for the Management of Crohn's Disease: A Systematic Review and Meta-analysis. Inflamm Bowel Dis 2015;21(7):1695–708.
69. Hu A, Kotze PG, Burgevin A, et al. Combination Therapy Does Not Improve Rate of Clinical or Endoscopic Remission in Patients with Inflammatory Bowel Diseases

Treated With Vedolizumab or Ustekinumab. Clin Gastroenterol Hepatol 2021; 19(7):1366–76.e2.

70. Feagan BG, Sandborn WJ, Gasink C, et al. Ustekinumab as Induction and Maintenance Therapy for Crohn's Disease. N Engl J Med 2016;375(20):1946–60.

71. Peluso I, Pallone F, Monteleone G. Interleukin-12 and Th1 immune response in Crohn's disease: pathogenetic relevance and therapeutic implication. World J Gastroenterol 2006;12(35):5606–10.

72. Hanauer SB, Sandborn WJ, Feagan BG, et al. IM-UNITI: Three-year Efficacy, Safety, and Immunogenicity of Ustekinumab Treatment of Crohn's Disease. J Crohns Colitis 2020;14(1):23–32.

73. Ollech JE, Normatov I, Peleg N, et al. Effectiveness of Ustekinumab Dose Escalation in Patients With Crohn's Disease. Clin Gastroenterol Hepatol 2021;19(1): 104–10.

74. Ghosh S, Gensler LS, Yang Z, et al. Ustekinumab Safety in Psoriasis, Psoriatic Arthritis, and Crohn's Disease: An Integrated Analysis of Phase II/III Clinical Development Programs. Drug Saf 2019;42(6):751–68.

75. Papp K, Gottlieb AB, Naldi L, et al. Safety Surveillance for Ustekinumab and Other Psoriasis Treatments From the Psoriasis Longitudinal Assessment and Registry (PSOLAR). J Drugs Dermatol 2015;14(7):706–14.

76. Biemans VBC, van der Woude CJ, Dijkstra G, et al. Ustekinumab is associated with superior effectiveness outcomes compared to vedolizumab in Crohn's disease patients with prior failure to anti-TNF treatment. Aliment Pharmacol Ther 2020;52(1):123–34.

Dual Advanced Therapies and Novel Pharmacotherapies for Moderately to Severely Active Crohn's Disease

Chung Sang Tse, MD*, Parambir S. Dulai, MBBS

KEYWORDS

• Dual biologic therapies • Combination biologics and small molecules • Clinical trials

KEY POINTS

• Dual advanced therapies (combination of biologics and/or small molecule therapies) have been used to treat refractory Crohn's disease and/or concomitant rheumatologic extraintestinal manifestations with a 30-60% efficacy, although adverse events (particularly infectious complications) can occur in nearly two-thirds of patients.

• Risankizumab demonstrated promising results for inducing and maintaining clinical and endoscopic response in phase 2 clinical trials, and its safety and efficacy are further explored in phase 3 placebo-controlled induction (completed, preliminary results reported) and maintenance studies (underway).

• Phase 2 induction studies of mirikizumab, ozanimod, and guselkumab have demonstrated varying degrees of efficacy in inducing clinical and/or endoscopic response with an acceptable safety profile; phase 3 trials of these agents are currently underway with anticipated study completion over the next 2-5 years.

INTRODUCTION

Over the past 2 decades, there have been tremendous advancements in the number of pharmacotherapies with increasingly specific therapeutic targets for patients with moderately to severely active Crohn's disease (CD).[1] Nevertheless, less than 50% of patients with CD have sustained benefit from existing Food and Drug Administration (FDA)-approved anti-TNF antagonists, anti-integrin, and anti-interleukin therapies[2,3]

Division of Gastroenterology, University of California, San Diego, 9500 Gilman Drive, MC 0956, La Jolla, CA 92093-0956, USA
* Corresponding author.
E-mail address: cstse@ucsd.edu
Twitter: @CSTseMD (C.S.T.)

Gastroenterol Clin N Am 51 (2022) 283–298
https://doi.org/10.1016/j.gtc.2021.12.005
0889-8553/22/© 2021 Elsevier Inc. All rights reserved.

and greater than 20% have refractory CD despite treatments with multiple biologic agents.[4]

In this review, we will explore the available evidence for the safety and efficacy of dual advanced therapies (DATs) that combine biologic (intravenous [IV] or subcutaneous [SQ]) and/or oral small molecule therapies in patients with CD, some of whom have concomitant rheumatologic disease/extraintestinal manifestation (EIM), based on published case series and small cohort studies.[5–9] We will also review the available data for emerging pharmacologic therapies in phase 2 or 3 clinical trials in patients with moderately to severely active CD. We intend to inform readers of novel treatments for CD that are of the most interest within the realm of clinical practice in treating refractory CD ± active rheumatologic symptoms.

DUAL ADVANCED THERAPY

Antitumor necrosis factor (TNF) antagonists (infliximab, adalimumab, and certolizumab pegol), anti-integrin (vedolizumab), and anti-interleukin (ustekinumab) were approved by the FDA between 1998 and 2016 for the treatment of adults with moderately to severely active CD. Golimumab, an anti-TNF antagonist, and tofacitinib, an oral pan-Janus kinase (JAK) inhibitor, are approved for the treatment of moderately to severely active ulcerative colitis (UC), but not for CD. Apremilast is an oral small molecule phosphodiesterase 4 used to treat psoriasis and psoriatic arthritis.[10] Off-label use of concomitant biologic and/or small molecule therapies has been reported in case series/small cohort studies of patients with refractory CD after inadequate response to multiple biologic therapies[5–9,11,12] or active rheumatologic symptoms[6,7,9] (Table 1).In a systematic review and meta-analysis of 10 studies (each with a study sample of ≥10 patients) of 211 patients with CD who had 279 trials of combination advanced therapy, the pooled clinical and endoscopic remission rates were 59% and 34%, respectively.[13] In the largest cohort study of patients with IBD treated with DAT, Glassner and colleagues[8] report 50 patients with IBD (31 CD, 18 UC, 1 indeterminate IBD) treated with 53 combinations of DAT at the Houston Methodist Hospital (see Table 1). Thirty-one patients with CD 34 were treated with 34 combinations of DAT (in 4 classes of biologic/small molecule therapies): vedolizumab and ustekinumab (n = 23), vedolizumab and anti-TNF (n = 5), tofacitinib and anti-TNF (n = 2), tofacitinib and ustekinumab (3), and adalimumab and apremilast (n = 1). One-fifth (20%, 6/31) of the patients with CD had concomitant rheumatologic disease (4 psoriasis, 2 psoriatic arthritis, and 2 ankylosing spondylitis). Before the initiation of DAT, 17% (n = 5) were in remission, 31% (n = 9) mild disease, 38% (n = 11) moderate disease, and 14% (n = 4) severe disease (by the Harvey-Bradshaw Index [HBI]). For the 5 patients with CD in remission at baseline, DAT was initiated for persistent rheumatologic symptoms from psoriatic arthritis or ankylosing spondylitis. The median duration of DAT was 8 months (interquartile range [IQR] 5.5–13 months) for the entire cohort of 50 patients with IBD (without specification by IBD subtype). Although on DAT, 16% (5/31) of patients with CD underwent surgery. Otherwise, the efficacy (clinical, endoscopic, biochemical response) and adverse events (AEs) rates were reported as an agglomerate for all the study patients without delineation by IBD subtype. As a cohort of IBD patients, there were increases in the rates of clinical remission (50% vs 14%, $P = .0018$; median follow-up 4 months, IQR 3–6 months), endoscopic remission (34% vs 6%, $P = .0039$; median follow-up 8 months, IQR 6–12 months), and decrease in C-reactive protein (CRP; 5.0 mg/dL to 2.4 mg/dL, $P = .002$; median follow-up 3 months, IQR 2–5 months) after the initiation of DAT compared with baseline.[8] A total of 26% (13/50) of patients with IBD experienced 23 AEs, the most common of which were enteric and sinopulmonary infections (14 cases), while on DAT after a mean duration of

Table 1
Dual advanced therapies (biologic or small molecules) for Crohn's disease in case series and cohort studies published from January 2018 to July 2021

Publication	Biologic/Small Molecule Combinations	Efficacy & Safety
Glassner et al,[8] 2020	50 patients with IBD (31 CD, 18 UC, 1 indeterminate IBD), for which the CD patients were treated with 34 combinations of DAT: • Vedolizumab and ustekinumab (n = 23) • Vedolizumab and anti-TNF (n = 5) • Tofacitinib and anti-TNF (n = 2) • Tofacitinib and ustekinumab (3) • Adalimumab and apremilast (n = 1)	• Efficacy: 5 patients with CD underwent surgery while on DAT. Otherwise, the efficacy of DAT for the cohort of 50 patients without delineation by IBD subtype: clinical remission increased from 14% to 50% ($P = .0018$), endoscopic remission increased from 6% to 34% ($P = .0039$), and CRP decreased from 5 mg/dL to 2.4 mg/dL ($P = .002$) from baseline to follow-up (median 8 mo, IQR 5.5–13 mo) • Safety: 23 AEs, of which 8 were serious AEs (no deaths) were reported in the cohort of 50 IBD patients (CD not specified)
Yang et al,[5] 2020	22 patients with refractory CD treated with 23 combinations of DAT: • Vedolizumab and ustekinumab (n = 8) • Vedolizumab and anti-TNF (n = 13) • Ustekinumab and anti-TNF (n = 3)	• Efficacy: 50% (12/24) had clinical response and 41% (10/24) had clinical remission, 43% had endoscopic improvement and 26% had endoscopic remission (by SES-CD). Mean CRP decreased from mean 17.0–9.0 ($P = .02$) across the study • Safety: 3 patients had AEs, drug-induced lupus, pneumonia, and 1 patient had recurrent basal cell skin cancer and infections (prior history of these conditions before DAT)
Kwapisz et al,[11] 2021	15 patients (14 CD, 1 UC) with medically refractory luminal disease: • Vedolizumab and anti-TNF (n = 8) • Ustekinumab and anti-TNF (n = 2) • Vedolizumab and ustekinumab (n = 5)	• Efficacy (not delineated between CD/UC): 73% (11/15) symptomatic improvement, 67% (10/15) corticosteroid dose reduction, and 20% (3/15) disease progression requiring surgery • Safety: 20% (n = 3) hospitalized for infections; 1 patient discontinued vedolizumab for postinfusion arthralgia

(continued on next page)

Table 1
(continued)

Publication	Biologic/Small Molecule Combinations	Efficacy & Safety
Privitera et al,[6] 2021	11 patients with active CD (n = 5) or active rheumatologic symptoms (n = 6): • Ustekinumab and anti-TNF (n = 5) • Ustekinumab and vedolizumab (n = 2) • Vedolizumab and anti-TNF (n = 3) • Vedolizumab and apremilast (n = 1)	• Efficacy: Of the patients with moderately active CD, 20% (1/5) had remission and 80% (4/5) had mild CD activity. Of the patients with severe psoriatic/spondyloarthritic symptoms, 50% (3/6) had remission and 50% (3/6) had mild rheumatologic symptoms. • Safety: 2 AEs, perianal abscess and drug-induced liver injury
Burer et al,[12] 2018	4 patients with CD treated with vedolizumab and anti-TNF: • Vedolizumab and infliximab (n = 2) • Vedolizumab and adalimumab (n = 2)	• Efficacy: All patients had clinical remission at the end of follow-up (range 12–20 mo); 50% (2/4) endoscopic remission and 25% (1/4) endoscopic improvement after a median of 14 mo • Safety: 1 patient (25%) had recurrence of polyarthritis after discontinuation of adalimumab
Mao et al,[7] 2018	4 patients with active CD (1 with active AS): • Vedolizumab and anti-TNF (n = 3) • Vedolizumab and ustekinumab (n = 1)	• Efficacy: 75% (3/4) achieved clinical remission; 25% (1/4) had esophageal CD flare despite resolution of AS symptoms • Safety: 1 patient with 2 episodes of uncomplicated *C difficile* infections; another patient with hand-foot-mouth disease and influenza
Fumery et al,[9] 2020	7 patients with IBD, including 5 CD (2 AS, 2 psoriasis): • Vedolizumab and anti-TNF (n = 1) • Ustekinumab and anti-TNF (n = 4)	• Efficacy: no clinical or endoscopic response in one patient with luminal and perianal CD (12 mo of golimumab and vedolizumab); clinical-biochemical remission with endoscopic response in another with CD and AS (30 mo of golimumab and ustekinumab); deep remission and improvement of AS in one patient (12 mo of etanercept and vedolizumab); CD deep remission without improvement of psoriasis in 2 patients (3–4 mo of ustekinumab and adalimumab/infliximab) • Safety: No adverse events reported

Abbreviations: AS, ankylosing spondylitis; CD, Crohn's disease; CD-PRO/SS, Crohn's Disease-Patient Reported Outcome Signs and Symptoms; CRP, C-reactive protein; DAT, dual biologic therapy; EIM, extraintestinal manifestation; HBI, Harvey-Bradshaw Index; IBD-U, indeterminate inflammatory bowel disease; IQR, interquartile range; PRO-2, two-item patient-reported outcome; SES-CD, Simplified Endoscopic Score-Crohn's disease; TNF, tumor necrosis factor; UC, ulcerative colitis.

Key: *Efficacy and safety outcomes were reported for all patients with IBD without delineation of response by IBD subtype.

5.1 ± 4.8 months.[8] Although no deaths were reported, 8 serious AEs requiring hospitalization (all related to infections/abscesses) were reported in 6 patients with IBD after a mean duration of DAT of 4.1 ± 3.6 months (see **Table 1**).[8] Overall, this retrospective cohort study suggests that combination biologic or small molecule therapy for IBD in patients with persistent CD or rheumatologic disease activity can be effective although side-effects, particularly infectious complications, can occur.

Yang and colleagues[5] describe the largest cohort study of patients with CD treated with DAT where clinical, biochemical, and endoscopic responses are reported (see **Table 1**). At the University of California, San Diego, and University of Calgary, 22 patients with refractory CD (phenotype 59% stricturing, 36% penetrating, and 50% with perianal fistulas; 91% had IBD-related surgeries) with treatment failure to 4 single biologic therapies ± immunomodulators previously were treated with 24 trials of DAT with 3 combinations of biologic therapy agents/classes (no small molecules): vedolizumab and ustekinumab (n = 8), vedolizumab and anti-TNF (n = 13), and ustekinumab and anti-TNF (n = 3). The median duration of DAT treatment was 274 days (IQR 191–365 days) with up to 1-year of follow-up. Half (50%) of the DAT trials had clinical improvement and 41% had clinical remission (by the 2-item patient-reported outcome [PRO2] measure); 43% had endoscopic improvement and 26% had endoscopic remission (by the Simple Endoscopic Score for Crohn's Disease [SES-CD] or explicitly stated); and the mean CRP decreased from 17.0 (IQR 11.0–24.0) to 9.0 (IQR 4.0–14.0) (P = .02) (see **Table 1**). Three patients had adverse experienced: drug-induced lupus (vedolizumab with adalimumab; adalimumab was discontinued), pneumonia (vedolizumab with ustekinumab), and a patient had basal cell skin cancer, recurrent *Clostridium difficile* infection, and Acinetobacter bacteremia (this patient had all 3 diseases before the initiation of vedolizumab and an anti-TNF agonist). Overall, dual biologic therapy was associated with clinical, biochemical, and endoscopic improvements in a subset of patients with refractory CD in this cohort.

Privitera and colleagues[6] describe the third largest cohort of patients with IBD (11 CD, 5 UC) treated with DAT at 9 Italian IBD referral centers (see **Table 1**). In the 11 patients with CD, DAT were initiated in 5 patients for treatment of moderately active CD (by HBI) and in 6 patients for severe EIM symptoms (by clinical judgment). Four combinations of DAT were used: anti-TNF with either ustekinumab (n = 5) or vedolizumab (n = 3); ustekinumab and vedolizumab (n = 2); and vedolizumab and apremilast (n = 1). Of the 5 patients for which DAT was initiated for moderately active CD, 2 did not have rheumatologic disease/symptoms and 3 had mild/inactive psoriatic disease at baseline, the DAT treatment ranged from 2 to 8 months, and after DAT induction (2 months), 4 of 5 patients had mild CD symptoms and 1 achieved remission. Of the 6 patients for which DAT was initiated for severe rheumatologic symptoms (5 spondyloarthritis and 1 psoriatic disease; baseline CD activity were equally distributed between remission, mild, moderate disease), the DAT treatment ranged from 5 to 19 months, and all patients achieved CD remission and had mild/remission of psoriatic/spondyloarthritic symptoms (equally divided) after 2 months of DAT. AEs were reported in 2 patients: perianal abscess (4 months of certolizumab ustekinumab) and drug-induced liver injury (19 months of apremilast and vedolizumab). Overall, in this cohort, DAT rapidly improved both intestinal and extraintestinal symptoms with few AEs in patients with CD ± concomitant rheumatologic symptoms (see **Table 1**).[6]

Kwapisz and colleagues, 2021,[11] describe the fourth largest cohort study of patients with IBD (14 CD, 1 UC) treated with DAT for the management of refractory luminal disease at the Mayo Clinic, Rochester (see **Table 1**). In this cohort, 3 combinations of dual biologic therapy classes were used (no small molecule agents): vedolizumab and anti-TNF (n = 8); ustekinumab and anti-TNF (n = 2); and vedolizumab and ustekinumab (n = 5). The median duration of dual biologic treatment was 6 months; the median follow-up time was 24 months. Most patients (73%, 11/15) had symptomatic improvement (by the Crohn's disease-patient reported outcome signs and symptoms [CD-PRO/SS] or partial Mayo score for UC) and 67% (10/15) had corticosteroid dose reduction, but 20% (3/15) had disease progression that required surgical management. There were 3 serious AEs that required hospitalization (Salmonella gastroenteritis, C difficile infection, and malnutrition), 4 infections treated with antibiotics, and vedolizumab was discontinued in a patient for postinfusion arthralgia (see **Table 1**).

Three additional published case series each with less than 10 patients are summarized in **Table 1**. Overall, DAT were associated with improved CD and/or rheumatologic disease activity in ~29% to 50% of patients, though infectious complications can occur in ~15% to 25% of patients.

NOVEL PHARMACOLOGIC THERAPIES IN PHASE 2 AND 3 CLINICAL TRIALS
Mirikizumab

Mirikizumab is a humanized IgG4 monoclonal antibody that targets IL-23p19 (p19 subunit of the IL23 cytokine).[14,15] The efficacy and safety of mirikizumab was evaluated in SERENITY, a phase 2, randomized, parallel-arm, placebo-controlled trial of 191 patients with moderately-to-severely active CD,[14,15] and VIVID, an ongoing phase 3 trial (ClinicalTrials.gov: NCT03926130) (**Table 2**).

In SERENITY, 191 patients were randomized 2:1:1:2 to dose-ranging IV mirikizumab (200 mg, 600 mg, or 1000 mg) or placebo at weeks 0, 4, and 8.[15] Clinical improvements were observed in patients treated (at all doses for CDAI, 42%–56%, P<.03; mirikizumab 600 mg and 1000 mg by PRO-2, 22%–28%, P<.05) as compared with placebo (23% and 6%, respectively) from baseline to week 12 (see **Table 2**).[14] Endoscopic response (SES-CD 50% reduction from baseline) rates were significantly higher (P<.01) at week 12 for patients treated with mirikizumab 600 mg (38%; 95% confidence interval [CI], 21–54) and 1000 mg (44%; 95% CI, 32–56) as compared with placebo (11%; 95% CI, 3–19).[14] Similarly, endoscopic remission (SES-CD <4 for ileocolonic CD or <2 for isolated ileal CD and no subscore >1) was statistically higher at week 12 for patients treated with mirikizumab 600 mg (15.6%, P = .03) and 1000 mg (20%, P = .009) as compared with placebo (1.6%).[14]

With regards to safety, treatment-emergent AEs rates were similar across all mirikizumab dose-ranging groups (58%–66%) and placebo (70%) (see **Table 2**). Similarly, serious AEs were similar across all mirikizumab-treated (3%–10%) and placebo (11%) groups.[14]

Overall, induction with mirikizumab had higher rates of overall clinical and endoscopic from baseline to week 12 as compared with placebo in the phase 2 SERENITY study. A phase 3 randomized placebo-active controlled trial with an estimated enrollment of 1150 patients is currently underway in the VIVID trial with an estimated completion date in April 2023 (ClinicalTrials.gov: NCT03926130).

Guselkumab

Guselkumab is a humanized IgG1 monoclonal antibody with selective antagonistic binding to IL-23.[16–19] The efficacy and safety of guselkumab was evaluated in GALAXI 1, a phase 2, multicenter, placebo-controlled dose-ranging study (200 mg, 600 mg, and 1200 mg IV at weeks 0, 4, and 8, respectively) of 250 patients with moderately to severely active CD with inadequate response to intolerance to corticosteroids, immunosuppressants, and/or biologic therapies (anti-TNF antagonists, vedolizumab) (see **Table 2**).[16–18]

Table 2
Updates on pharmacologic therapies in phase 2 or 4 clinical trials for moderate to severely active Crohn's disease published from January 2018 to July 2021

Class	Pharmacotherapy	Trials, Phases	Mechanism; Administration	Updates
Anti-Interleukin	Mirikizumab[14,15]	SERENITY (phase 2), VIVID (phase 3, ongoing)	Humanized IgG4 monoclonal antibody with selective binding to the p19 subunit of IL-23; IV and SQ	• Efficacy (clinical): Clinical improvements (CDAI and PRO-2) were observed in the mirikizumab 600 mg (35%–53%) and 1000 mg (22%–28%) groups as compared with placebo (6%–23%; $P<.05$) from baseline to week 12.[14,15] • Efficacy (endoscopic): A higher portion of patients achieved 50% reduction in SES-CD scores at week 12 (from baseline) in the mirikizumab 600 mg (38%) and 1000 mg (44%) groups compared with placebo (11%; $P<.01$). Similarly, endoscopic remission were observed in 16% and 20% of patients in the mirikizumab 600 mg and 1000 mg groups, respectively, compared with 2% in the placebo group ($P = .03$).[14] • Safety: Similar frequencies of treatment-emergent AEs (58%–66%) and serious AEs (0%–9%) were observed across mirikizumab treatment groups and in the placebo group (70% and 11%, respectively)[14]
	Guselkumab[16–18]	GALAXI 1 (phase 2)	Humanized IgG1 monoclonal antibody with selective binding to IL-23; IV	• Efficacy (clinical): Guselkumab-treated patients had higher rates of clinical remission (CDAI score < 150; 20%, 42%, and 54%) at weeks 4, 8, and 12, respectively, as compared with placebo (12%, 16%, 16%; $P = .001$)[16,17] • Efficacy (biochemical): Reductions in CRP (median −2.2 mg/L) and fecal calprotectin (median −176 μg/g) were numerically greater in guselkumab-treated patients compared with the placebo group (0.0 mg/L and 20 μg/g) from baseline to week 12 (P-values not presented)[17]

(continued on next page)

Table 2
(continued)

Class	Pharmacotherapy	Trials, Phases	Mechanism; Administration	Updates
				• Efficacy (endoscopic): Numerically more guselkumab-treated patients had reductions in SES-CD ((LS mean −4.6 vs −0.5), endoscopic healing (17% vs 4%) and endoscopic remission (14% vs 4%) from baseline to week 12 as compared with placebo (*P*-values not presented).[19] • The early trend for achievement of clinical,[17] biochemical,[18] and endoscopic[19] response were observed in the overall guselkumab-treated population, as well as subgroups with refractory disease to biologic or conventional therapies (corticosteroid, immunosuppressant). • Safety: In the guselkumab 200, 600, 1200 mg IV, and placebo treatment groups, serious AEs occurred in 4%, 4%, 2%, and 4%, and serious infections occurred in 2%, 0%, 0%, and 0% of patients, respectively. There were no reported deaths, active tuberculosis, serious hypersensitivity reactions, or malignancies.[16]
	Risankizumab[20–23]	Phase 2 extended open-label studies; FORTIFY (phase 3); ADVANCE and MOTIVATE (phase 3)	Humanized IgG1 monoclonal antibody with selective binding to the p19 subunit of IL-23; IV induction and SQ maintenance	• Efficacy (clinical): In the extended open-label study (up to 206 wk), 77% (23/30 of responders; 35%, 23/65, with nonresponder imputation) had clinical remission (CDAI <150).[21] In the phase 3 studies, significantly more (all *P*<.05) of risankizumab-induced patients (17%–21%, 28%–38%, and 35%–45%) had clinical remission at weeks 4, 8, and 12, respectively, as compared with the placebo group (8%–11%, 13%–17%, 19%–25%).[22] • Efficacy (endoscopic): In the extended open-label study (up to 206 wk), 59% (23/39 of responders; 35%, 23/39, with nonresponder imputation) had endoscopic remission (CDEIS ≤4, or ≤2 for isolated

| Sphingosine-1-Phosphate | Ozanimod[2] | STEPSTONE (phase 2, uncontrolled) | S1P subtype 1 and 5 receptor modulator; oral capsule | • Efficacy: Clinical remission (CDAI <150 points) was achieved in 39% (27/69) of patients after 12 wk of ozanimod, as well as decreases in SES-CD, CDAI, PRO2, GHAS, and RHI scores in an uncontrolled trial (n = 69).[2]
• Safety: Discontinuation of ozanimod due to AEs occurred in 16% (11/69) of patients. The most common AEs were CD flare (26%, 18/69) and abdominal pain (15%, 10/69) of patients.[2] |

Crohn's ileitis).[21] In the phase 3 studies, significantly more patients achieved endoscopic remission in the risankizumab-treated groups compared with placebo (20%–24% vs 4%–9%, $P<.001$).[23]

• Safety: Serious AEs and discontinuations due to AEs were observed/occurred in 35% (23/65) and 32% (21/65) of patients in the extended open-label study.[21] The most common AEs (20%–31%) were nasopharyngitis, gastroenteritis, and fatigue.[21] There were no reported tuberculosis infections, malignancies, or death.[20–23]

(continued on next page)

Table 2 (continued)				
Class	Pharmacotherapy	Trials, Phases	Mechanism; Administration	Updates
Janus Kinase Inhibitor	Upadacitinib[27,28]	CELEST (phase 2)	Oral JAK kinase inhibitor with JAK1 selectivity; oral	• Efficacy (induction, week 12/16): Dose-response endoscopic remission was observed in upadacitinib-treated patients, with the highest rates observed in patients who received upadacitinib 24 mg twice-daily (22%, *P*<.01), compared with placebo (0%). Clinical remission rates did not differ between patients who received upadacitinib (11%–27%) and placebo (14%, *P*>.4). A transcriptomics substudy found that upadacitinib reversed the overexpression of inflammatory fibroblasts after 12–16 wk. • Efficacy (maintenance, week 52): a higher proportion of patients who received upadacitinib 12 mg twice-daily were in clinical remission as compared with those who received upadacitinib 3 mg twice-daily (52%–73% vs 29%–41%, *P*<1), but the rates of endoscopic remission were not different between the dose-ranging groups. • Safety: AEs were the most common in the upadacitinib 12 mg twice-daily group (81% any AEs, 28% serious AEs, and 25% AEs that led to discontinuation of treatment). Significantly higher increases in the total cholesterol, high-density lipoprotein, and low-density lipoprotein levels were observed in patients who received upadacitinib 12 mg and 24 mg twice-daily as compared with placebo from baseline to week 16. There were no deaths or tuberculosis infections reported.

Abbreviations: AE, adverse event; CDAI, Crohn's disease activity index; CRP, C-reactive protein; FACIT, Functional Assessment of Chronic Illness Therapy; GHAS, Geboes Histology Activity Score; IgG, immunoglobulin; IL, interleukin; IV, intravenous; JAK, Janus kinase; LS, least square; MAdCAM-1, mucosal addressin cell adhesion molecule-1; PRO-2, two-item patient-reported outcome; RHI, Robart's Histopathology Index; SES-CD, Simple Endoscopic Score for Crohn's Disease; S1P, sphingosine 1-phosphate; SD, standard deviation; SES-CD, Simple Endoscopic Score for Crohn's Disease; SQ, subcutaneous.

A higher proportion of guselkumab-treated patients achieved clinical remission (CDAI score < 150; 20%, 42%, and 54%) at weeks 4, 8, and 12, respectively, as compared with placebo (12%, 16%, 16%; P = .001) (see **Table 2**).[17] A higher and increasing proportion of guselkumab-treated patients had clinical response (CDAI decrease by ≥100 from or CDAI <150), from 44.0% to 56.0% to 66.0% at weeks 4, 8, and 12, respectively, as compared with placebo (26%, 26%, 24%; P<.001).[16,17]

Similarly, a higher proportion of guselkumab-treated patients had clinical-biomarker response (clinical response and CRP/fecal calprotectin reduced by ≥50% from baseline) that increased from weeks 4, 8, and 12 (26% to 43% to 48%) as compared with placebo (14%, 10%, 8%; P<.001).[17] Guselkumab-treated patients, as compared with placebo, had greater reductions in CRP (median −2.2 mg/L vs 0.0 mg/L; normalization in 35% vs 19%) and fecal calprotectin (median −176 μg/g vs 20 μg/g; normalization in 33% vs 27% placebo) from baseline to week 12 (P-values not reported) (see **Table 2**).[18]

A higher proportion of guselkumab-treated patients achieved endoscopic response (SES-CD decrease by ≥50% from baseline or SES-CD ≤2), endoscopic healing (absence of mucosal ulcerations), and endoscopic remission (SES-CD≤2), 37%, 17%, and 14%, respectively, as compared with placebo (12%, 4%, 4%) at week 12 based on video ileocolonoscopies read by masked central readers (P-values not presented) (see **Table 2**).[19] Guselkumab-treated patients had numerically greater reductions in SES-CD scores compared with the placebo group from baseline to week 12 (least square [LS] mean −4.6 vs −0.5); however, a dose-response relationship with guselkumab was not demonstrated for the clinical or endoscopic outcomes.[19]

With regards to safety, guselkumab-treated patients had similar rates of overall AEs (40%–52%) and serious AEs (2%–4%) as compared with the placebo group (57% and 4%, respectively) through week 12.[16] The overall discontinuation rate through week 12 was low (4%).[16] There were no reported deaths, tuberculosis, or serious hypersensitivity reactions.[16]

Overall, induction with guselkumab had higher rates of overall clinical remission, clinical-biomarker response, and clinical response as early as week 4 that continued to increase in proportion through week 12 as compared with placebo; however, a dose-response relationship was not apparent within the range of doses tested. A small phase 3, open-label study (estimated enrollment of 25 patients) is currently underway with anticipated completion in 2025 (ClinicalTrials.gov: NCT04397263).

Risankizumab

Risankizumab is a humanized monoclonal IgG1 antibody targeting the IL-23 p19 subunit that received FDA approval for the treatment of moderate-to-severe plaque psoriasis in April 2019.[20–23] The efficacy and safety of risankizumab in patients with moderately to severely active CD was evaluated in a phase 2 open-label extension study[20] and three phase 3 trials, FORTIFY, ADVANCE, and MOTIVATE (see **Table 2**).[21–23]

In the phase 2 open-extension trial of risankizumab, 101 patients who did not achieve deep remission by week 12 of the original phase 2 study[24] (33 from the placebo group, 23 from the risankizumab 200 mg group, and 34 from the risankizumab 600 mg group) received an additional 12 weeks of open-label risankizumab 600 mg, then patients who achieved deep remission/clinical remission by week 26 proceeded to the 52-week maintenance trial (risankizumab 180 mg SQ every 8 weeks).[20] In this open-extension trial at week 26, 54% (55/101) were in clinical remission (CDAI <150) and 6% (6/101) had clinical-endoscopic remission (see **Table 2**). Of the 62 patients who remained in the maintenance trial (including 1 patient who did not achieve clinical remission but continued to maintenance trial due to protocol deviation) at week

52, 71% achieved clinical remission, 35% endoscopic remission (CDEIS ≤4, or ≤2 for isolated Crohn's ileitis), 29% clinical-endoscopic remission, and 24% mucosal healing (absence of mucosal ulceration) (see **Table 2**).[20] Endoscopic outcomes were assessed by masked central reading of ileocolonoscopies.[20,21]

In the final results from the open-label extension phase 2 study, which continued till the closure of Study M15-898 at week 206, 65 patients who achieved clinical response (reduction of CDAI ≥100 from baseline) without clinical remission (CDAI <150) at week 26/52 proceeded to receive risankizumab 180 mg SQ every 8 weeks (4 patients received reinduction of risankizumab 600 mg IV every 4 weeks for 3 doses at week 26/52).[21] At week 206, clinical remission was observed in 77% (23/30; 35%, 23/65, with nonresponder imputation) and endoscopic remission in 59% (23/39; 35%, 23/39, with nonresponder imputation) of patients (see **Table 2**).[21] Overall, the open-label extension study of risankizumab supported the efficacy of selective IL-23 blockade for the treatment of moderately to severely active CD.[21]

ADVANCE and MOTIVATE are active phase 3, double-blind, randomized, placebo-controlled trials with 850 and 569 patients, respectively, with moderately to severely active CD with inadequate response or intolerance to conventional and/or biologic treatments. Patients were randomized to 2:2:1 or 1:1:1 of risankizumab 600 mg IV, 1200 mg IV, or placebo as induction therapy in ADVANCE and MOTIVATE, respectively.[22,23] At weeks 4, 8, and 12, significantly more (all $P<.05$) patients achieved clinical remission in the risankizumab 600 mg (17%–21%, 28%–35%, 35%–45% by CDAI <150 or PRO-2 stool frequency subscore [SFS] ≤2.8 and abdominal pain subscore [APS] ≤1 with neither worse than baseline) and 1200 mg groups (18%–21%, 30%–38%, 39%–42% by CDAI or PRO-2 criteria) as compared with placebo (8%–11%, 13%–17%, 19%–25%) (see **Table 2**).[22] At week 12, 19% to 24% ($P<.001$) and 20% to 24% ($P<.001$) of patients in the risankizumab 600 mg and 1200 mg groups, respectively, achieved endoscopic remission (SES-CD≤4) as compared with 4% to 9% in the placebo group (see **Table 2**).[23]

FORTIFY is a phase 3 placebo-controlled induction study of risankizumab in 931 patients with moderately to severely active CD that was completed in April 2021. Preliminary results are available from the sponsor's center news center.[25]

With regards to safety, overall AEs and serious AEs were reported in 92% (60/65) and 35% (23/65) in the phase 2 extended open-label study.[21] In the extended open-label study, 32% (21/65) patients prematurely discontinued risankizumab, including 9% (6/65) that were AE-related (see **Table 2**).[21] The most common AEs were nasopharyngitis (31%), gastroenteritis (23%), and fatigue (20%).[21] No tuberculosis infections, malignancies, or death were observed in the risankizumab open-label study or extended open-label study.[20,21]

Overall, phase 2 and 3 trials support the efficacy of risankizumab induction therapy for clinical and endoscopic response, and phase 3 trials maintenance trials are completed/underway to provide additional data on its safety and efficacy in patients with moderately to severely active CD.

Ozanimod

Ozanimod is an oral agent that selectively binds sphingosine-1-phosphate (S1P) receptor subtypes 1 and 5[2] that was recently approved by the FDA for treatment of patients with moderately to severely active UC in May 2021.[2,26] For CD, the safety and efficacy of ozanimod 1 mg oral capsule was evaluated in STEPSTONE, a phase 2, uncontrolled, multicenter trial of 69 patients with moderately to severely active CD[2] (see **Table 2**). Ozanimod was administered in a 7-day escalation protocol (0.25 mg daily for 4 days and then 0.5 mg daily for 3 days) then 1 mg daily.[2]

Clinical, endoscopic, and histologic improvement were observed based on decreases in the mean SES-CD (−2.2, SD 6.0), CDAI (−130, SD 104), PRO2 (−66, SD 65), global histologic disease activity score (GHAS; −5.9, SD 11.0), and Robarts histologic index (RHI; −10.6, SD 25.1) scores from baseline to week 12[2] (see **Table 2**). Clinical remission (CDAI <150 points) was achieved in 39% (27/69) of patients.[2]

With regards to safety in the phase 2 uncontrolled trial for ozanimod in patients with moderately to severely active CD (n = 69), the most common treatment-emergent AEs were CD flare (26%), abdominal pain (15%), lymphopenia (13%), arthralgia (13%), and nausea (12%) (see **Table 2**).[2] Ozanimod was discontinued in 16% (11/69) of patients who experienced treatment-emergent AEs.[2] There were no clinically important changes in heart rate were observed at treatment initiation.[2]

Overall, clinical, endoscopic, and histologic improvements were observed in STEP-STONE, a phase 2 uncontrolled trial of ozanimod. A phase 3 placebo-controlled induction study of ozanimod 1 mg is underway with estimated enrollment of 600 patients with moderately to severely active CD and anticipated completion in 2023 (Clinical-Trials.gov: NCT03440372). A phase 3 open-label extension study of ozanimod 1 mg × 48 weeks is underway with estimated enrollment of 1200 patients and anticipated to be completed in 2026 (ClinicalTrials.gov: NCT03467958).

Upadacitinib

Upadacitinib is an oral JAK1 inhibitor that received FDA approval for treatment of adults with moderate to severe rheumatoid arthritis in August 2019.[27,28] In CD, the efficacy and safety of upadacitinib was evaluated in CELEST, a phase 2, randomized placebo-dose ranging trial (3 mg, 6 mg, 12 mg, or 24 mg twice-daily; or 24 mg once-daily) in 220 patients with moderately to severely active CD refractory/intolerant to immunosuppressants or anti-TNF antagonists[27] (see **Table 2**).

Postinduction (week 12/16), the rates of clinical remission (average daily SFS 1.5 and APS 1.0, with neither worse than the baseline value) were not significantly different (P>.4) between upadacitinib-treated (11%–27%) and placebo 14% groups, and a dose-response association was also not observed[27] (see **Table 2**). Dose-response relationship for endoscopic remission (SES-CD ≤4 and a ≥2-point reduction from baseline, with no subscore >1) was observed in 10% (P< .1), 8% (P-value not reported), 8% (P< .1), 22% (P<.01), and 14% (P<.05) of patients treated with upadacitinib 3 mg, 6 mg, 12 mg, 24 mg twice-daily, and 24 mg once-daily, respectively, versus 0% in the placebo group (see **Table 2**).[27] A total of 180 patients completed the induction period and were rerandomized to upadacitinib 3 mg, 6 mg, 12 mg twice-daily, or 24 mg once-daily, in the maintenance period. At week 52, 52% to 73% of patients in the upadacitinib 12 mg twice-daily group were in clinical remission, as compared with 29% to 41% in the upadacitinib 3 mg twice-daily group (P<.1); clinical remission rates were not different in the other dose-ranging groups (see **Table 2**).[27] At week 52, the rates of endoscopic response were not different between the dose-ranging groups.[27]

With regards to safety, higher incidences of AEs occurred with the higher doses of upadacitinib (≥12 mg twice-daily; see **Table 2**).[27] Serious AEs occurred in 5% to 28% upadacitinib-treated patients, with the highest incidence in the 12 mg twice-daily group (28%, 10/36).[27] Similarly, 3% to 25% of patients had AEs that led to the discontinuation of upadacitinib, with highest incidence occurring in patients treated with 12 mg twice-daily (25%, 9/26) (see **Table 2**). Moreover, at week 16, patients who received upadacitinib 12 mg twice-daily and 24 mg twice-daily had significantly higher increases in the total cholesterol (mean 0.44, SD 0.9, $P<.05$; mean 0.70, SD 0.68, $P<.001$), high-density lipoprotein (mean 0.15, SD 0.28, $P<.1$; mean 0.48, SD 0.47, $P<.001$), and low-density lipoprotein (mean 0.43, SD 0.69, $P<.01$; mean 0.42, SD 0.48, $P<.01$) cholesterol levels compared with patients in the placebo group (mean −0.10, SD 0.68; mean −0.02, SD 0.34; mean −0.01, SD 0.47, respectively). There were no deaths or tuberculosis occurred in the 52-week study.[27]

Overall, a dose-response relationship for endoscopic remission was demonstrated in the phase 2 ozanimod induction study, CELEST, though its efficacy for achieving clinical remission was not observed. A phase 3 placebo-controlled induction study is currently underway to further explore the efficacy and safety of upadacitinib induction, with estimated enrollment of 501 patients and study completion in February 2022 (ClinicalTrials.gov: NCT03345849).

A transcriptomics substudy was conducted in 74 patients from the CELEST study who had endoscopic remission but persistent mucosa inflammation at week 12 or 16 (postinduction).[28] In areas with mucosal inflammation, treatment with upadacitinib was observed to be associated with the reversal in the overexpression of inflammatory fibroblast (SOX6, PTGDR2, and PDGFD), interferon-γ effector (IFNG, TBX21, and GZMH), and acute inflammatory markers (CHI3L1, OSM, and S100A8) in anti-TNF refractory patients from baseline to week 12/16 (see **Table 2**).[28] Conversely, the transcriptomes of noninvolved intestinal areas did not differ between baseline and postinduction. This suggests that upadacitinib modulates mucosal inflammatory molecular pathways as a mechanism by which JAK1 inhibition may be effective in patients with CD and refractory to anti-TNF therapy.[28]

SUMMARY

In summary, in patients with refractory CD and/or active EIMs (eg, ankylosing spondylitis) or rheumatologic diseases (eg, psoriatic arthritis) despite the use of single biologic or small molecule agents may benefit from a combination of DAT. Several novel pharmacotherapies with more specific mechanistic targets (eg, interleukin-23, Janus kinase inhibitor subtypes, and sphingosine-1-phosphate) have shown promising results in phase 2 clinical trials and multiple phase 3 studies are currently underway with anticipation of completion over the next 5 years. Pharmacologic therapies with improved efficacy, safety, and tolerability are active areas for research and development to address lingering unmet needs for patients with moderately to severely active CD.

CLINICS CARE POINTS

- Dual advanced therapies (combination of biologics and/or small molecule therapies) have been used to treat refractory Crohn's disease and/or concomitant rheumatologic extraintestinal manifestations with a 30% to 60% efficacy, although adverse events (particularly infectious complications) can occur in nearly two-thirds of patients.

- Risankizumab demonstrated promising results for inducing and maintaining clinical and endoscopic response in phase 2 clinical trials, and its safety and efficacy are further explored in phase 3 placebo-controlled induction (completed, preliminary results reported) and maintenance studies (underway).

- Phase 2 induction studies of mirikizumab, ozanimod, and guselkumab have demonstrated varying degrees of efficacy in inducing clinical and/or endoscopic response with an acceptable safety profile; phase 3 trials of these agents are currently underway with anticipated study completion over the next 2 to 5 years.

DISCLOSURE

P.S. Dulai: Consulting and/or grant support from Takeda, Abbvie, Janssen, Pfizer, Gilead, BMS, Lily, Novartis, Scipher, and Prometheus. C.S. Tse has nothing to disclose.

REFERENCES

1. Feuerstein JD, Ho EY, Shmidt E, et al. AGA clinical practice guidelines on the medical management of moderate to severe luminal and perianal fistulizing crohn's disease. Gastroenterology 2021;160(7):2496–508.
2. Feagan BG, Sandborn WJ, Danese S, et al. Ozanimod induction therapy for patients with moderate to severe Crohn's disease: a single-arm, phase 2, prospective observer-blinded endpoint study. Lancet Gastroenterol Hepatol 2020;5(9): 819–28.
3. Rutgeerts P, Gasink C, Chan D, et al. Efficacy of Ustekinumab for Inducing Endoscopic Healing in Patients With Crohn's Disease. Gastroenterology 2018;155(4): 1045–58.
4. Shi HY, Ng SC. The state of the art on treatment of Crohn's disease. J Gastroenterol 2018;53(9):989–98.
5. Yang E, Panaccione N, Whitmire N, et al. Efficacy and safety of simultaneous treatment with two biologic medications in refractory Crohn's disease. Aliment Pharmacol Ther 2020;51(11):1031–8.
6. Privitera G, Onali S, Pugliese D, et al. Dual Targeted Therapy: A Possible Option for the Management of Refractory Inflammatory Bowel Disease. J Crohn's Colitis 2020;15(2):335–9.
7. Mao EJ, Lewin S, Terdiman JP, et al. Safety of dual biological therapy in Crohn's disease: a case series of vedolizumab in combination with other biologics. BMJ Open Gastroenterol 2018;5(1):e000243.
8. Glassner K, Oglat A, Duran A, et al. The use of combination biological or small molecule therapy in inflammatory bowel disease: A retrospective cohort study. J Dig Dis 2020;21(5):264–71.
9. Fumery M, Yzet C, Brazier F. Letter: combination of biologics in inflammatory bowel diseases. Aliment Pharmacol Ther 2020;52(3):566–7.
10. Fala L. Otezla (Apremilast), an oral PDE-4 inhibitor, receives FDA approval for the treatment of patients with active psoriatic arthritis and plaque psoriasis. Am Health Drug benefits 2015;8(Spec Feature):105.
11. Kwapisz L, Raffals LE, Bruining DH, et al. Combination Biologic Therapy in Inflammatory Bowel Disease: Experience From a Tertiary Care Center. Clin Gastroenterol Hepatol 2021;19(3):616–7.
12. Buer LCT, Høivik ML, Warren DJ, et al. Combining Anti-TNF-α and Vedolizumab in the Treatment of Inflammatory Bowel Disease: A Case Series. Inflamm Bowel Dis 2018;24(5):997–1004.
13. Ahmed W, Galati J, Kumar A, et al. Dual Biologic or Small Molecule Therapy for Treatment of Inflammatory Bowel Disease: A Systematic Review and Meta-analysis. Clin Gastroenterol Hepatol 2021. https://doi.org/10.1016/j.cgh.2021.03.034.
14. Sands BES WJ, Peyrin-Biroulet L, Higgins P, et al. OP108 Efficacy and Safety of Mirikizumab After 52-Weeks Maintenance Treatment in Patients with Moderate-To-Severe Crohn's Disease. Gastroenterology 2021. Nov 5;S0016-5085(21) 03725-2.
15. Sandborn WJ, Sands BE, Hindryckx P, et al. S0705Evaluationof Symptom Improvement During Induction in Patients With Crohn's Disease Treated With Mirikizumab. Am Coll Gastroenterol 2020;115:S354.

16. Sandborn WJ, Chan DJ J, Lang G, et al, on behalf of the GALAXI 1 Investigators. OP089 The efficacy and safety of guselkumab induction therapy in patients with moderately to severely active Crohn's disease: week 12 interim analyses from the phase 2 GALAXI 1 study. United European Gastroenterology Journal 2020;Vol. 8(8S):8–142.

17. Danese S, Sandborn WJ, Feagan BG, et al. OP28 The effect of guselkumab induction therapy on early clinical outcome measures in patients with Moderately to Severely Active Crohn's Disease: Results from the phase 2 GALAXI 1 study. J Crohn's Colitis 2021;15(Supplement_1):S027–8.

18. Sands BE, Danese S, Andrews JM, et al. Fr532 The effect of guselkumab induction therapy on inflammatory biomarkers in patients with moderately to severely active crohn's disease: week 12 results from the phase 2 GALAXI 1 Study. Gastroenterology 2021;160(6, Supplement). S-350-S-351.

19. D'Haens G, Rubin DT, Panes J, et al. 455 The effect of guselkumab induction therapy on endoscopic outcome measures in patients with moderately to severely active crohn's disease: week 12 results from the phase 2 GALAXI 1 Study. Gastroenterology 2021;160(6, Supplement):S-91.

20. Feagan BG, Panes J, Ferrante M, et al. Risankizumab in patients with moderate to severe Crohn's disease: an open-label extension study. Lancet Gastroenterol Hepatol 2018;3(10):671–80.

21. Ferrante M, Feagan BG, Panés J, et al. OP27 Long-term safety and efficacy of risankizumab treatment in patients with Crohn's disease: Final results from the Phase 2 open-label extension study. J Crohn's Colitis 2020;14(Supplement_1): S024–5.

22. Schreiber S, Ferrante M, Panaccione R, et al. OP26 Risankizumab induces early clinical remission and response in patients with Moderate-to-Severe Crohn's Disease: Results from the phase 3 ADVANCE and MOTIVATE studies. J Crohn's Colitis 2021;15(Supplement_1):S026–7.

23. Bossuyt P, Ferrante M, Baert F, et al. OP36 Risankizumab therapy induces improvements in endoscopic endpoints in patients with Moderate-to-Severe Crohn's Disease: Results from the phase 3 ADVANCE and MOTIVATE studies. J Crohn's Colitis 2021;15(Supplement_1):S033–4.

24. Feagan BG, Sandborn WJ, D'Haens G, et al. Induction therapy with the selective interleukin-23 inhibitor risankizumab in patients with moderate-to-severe Crohn's disease: a randomised, double-blind, placebo-controlled phase 2 study. Lancet 2017;389(10080):1699–709.

25. AbbVie. Phase 3 Maintenance Results Show Patients with Crohn's Disease Receiving Risankizumab (SKYRIZI®) Achieved Endoscopic Response and Clinical Remission at One Year. AbbVie Inc. Updated 2 June 2021. 2021. Available at: https://news.abbvie.com/news/press-releases/phase-3-maintenance-results-show-patients-with-crohns-disease-receiving-risankizumab-skyrizi-achieved-endoscopic-response-and-clinical-remission-at-one-year.htm. Accessed September 11, 2021.

26. Bristol-Myers Squibb Company. Zeposia Prescribing Information. Zeposia U.S. Product Information. Princeton, N.J.: Bristol-Myers Squibb Company; 2021.

27. Sandborn WJ, Feagan BG, Loftus EV Jr, et al. Efficacy and Safety of Upadacitinib in a Randomized Trial of Patients With Crohn's Disease. Gastroenterology 2020; 158(8):2123–38.e8.

28. Aguilar D, Revilla L, Garrido-Trigo A, et al. Randomized Controlled Trial Substudy of Cell-specific Mechanisms of Janus Kinase 1 Inhibition With Upadacitinib in the Crohn's Disease Intestinal Mucosa: Analysis From the CELEST Study. Inflamm Bowel Dis 2021. https://doi.org/10.1093/ibd/izab116.

Therapeutic Drug Monitoring of Biologics in Crohn's Disease

Laurie B. Grossberg, MD*, Adam S. Cheifetz, MD,
Konstantinos Papamichael, MD, PhD

KEYWORDS

- Therapeutic drug monitoring (TDM) • Biologics • Anti-TNF • Crohn's disease

KEY POINTS

- Reactive therapeutic drug monitoring (TDM) is considered standard of care for optimizing biologics in inflammatory bowel disease (IBD) including Crohn's disease (CD).
- Preliminary data show that proactive TDM for optimizing biologics is associated with more favorable outcomes in IBD.
- TDM can efficiently guide therapeutic decisions in specific clinical scenarios including treatment deescalation, optimized monotherapy with an antitumor necrosis factor, and following a drug holiday.
- Higher biological drug concentrations are associated with favorable therapeutic outcomes in specific IBD populations or phenotypes, including pediatrics, perianal fistulizing CD, small bowel CD, and following an ileocolonic resection for CD.
- The future of TDM aims toward personalized medicine with the use of rapid assays, pharmacogenomics, and pharmacokinetic dashboards.

INTRODUCTION

Crohn's disease (CD) is a chronic inflammatory bowel disease (IBD) that is characterized by transmural inflammation that can affect any part of the gastrointestinal tract, leading to complications such as fibrotic strictures, fistulas, and abscesses.[1] Biological therapies including antitumor necrosis factor (TNF) agents (infliximab, adalimumab, certolizumab, and associated biosimilars), antiintegrin therapies (natalizumab, vedolizumab), and an anti-interleukin-12/23 monoclonal antibody (ustekinumab) have revolutionized the care of patients with moderate-to-severe CD.[2]

Therapeutic drug monitoring (TDM) refers to the measurement of a drug concentration or its metabolite to optimize efficacy and reduce toxicity and is a means of personalized patient care. Historically, providers have used TDM in IBD to measure

Division of Gastroenterology, Center for Inflammatory Bowel Diseases, Beth-Israel Deaconess Medical Center, Harvard Medical School, 330 Brookline Ave, Boston, MA 02215, USA
* Corresponding author.
E-mail address: lgrossbe@bidmc.harvard.edu

Gastroenterol Clin N Am 51 (2022) 299–317
https://doi.org/10.1016/j.gtc.2021.12.007
0889-8553/22/© 2022 Elsevier Inc. All rights reserved.

cyclosporine concentrations in ulcerative colitis (UC) and to measure thiopurine metabolites.[3] More recently, TDM in CD primarily refers to checking biological drug concentrations and antidrug antibodies (ADAs). The data show that higher drug concentrations are associated with improved outcomes, including clinical, biochemical, endoscopic, and histologic remission.[4] In addition, the presence of adequate drug concentrations decreases the risk of relapse, hospitalization, surgery, and ADAs.[4–6] On the other hand, low drug concentrations are associated with ADAs and poor response or loss of response to treatment.[4,5] Therefore, the role of TDM in the treatment of CD has become a prominent topic in IBD research.

This review summarizes the role of TDM of biologics in CD, focusing more on data from prospective studies and randomized controlled trials (RCTs). In addition, the authors address the use of TDM in specific clinical scenarios including treatment deescalation, optimized monotherapy with anti-TNF, and following a drug holiday and in specific populations or phenotypes including pediatrics, perianal and small bowel CD, and following ileocolonic resection for CD. Finally, future directions of TDM of biologics are briefly described.

THERAPEUTIC DRUG MONITORING OF BIOLOGICS IN CROHN'S DISEASE

Reactive TDM refers to the measurement of drug concentrations and ADAs in the setting of active IBD symptoms or findings of disease activity on biochemical, radiologic, or endoscopic evaluation. Reactive TDM is considered the standard of care and is recommended by current guidelines, as it has rationalized the management of treatment failure and is more cost-effective than empirical dose escalation.[6,7] Proactive TDM refers to the practice of checking drug concentrations and ADAs with the goal of optimizing therapy to a target trough concentration in order to reduce risk of poor outcomes. Preliminary data, mostly from retrospective studies, comparing proactive versus empirical treatment optimization and/or reactive TDM, show that proactive TDM is beneficial in patients with IBD.[8–11] However, its use in clinical practice is currently considered controversial, as there are only limited data from prospective studies and RCTs.[12–17]

Two RCTs, TAXIT (Trough Concentration Adapted Infliximab Treatment) and TAILORIX (A Study investigating Tailored Treatment With Infliximab for Active Crohn's Disease), assessed proactive TDM of maintenance infliximab in patients with IBD.[13,14] In the TAXIT trial, patients receiving infliximab were first optimized to drug trough concentrations of 3 to 7 μg/mL, and then randomized 1:1 to receive further dosing based on clinical judgment or trough concentrations. The primary endpoint assessing the proportion of patients in clinical remission in each treatment arm did not reach statistical significance (66% in the clinical dosing group vs 69% in the TDM group, $P = .686$). However, more patients with CD achieved clinical remission during the dose optimization phase (85% after optimization vs 65% before escalation, $P = .020$) and had significant reductions in C-reactive protein (CRP) (3.2 vs 4.3 mg/L, $P < .001$). In addition, more patients in the clinically based group relapsed during the maintenance phase (17% vs 7%, $P = .018$), had suboptimal trough concentrations, and developed antibodies to infliximab (ATI) compared with those in the TDM arm. One major criticism of this study is that the early optimization for all patients and short-term follow-up may have influenced the outcomes and lessened the differences seen between the 2 treatment arms.[13] In the TAILORIX study, 122 biologic-naïve patients with CD received infliximab induction treatment in combination with an immunosuppressant. At week 14, patients were assigned to 3 maintenance arms: 2 based on biomarker and trough concentration dose intensification by either 2.5 mg/kg or 5 mg/

kg, and the third arm was clinically based on dose intensification from 5 mg/kg to 10 mg/kg. There was no difference between the 3 treatment arms in achieving corticosteroid-free clinical remission between weeks 22 through 54 with no ulcers at week 54 (47% vs 38% vs 40%, $P = .50$).[14] There were several limitations in study design including that patients were only able to start dose intensification at week 14, and changes could not be made again until 8 weeks later unless infliximab concentrations were very low less than 1 μg/mL. Importantly, patients in the control group were able to receive more liberal dose intensification, even in the absence of elevated biomarkers (as opposed to the interventional groups). Moreover, only 14% of patients actually underwent dose optimization based on infliximab trough concentrations in the combined intervention groups. In the end, the drug concentrations in all 3 groups were similar.

On the other hand, the PRECISION (Precision Dosing of Infliximab Versus Conventional Dosing of Infliximab) trial showed a benefit for proactive TDM in patients with IBD on infliximab in clinical remission compared with standard-of-care dosing.[15] In this study, a Bayesian pharmacokinetic model was applied to determine optimal dosing regimens. The model incorporated patient data including gender, body weight, drug and ADA concentrations, serum CRP, and albumin. Eighty patients (66 CD, 14 UC) were enrolled, and after 1 year, more patients in the precision group were in clinical remission compared with the control group (88% vs 64%, $P = .017$). At 1 year, patients in the precision group had also lower fecal calprotectin values (47 mg/g vs 144 mg/g, $P = .031$).[15] In this study, endoscopic evaluation was not performed; however, the difference detected in fecal calprotectin does provide some objective evidence of efficacy. In addition, a low target trough of 3 mg/mL was used.

In the NOR-DRUM (NORwegian DRUg Monitoring study) RCT, Syversen and colleagues assessed the effect of TDM versus standard therapy during infliximab induction on disease remission in 411 patients with chronic immune-mediated inflammatory diseases.[16] The results showed that 50.5% in the TDM group versus 53% in the standard therapy group achieved remission at week 30 ($P = .78$). Although this study did not support the use of TDM, it was not tailored to patients with IBD and there was not statistical power to test each group separately.[16] In addition, the maintenance infliximab target range was 3 to 8 mg/L, which is lower than what was previously suggested.[5,6]

In a more recent prospective study, an ultraproactive TDM strategy was applied using point-of-care testing (POCT) in patients with IBD on infliximab maintenance treatment.[17] Patients at one center were treated with the ultraproactive TDM algorithm, and patients at the other center received reactive TDM. In the ultraproactive group, a POCT was used before infusion, and if concentrations were less than 3 μg/mL, the dose interval was shortened by 2 weeks. If the POCT before the next infusion showed trough concentrations less than 3 μg/mL, the dose was optimized. A total of 187 patients were included, and at 1 year there was no difference in infliximab failure (19% vs 10%, $P = .08$) or sustained clinical remission (75% vs 83%, $P = .17$) between the ultraproactive group and the reactive TDM group, respectively.[17] Limitations of this study include that data in the reactive group were analyzed retrospectively, no serum samples were available in the reactive cohort to compare the pharmacologic data between the 2 cohorts, and there was no standardized assessment of mucosal remission. Data were only available in 38% of patients and prone to selection bias.[17]

In the PAILOT (Pediatric Crohn's Disease Adalimumab Level-based Optimization Treatment) RCT, 78 biologic-naïve pediatric patients with CD who responded to adalimumab induction were randomized to receive proactive TDM or reactive TDM for 72 weeks. This study showed that proactive TDM with optimization of adalimumab trough concentrations to concentrations greater than 5 μg/mL led to higher rates of sustained corticosteroid-free clinical remission (82% vs 48%, P = .002) and sustained corticosteroid-free remission, normal CRP, and normal fecal calprotectin (42% vs 12%, P = .003) compared with reactive monitoring in patients with loss of response (P = .001).[12]

Several prospective association studies support the use of TDM in CD. The PANTS (Personalized Anti-TNF Therapy in Crohn's Disease) study was a multicenter, prospective observational cohort study of patients with CD who received treatment with infliximab (n = 955) or adalimumab (n = 655). The only factor associated with nonresponse was a low drug concentration at week 14 (infliximab, odds ratio [OR]: 0.35; 95% confidence interval [CI]: 0.20 to 0.62; P = .00038 and adalimumab, OR: 0.13; 95% CI: 0.06 to 0.23; P < .0001). The optimal week 14 concentrations associated with remission at weeks 14 and 54 were 7 mg/L for infliximab and 12 mg/L for adalimumab. Furthermore, low week-14 concentrations were associated with subsequent development of ADAs.[18] In one study assessing 100 patients with active CD, higher vedolizumab concentrations at weeks 2, 10, and 22 in patients were associated with lower simplified endoscopic activity scores for CD. Higher vedolizumab concentrations at week 22 were associated with higher rates of endoscopic remission at week 26. A vedolizumab concentration of 10.5 mg/L at week 22 discriminated patients with and without endoscopic response at week 26.[19] Walshe and colleagues investigated the association between ustekinumab concentrations and clinical and biochemical outcomes in patients with CD. The study showed significant correlations between week 6 ustekinumab concentrations and baseline albumin [rho (r) = 0.644, 95% CI: 0.304–0.839, P < .001] and baseline calprotectin (r = −0.678, 95% CI: −0.873 to −0.296, P < .001). Week 6 ustekinumab concentrations correlated with week 12 Crohn's disease activity index (r = −0.513, 95% CI: −0.796 to −0.046, P < .01) and CRP (r = −0.578, 95% CI: −0.808 to −0.194, P < .01).[20] These studies suggest that early TDM and treat-to-target approaches may be helpful to improve outcomes for patients with CD treated with vedolizumab or ustekinumab.

THERAPEUTIC DRUG MONITORING IN SPECIFIC CLINICAL SCENARIOS
Deescalation of Therapy

TDM may also be valuable in deescalating treatment of patients who are in remission on treatment. Advantages of dose deescalation include decreased costs and patient convenience if dose intervals can be increased. The TAXIT RCT showed that dose reduction in patients with IBD and supraoptimal infliximab trough concentrations (>7 μg/mL) did not lead to flares or an increase of inflammatory markers but did result in significant cost savings.[13] Allegretti and colleagues performed a pilot study of dose deescalation in patients with CD in clinical remission (Harvey-Bradshaw Index [HBI] ≤ 2 for at least 6 months before enrollment) treated with infliximab for at least 1 year. Subjects were eligible to undergo one dose deescalation from 10 or 7.5 mg/kg to 5 mg/kg or from 5 mg/kg to 3 mg/kg if their baseline trough concentration was greater than 10 μg/L with no interval adjustment. Patients were followed-up through 3 infusions after deescalation. Fifty-two patients were screened, of which 55.7% (29) were eligible, and 19 patients agreed to deescalation (13 decreased to 5 mg/kg and 6–3 mg/kg). The mean baseline trough was 24.6 μg/mL, and after 3 addition infusions the mean trough was 11.2 μg/mL. Of the 19 patients, all had HBI scores of 0 to 1, and only 3 required reescalation to original dosing (2 due to low level ATI and 1 due to joint pain).[21] This study suggests that dose deescalation is possible, even to doses as low as 3 mg/kg in patients with high trough concentrations (>10 μg/mL). However, this was a single-center study with small numbers and short-term follow-up. Other studies assessing the role of TDM in deescalation include patients with both CD and UC. Petitcollin and colleagues evaluated the probability of relapse after dose deescalation of infliximab in patients with IBD.[22] The study found infliximab trough concentrations of less than 5.7 µg/mL before deescalation and infliximab trough concentrations of less than 2.4 µg/mL after deescalation to independently predict relapse.[22] Similarly, another study assessed patients with IBD undergoing dose deescalation of infliximab based on clinical remission or clinical remission with infliximab trough concentration greater than 7 mg/L.[23] The results demonstrated that trough concentration–based deescalation was associated with reduced risk of relapse (hazard ratio [HR]: 0.45; 95% CI: 0.22–0.90, $P = .024$). The median trough concentration associated with relapse after deescalation was 3.9 mg/L versus 5.95 mg/L among the patients who did not relapse.[23] Furthermore, Amiot and colleagues found that TDM-based management was more accurate in preventing relapse than blind management of infliximab during deescalation.[24] For adalimumab, one study found higher trough concentrations (>12.2 µg/mL) to be associated with successful deescalation in patients with IBD.[25] Although these studies were all single-center studies and have limitations, the results all do suggest that TDM should be performed before deescalation, and considered following deescalation in order to prevent relapse.

Optimized Monotherapy

The benefit of combination therapy with an anti-TNF agent and an immunomodulator (IMM) in the treatment of CD must be balanced with the potential increased risks of infection and malignancy.[26] In the pivotal SONIC (The Study of Biologic and Immunomodulator Naïve Patients in Crohn's Disease) RCT, patients with moderate-to-severely active CD treated with infliximab in combination with azathioprine were more likely to achieve corticosteroid-free remission and endoscopic healing compared with either drug alone at week 26.[27] However, subsequent studies showed that IMM may increase the exposure of anti-TNF therapy and reduce the risk of immunogenicity.[28,29] Therefore, recent research has sought to answer whether the benefit of combination therapy is related to the synergistic effect of both drugs together or due to pharmacokinetics. Colombel and colleagues performed a post hoc analysis of the SONIC trial to assess the benefit of combination therapy versus monotherapy and found that combination therapy was associated with higher serum infliximab concentrations.[30] The study showed that within quartiles of serum infliximab concentrations there was no difference in corticosteroid-free clinical remission at week 26 in the monotherapy versus combination therapy group in the higher quartiles.[30] These data suggest that as long as infliximab concentrations are adequate, combination therapy may not be necessary. A recent retrospective study showed that there was no differences in infliximab retention rates at 1 year, steroid use at 1 year, or mucosal healing at the end of follow-up for patients receiving optimized monotherapy based on proactive TDM versus combination therapy.[31] Another retrospective study compared outcomes of patients receiving infliximab monotherapy with proactive TDM at week 10, infliximab monotherapy without proactive TDM (standard of care), and combination therapy for infliximab with an IMM.[32] The results revealed that patients who received monotherapy with proactive TDM at week 10 were less likely to discontinue infliximab compared with patients receiving monotherapy without TDM ($P = .04$); however, there was no difference between monotherapy with proactive TDM and combination therapy.[32] These preliminary studies suggest that optimized monotherapy based on proactive may be an alternative to combination therapy with an IMM, although prospective data are lacking.

Drug Holiday

Another application for TDM is reintroduction of biological therapy after a drug holiday. In a large retrospective study, Baert and colleagues assessed patients with IBD restarting infliximab after a median 15-month drug holiday. In this study, the absence of ATI on an early sample after reexposure was associated with short-term responses and safe reintroduction of therapy.[33] In a recent retrospective study, Normatov and colleagues assessed early TDM in patients restarting infliximab after more than or equal to 6-month drug holiday. In this study patients were divided into 2 groups: one that checked TDM 1 to 3 weeks after first reinduction (TDM group) dose and those who did not (non-TDM group). The study found that there was no significant difference in infusion reactions between the antibody negative TDM group and the non-TDM group. However, more severe infusion reactions, defined as those necessitating treatment cessation due to significant cardiovascular or respiratory symptoms, occurred in the non-TDM group.[34] These studies imply that checking TDM early in reinduction after a drug holiday may be helpful in predicting response and the likelihood of an infusion reaction, but prospective validation of these data along with additional studies with other biologics are needed.

THERAPEUTIC DRUG MONITORING IN SPECIFIC POPULATIONS OR PHENOTYPES OF CROHN'S DISEASE

Numerous exposure-response relationship studies have shown that higher biological drug concentrations are associated with higher rates of favorable therapeutic outcomes in patients with IBD.[4,5] This is also true for specific populations or phenotypes of CD, including patients with perianal fistulizing disease, small bowel CD, or those with an ileocolonic resection (**Table 1**)[35–43] as well as the pediatric population (**Table 2**).[44–58]

Perianal Fistulizing Crohn's Disease

Although current guidelines suggest target infliximab maintenance trough concentrations of greater than 5 μg/mL,[6] data suggest that higher trough concentrations may be beneficial in patients with CD and perianal fistula.[35,36,41,42] A post hoc analysis of the ACCENT II (A Randomized, Double-blind, Placebo-controlled Trial of Anti-TNF Chimeric Monoclonal Antibody [Infliximab; REMICADE Janssen Biotech, Inc, Malvern, PA, USA] in the Long-term Treatment of Patients with Fistulizing Crohn's Disease) including patients with active fistulizing CD (n = 282, during induction and n = 139 patients during maintenance therapy) showed that higher drug concentrations at week 6 and week 14 were associated with composite remission at week 14 defined as complete fistula closure and CRP normalization. Moreover, infliximab concentrations greater than or equal to 15 μg/mL and greater than or equal to 6.1 μg/mL at weeks 6 and 14, respectively, were associated with composite remission at week 14.[35] Yarur and colleagues assessed patients with CD and perianal fistula treated with infliximab for at least 24 weeks. Patients with fistula healing had higher median maintenance infliximab concentrations compared with those with ongoing active fistulas (15.8 vs 4.4 μg/mL, $P < .0001$). Infliximab concentrations greater than or equal to 10.1 μg/mL predicted fistula closure.[41] Similarly, a pediatric multicenter cohort study showed that an infliximab concentration of 12.7 μg/mL at week 24 best predicted fistula healing.[42] A recent cross-sectional retrospective multicenter study including perianal fistulizing CD on maintenance infliximab or adalimumab with drug concentrations within 6 month of perianal MRI showed that patients with radiological remission compared with those with active disease had higher median infliximab (7.4 vs

Table 1
Exposure-outcome relationship data of biologics in specific populations with Crohn's disease

Study Type	Drug (Treatment Time Point)	Cut-Off, µg/mL	Therapeutic Outcome (Time Point)	TDM Assay	Ref.
Perianal Fistulizing CD					
Post hoc analysis of ACCENT II	IFX (week 2)	≥20.2	Complete fistula response & CRP normalization (week 14)	ELISA	Papamichael et al,[35] 2021
	IFX (week 6)	≥15			
	IFX (week 14)	≥7.2			
Retrospective	IFX (week 2)	>9.2	Fistula response (week 14 or 30)	ELISA	Davidov et al,[43] 2017
	IFX (week 6)	>7.2	Fistula response (week 14)		
	IFX (week 6)	>8.6	Fistula response (week 30)		
Retrospective[a]	IFX (week 14)	>12.7	Fistula response (week 24)	ELISA	El-Matary et al,[42] 2019
Retrospective	IFX (maintenance)	>10.1	Fistula healing	HMSA	Yarur et al,[41] 2017
Retrospective	IFX (maintenance)	≥5	Fistula closure	ELISA	Strik et al,[40] 2019
	ADM (maintenance)	≥5.9			
Retrospective	IFX (maintenance)	>6.8	Fistula healing	ELISA	Plevris et al,[39] 2020
	IFX (maintenance)	>9.8	Fistula closure		
	ADM (maintenance)	>7.1	Fistula healing or closure		
Retrospective	IFX (maintenance)	≥4	Radiological healing	ELISA/HMSA	De Gregorio et al,[36] 2021
		≥6.5	Radiological remission		
	ADM (maintenance)	≥7.2	Radiological healing		
		≥9.7	Radiological remission		

(continued on next page)

Table 1
(continued)

Study Type	Drug (Treatment Time Point)	Cut-Off, µg/mL	Therapeutic Outcome (Time Point)	TDM Assay	Ref.
Ileocolonic resection for CD					
Retrospective	IFX (maintenance)	<1.8	Significant endoscopic POR	ELISA	Fay et al,[37] 2017
Small bowel CD					
Retrospective	IFX (maintenance)	>5	Endoscopic remission	ELISA	Takenaka et al,[38] 2021
	ADM (maintenance)	>14			
	UST (maintenance)	>4			

Abbreviations: ADM, adalimumab; CD, Crohn's disease; CRP, C-reactive protein; ELISA, enzyme-linked immunosorbent assay; HMSA, homogeneous mobility shift assay; POR, postoperative recurrence; Ref., reference; IFX, infliximab; TDM, therapeutic drug monitoring; UC, ulcerative colitis.

ACCENT II: A Randomized, Double-blind, Placebo-controlled Trial of Anti-TNFa Chimeric Monoclonal Antibody (Infliximab; REMICADE janssen biotech, Inc, Malvern, PA) in the Long-term Treatment of Patients with Fistulizing Crohn's Disease.

[a] Pediatric.

Table 2
Exposure-outcome relationship data of infliximab or adalimumab in pediatric population with Crohn's disease

Study Type	Drug (Treatment Time Point)	Cut-Off, μg/mL	Therapeutic Outcome (Time Point)	TDM Assay	Ref.
Retrospective	IFX (week 2) IFX (week 6)	>9.2 >2.2	Clinical remission (week 14) Drug retention beyond 1 y of treatment	ELISA	Ungar et al,[46] 2018
Prospective	IFX (week 2) IFX (week 6) IFX (week 6)	≥26.7 ≥15.9 ≥18	Clinical response (week 14) Clinical response (week 14) CRP<.5 mg/dL	ELISA	Clarkston et al,[49] 2019
Retrospective	IFX (week 6)	>8.3	Clinical remission (week 14)	ELISA	Courbette et al,[58] 2020
Retrospective[a]	IFX (week 6) IFX (week 14) IFX (maintenance)	>9.8 >2 >1.6	CRP <.5 mg/dL ESR <18 mm/h ESR <18 mm/h	ELISA	Choi et al,[55] 2019
Prospective	IFX (week 10)	≥9.1	Drug retention (week 52)	HMSA	Stein et al,[56] 2016
Prospective[a]	IFX (week 14)	>5.5	Clinical remission (week 54)	HMSA	Singh et al,[50] 2014
Prospective[a]	IFX (week 14)	>3.1	Sustained clinical remission	ELISA	Naviglio et al,[48] 2019
Prospective	IFX (week 14)	>11.5	FC < 100 μg/g (week 14)	ELISA	Colman et al,[44] 2021
Retrospective[a]	IFX (week 14)	>4.6	Clinical & biochemical remission (week 52)	ELISA	van Hoeve et al,[45] 2019
Retrospective	IFX (maintenance)	≥2.5	Relapse after drug withdrawal for remission	ELISA	Kang et al,[57] 2018
Retrospective	IFX (maintenance)	>4.9 >5	Biochemical remission Mucosal healing	ELISA	Kang et al,[52] 2019
Retrospective[a]	IFX (maintenance)	>5.4	Endoscopic remission	ELISA	van Hoeve et al,[51] 2018
Prospective	ADM (week 4) ADM (week 4)	>22.5 >12.5	Steroid-free clinical & biomarker remission (week 24)	ELISA	Rinawi et al,[47] 2021

(continued on next page)

Table 2
(continued)

Study Type	Drug (Treatment Time Point)	Cut-Off, µg/mL	Therapeutic Outcome (Time Point)	TDM Assay	Ref.
Retrospective[a]	ADM (week 4)	>13.9	Clinical remission (week 52 or 82)	ELISA	Lucafò et al,[54] 2021
	ADM (week 22)	>7.5	Clinical remission (week 52)		
	ADM (week 22)	>10.5	Clinical remission (week 82)		
Prospective	ADM (week 16)	>8.8	Mucosal healing	ELISA	Choi et al,[53] 2020

Abbreviations: ADM, adalimumab; CD, Crohn's disease; CRP, C-reactive protein; ELISA, enzyme-linked immunosorbent assay; FC, fecal calprotectin; HMSA, homogeneous mobility shift assay; IFX, infliximab; Ref, reference; TDM, therapeutic drug monitoring; UC, ulcerative colitis.

[a] Both CD and UC.

3.9 µg/mL, $P < .05$) or adalimumab (9.8 vs 6.2 µg/mL, $P = .07$) concentrations, respectively. It also identified that the optimal infliximab and adalimumab concentrations were 6.5 µg/mL and 9.7 µg/mL for radiological remission, respectively.[36] Besides this study, there are only 2 other rather small retrospective studies that also found that higher drug concentrations were associated with positive fistula response (see Table 1).[39,40]

Ileocolonic Resection for Crohn's Disease

Current guidelines recommend using anti-TNF therapy in patients with CD with surgically induced remission.[59,60] Few studies evaluating TDM following ileocolonic resection suggest higher drug concentrations and lack of ADAs are associated with less disease recurrence. In the PREVENT (Prospective, Multicenter, Randomized, Double-Blind, Placebo-Controlled Trial Comparing REMICADE [infliximab] and Placebo in the Prevention of Recurrence in Crohn's Disease Patients Undergoing Surgical Resection Who Are at an Increased Risk of Recurrence) RCT, patients with CD who underwent ileocolonic resection received infliximab or placebo for 200 weeks. The results showed that a significantly lower number of patients receiving infliximab had endoscopic recurrence compared with placebo ($P < .001$). Of the patients receiving infliximab, the proportion that developed endoscopic recurrence decreased with increasing infliximab concentration, and endoscopic recurrence was seen in a higher proportion of patients who had ATI.[61] Fay and colleagues also found that higher median trough concentrations of infliximab were observed in patients without endoscopic recurrence.[37] Infliximab trough concentrations (median, 2.4 µg/mL vs 1.1 µg/mL, $P = .008$) and the presence of ATI (5.6% vs 71.4%, $P = .0001$) were associated with risk of significant endoscopic relapse.[37] Studies evaluating adalimumab for postoperative prophylaxis show conflicting data. Wright and colleagues demonstrated that there was no significant difference between adalimumab concentrations in patients who achieved endoscopic remission versus disease recurrence; however, drug concentrations were drawn irrespective of the timing of the last dose.[62] Therefore, the data may not represent comparison of trough concentrations between the 2 groups. On the other hand, 2 other studies show that low serum trough concentrations are associated with recurrence. Bodini and colleagues found that lower adalimumab concentrations were lower for patients with clinical or endoscopic recurrence than those in remission (7.5 [4.4–9.8] versus 13.9 [8.9–23.6] µg/mL, respectively, $P < .01$).[63] In another small study, the median serum adalimumab concentration was higher in patients without recurrence compared with those with endoscopic recurrence, defined as Rutgeerts score greater than or equal to i2 (7.95 µg/mL vs 3.25 µg/mL, respectively, $P = .004$). Furthermore, 86% of patients with an adalimumab trough concentration less than 4.2 µg/mL had recurrence compared with 15% of patients with concentrations greater than or equal to 4.2 µg/mL ($P = .025$).[64] These studies suggest that proactive TDM may be helpful in preventing disease recurrence in patients with CD following ileocolonic resection.

Small Bowel Crohn's Disease

To date, only one study specifically assessed the association between biological drug concentrations and endoscopic remission in patients with small bowel CD. In this cross-sectional study at a single tertiary care center, 143 patients with small bowel CD (66 on infliximab, 44 on adalimumab, and 33 on ustekinumab) were evaluated to determine the relationship between drug concentrations and endoscopic remission of small bowel CD using balloon-assisted enteroscopy. The findings show that concentrations of infliximab greater than 5 µg/mL, adalimumab greater than 14 µg/mL, and ustekinumab greater than 4 μg/mL best predicted endoscopic remission of small bowel lesions. Patients who achieved these concentrations compared with those with lower drug concentrations were 5.3, 9.4, and 14 times more likely to achieve endoscopic remission of small bowel CD for infliximab, adalimumab, and ustekinumab, respectively.[38]

Pediatric Crohn's Disease

TDM research in pediatric CD has also demonstrated exposure-response relationships between biological drug trough concentrations and favorable clinical outcomes including clinical response and remission, biochemical remission, mucosal healing, and drug retention (see **Table 2**).[44–58] In pediatric patients, research shows that a lower body weight is associated with increased clearance of infliximab, and younger pediatric patients are less likely to respond to infliximab.[65,66] Jongsma and colleagues assessed infliximab concentrations in 110 patients younger than 10 years and compared with 105 patients aged 10 years and older. The results show that most of the patients younger than 10 years (72%) had low trough concentrations less than 5.4 μg/mL. After 1 year, patients younger than 10 years required a significantly higher dose per 8 weeks compared with patients older than 10 years (9.0 mg/kg vs 5.5 mg/kg, $P < .001$).[67] This study suggests that patients younger than 10 years may need more than 5 mg/kg every 8 weeks of infliximab to achieve adequate concentrations. In a systematic review of the literature, similar data show that young children (<11 years) are more likely to require doses greater than 5 mg/kg or a shortening of interval between infliximab infusions in order to achieve adequate trough concentrations greater than 3 μg/mL.[68] In addition, the study also proposes consideration of intensified infliximab regimens in patients with high disease severity, low albumin, or those receiving infliximab monotherapy. Frequent proactive trough concentration measurements are advised for patients receiving monotherapy and those younger than 11 years.[68] Similar to adult patients, anti-TNF dose optimization has been shown to overcome ADAs in pediatric patients. In a retrospective study evaluating patients with IBD receiving infliximab or adalimumab, 58 patients developed ADAs. Of these patients, 28 underwent dose optimization and more than half (54%) had undetectable ADAs on follow-up.[69] Based on these results, the investigators suggest attempts at rescuing anti-TNF therapy with further dose optimization when ADA levels are less than 10 U/mL. Regarding the role of proactive TDM in the pediatric population, the PAILOT RCT, as discussed previously, suggested a benefit of proactive TDM over reactive TDM to maintain corticosteroid-free clinical remission in pediatric patients treated with adalimumab.[12] In a recent quality improvement project, infliximab order sets included a measurement of infliximab drug concentration at the fourth dose.[70] If a low drug concentration (<5 μg/mL) resulted, then a change in the therapy plan was recommended to achieve concentrations greater than 5 μg/mL. This initiative increased sustained remission rates in patients with an increase from 62% during early data collection in 2016 to 75% by January 2018.[70]

FUTURE DIRECTIONS OF THERAPEUTIC DRUG MONITORING

Future directions striving toward a more personalized application of TDM include the use of pharmacogenomics, point-of-care assays, and pharmacokinetic dashboards.

Pharmacogenomics refer to the study of how a person's genetic makeup influences response to medications. Recently this concept has been applied to treatment with anti-TNF therapy in IBD. A study by Salvador-Martín and colleagues assessed 154 children with IBD treated with infliximab or adalimumab and the associations between DNA polymorphisms and anti-TNF trough concentrations. The results show that variants rs5030728 (TLR4) and rs11465996 (LY96) were associated with subtherapeutic infliximab concentrations, whereas rs3397 (TNFRSF1B) was associated with subtherapeutic adalimumab concentrations. On the other hand, the variant rs1816702 (TLR2) was associated with supratherapeutic concentrations of adalimumab.[71] A genome-wide association study using the PANTS population showed that the HLA-DQA1*05 allele increased the rate of immunogenicity (HR = 1.90; 95% CI: 1.60–2.25; P = 5.88 x 10^{-13}). The association was found for both patients treated with infliximab and adalimumab with and without an IMM.[72] In another retrospective review, 262 patients with CD or UC treated with infliximab were screened for HLA-DQA1*05A>G (rs2097432). In this study, 79% of patients who had ATI carried at least one variant allele. Overall, the risk of ATI formation was higher in HLA-DQA1*05A>G carriers (HR = 7.29; 95% CI: 2.97–17.191, P = 1.46 × 10^{-5}). Carrier status was also associated with and increased likelihood of loss of response (adjusted HR = 2.34, 95% CI: 1.41–3.88, P = .001) and drug discontinuation (HR = 2.27, 95% CI: 1.46–3.43, P = 2.53 × 10^{-4}).[73] These data suggest that genotyping DNA variants before treatment with anti-TNF therapy may be valuable in tailoring treatment and personalized TDM to identify patients who would benefit more from proactive TDM and combination therapy.

Point-of-care assays are devices that provide clinical information without the need for a laboratory and can be performed on-site and provide rapid results. Over the last few years, several assays for POCT have been developed to detect both drug concentrations and/or the presence of ADAs.[74–79] Additional research validating their use and prospective studies assessing their utility in clinical practice are needed.

Pharmacokinetic models for individualized infliximab dosing are now being established to personalize treatment of patients with IBD. These dashboard models incorporate patient factors that affect clearance of infliximab and individual target trough concentrations. Doses can then be adjusted according to previously measured concentrations to maintain adequate drug concentrations. Several studies have assessed pharmacokinetic models specifically in IBD.[15,80–82] In the PRECISION RCT, the dashboard approach led to improved rates of clinical remission compared with standard-of-care dosing.[15] In pediatric CD, one study assessed the use of a pharmacokinetic dashboard and found that the standard-of-care dosing of infliximab was recommended in only 22% of patients and most of the patients required more aggressive infliximab dosing, suggesting these algorithms may be helpful in contributing to drug durability.[80]

SUMMARY

TDM of biologics can be a valuable tool when treating patients with IBD, including specific populations and phenotypes of CD such as the children and patients with perianal fistulizing and small bowel CD and those with an ileocolonic resection. In addition to reactive TDM, TDM may also have value in specific clinical scenarios including proactive TDM, dose deescalation, resuming drug after a prolonged holiday, and optimizing monotherapy as an alternative of combination treatment with an IMM. However, more data from well-designed prospective studies and RCTs are needed to evaluate the role of TDM in these situations. The future of TDM is exciting, as innovative research and new technologies including pharmacokinetic dashboards, pharmacogenomics, and POCT will allow for a more personalized approach to IBD care.

DISCLOSURE

A.S. Cheifetz reports consultancy fees from Janssen, Abbvie, Artugen, Procise, Prometheus, Arena, Grifols, Bacainn, and Bristol Myers Squibb. K. Papamichael reports lecture fees from Mitsubishi Tanabe Pharma and Physicians Education Resource LLC; consultancy fees from Prometheus Laboratories Inc; and scientific advisory board fees from ProciseDx Inc and Scipher Medicine Corporation. L.B. Grossberg has no disclosures to report.

REFERENCES

1. Roda G, Chien Ng S, Kotze PG, et al. Crohn's disease. Nat Rev Dis Primer 2020; 6(1):22.
2. Katsanos KH, Papamichael K, Feuerstein JD, et al. Biological therapies in inflammatory bowel disease: Beyond anti-TNF therapies. Clin Immunol 2019;206:9–14.
3. Bruns T, Stallmach A. Drug monitoring in inflammatory bowel disease: helpful or dispensable? Dig Dis 2009;27(3):394–403.
4. Papamichael K, Cheifetz AS, Melmed GY, et al. Appropriate therapeutic drug monitoring of biologic agents for patients with inflammatory bowel diseases. Clin Gastroenterol Hepatol 2019;17(9):1655–68.e3.
5. Cheifetz AS, Abreu MT, Afif W, et al. A comprehensive literature review and expert consensus statement on therapeutic drug monitoring of biologics in inflammatory bowel disease. Am J Gastroenterol 2021;116(10):2014–25.
6. Feuerstein JD, Nguyen GC, Kupfer SS, et al. American Gastroenterological Association Institute Guideline on Therapeutic Drug Monitoring in Inflammatory Bowel Disease. Gastroenterology 2017;153(3):827–34.
7. Steenholdt C, Brynskov J, Thomsen OØ, et al. Individualised therapy is more cost-effective than dose intensification in patients with Crohn's disease who lose response to anti-TNF treatment: a randomised, controlled trial. Gut 2014; 63(6):919–27.
8. Papamichael K, Juncadella A, Wong D, et al. Proactive Therapeutic drug monitoring of adalimumab is associated with better long-term outcomes compared with standard of care in patients with inflammatory bowel disease. J Crohns Colitis 2019;13(8):976–81.
9. Vaughn BP, Martinez-Vazquez M, Patwardhan VR, et al. Proactive therapeutic concentration monitoring of infliximab may improve outcomes for patients with inflammatory bowel disease: results from a Pilot Observational Study. Inflamm Bowel Dis 2014;20(11):1996–2003.
10. Papamichael K, Vajravelu RK, Vaughn BP, et al. Proactive infliximab monitoring following reactive testing is associated with better clinical outcomes than reactive testing alone in patients with inflammatory bowel disease. J Crohns Colitis 2018; 12(7):804–10.
11. Papamichael K, Chachu KA, Vajravelu RK, et al. Improved Long-term Outcomes of patients with inflammatory bowel disease receiving proactive compared with reactive monitoring of serum concentrations of infliximab. Clin Gastroenterol Hepatol 2017;15(10):1580–8.e3.
12. Assa A, Matar M, Turner D, et al. Proactive Monitoring of adalimumab trough concentration associated with increased clinical remission in children with Crohn's Disease Compared With Reactive Monitoring. Gastroenterology 2019;157(4): 985–96.e2.
13. Vande Casteele N, Ferrante M, Van Assche G, et al. Trough concentrations of infliximab guide dosing for patients with inflammatory bowel disease. Gastroenterology 2015;148(7):1320–9.e3.
14. D'Haens G, Vermeire S, Lambrecht G, et al. Increasing infliximab dose based on symptoms, biomarkers, and serum drug concentrations does not increase

clinical, endoscopic, and corticosteroid-free remission in patients with active luminal Crohn's Disease. Gastroenterology 2018;154(5):1343–51.e1.

15. Strik AS, Löwenberg M, Mould DR, et al. Efficacy of dashboard driven dosing of infliximab in inflammatory bowel disease patients; a randomized controlled trial. Scand J Gastroenterol 2021;56(2):145–54.

16. Syversen SW, Goll GL, Jørgensen KK, et al. Effect of Therapeutic Drug Monitoring vs Standard Therapy During Infliximab Induction on Disease Remission in Patients With Chronic Immune-Mediated Inflammatory Diseases: A Randomized Clinical Trial. JAMA 2021;325(17):1744–54.

17. Bossuyt P, Pouillon L, Claeys S, et al. Ultra-proactive therapeutic drug monitoring of infliximab based on point-of-care-testing in inflammatory bowel disease: results of a pragmatic trial. J Crohns Colitis 2021. https://doi.org/10.1093/ecco-jcc/jjab127. jjab127.

18. Kennedy NA, Heap GA, Green HD, et al. Predictors of anti-TNF treatment failure in anti-TNF-naive patients with active luminal Crohn's disease: a prospective, multicentre, cohort study. Lancet Gastroenterol Hepatol 2019;4(5):341–53.

19. Löwenberg M, Vermeire S, Mostafavi N, et al. Vedolizumab Induces Endoscopic and Histologic Remission in Patients With Crohn's Disease. Gastroenterology 2019;157(4):997–1006.e6.

20. Walshe M, Borowski K, Boland K, et al. Ustekinumab induction concentrations are associated with clinical and biochemical outcomes at week 12 of treatment in Crohn's disease. Eur J Gastroenterol Hepatol 2021. https://doi.org/10.1097/MEG.0000000000002116.

21. Allegretti JR, Canakis A, McClure E, et al. Infliximab De-escalation in patients with Crohn's Disease in clinical remission is safe and well-tolerated. Inflamm Bowel Dis 2021. https://doi.org/10.1093/ibd/izab131. izab131.

22. Petitcollin A, Brochard C, Siproudhis L, et al. Pharmacokinetic Parameters of Infliximab Influence the Rate of Relapse After De-Escalation in Adults With Inflammatory Bowel Diseases. Clin Pharmacol Ther 2019;106(3):605–15.

23. Lucidarme C, Petitcollin A, Brochard C, et al. Predictors of relapse following infliximab de-escalation in patients with inflammatory bowel disease: the value of a strategy based on therapeutic drug monitoring. Aliment Pharmacol Ther 2019;49(2):147–54.

24. Amiot A, Hulin A, Belhassan M, et al. Therapeutic drug monitoring is predictive of loss of response after de-escalation of infliximab therapy in patients with inflammatory bowel disease in clinical remission. Clin Res Hepatol Gastroenterol 2016;40(1):90–8.

25. Aguas Peris M, Bosó V, Navarro B, et al. Serum Adalimumab levels predict successful remission and safe deintensification in inflammatory bowel disease patients in clinical practice. Inflamm Bowel Dis 2017;23(8):1454–60.

26. Hanauer SB. Risks and benefits of combining immunosuppressives and biological agents in inflammatory bowel disease: is the synergy worth the risk? Gut 2007;56(9):1181–3.

27. Colombel JF, Mantzaris GJ, Rachmilewitz D, et al. Infliximab, Azathioprine, or Combination Therapy for Crohn's Disease. N Engl J Med 2010;362(15):1383–95.

28. Brandse JF, Mould D, Smeekes O, et al. A Real-life Population Pharmacokinetic Study Reveals Factors Associated with Clearance and Immunogenicity of Infliximab in Inflammatory Bowel Disease. Inflamm Bowel Dis 2017;23(4):650–60.

29. Vermeire S, Noman M, Van Assche G, et al. Effectiveness of concomitant immunosuppressive therapy in suppressing the formation of antibodies to infliximab in Crohn's disease. Gut 2007;56(9):1226–31.

30. Colombel J-F, Adedokun OJ, Gasink C, et al. Combination therapy with infliximab and azathioprine improves infliximab pharmacokinetic features and efficacy: a post hoc analysis. Clin Gastroenterol Hepatol Off Clin Pract J Am Gastroenterol Assoc 2019;17(8):1525–32.e1.

31. Drobne D, Kurent T, Golob S, et al. Optimised infliximab monotherapy is as effective as optimised combination therapy, but is associated with higher drug consumption in inflammatory bowel disease. Aliment Pharmacol Ther 2019;49(7): 880–9.

32. Lega S, Phan BL, Rosenthal CJ, et al. Proactively Optimized Infliximab Monotherapy Is as Effective as Combination Therapy in IBD. Inflamm Bowel Dis 2019; 25(1):134–41.

33. Baert F, Drobne D, Gils A, et al. Early trough levels and antibodies to infliximab predict safety and success of reinitiation of infliximab therapy. Clin Gastroenterol Hepatol Off Clin Pract J Am Gastroenterol Assoc 2014;12(9):1474–81.e2 [quiz: e91].

34. Normatov I, Fluxa D, Wang JD, et al. Real world experience with proactive therapeutic drug monitoring during infliximab reintroduction. Crohns Colitis 2021; 360. https://doi.org/10.1093/crocol/otab048. otab048.

35. Papamichael K, Vande Casteele N, Jeyarajah J, et al. Higher postinduction infliximab concentrations are associated with improved clinical outcomes in fistulizing Crohn's Disease: an ACCENT-II Post Hoc Analysis. Am Coll Gastroenterol 2021; 116(5):1007–14.

36. De Gregorio M, Lee T, Krishnaprasad K, et al. Higher anti-tumour necrosis factor-α levels correlate with improved radiological outcomes in Crohn's perianal fistulas. Clin Gastroenterol Hepatol 2021. https://doi.org/10.1016/j.cgh.2021.07. 053. S154235652100865X.

37. Fay S, Ungar B, Paul S, et al. The association between drug levels and endoscopic recurrence in postoperative patients with Crohn's Disease treated with tumor necrosis factor inhibitors. Inflamm Bowel Dis 2017;23(11):1924–9.

38. Takenaka K, Kawamoto A, Hibiya S, et al. Higher concentrations of cytokine blockers are needed to obtain small bowel mucosal healing during maintenance therapy in Crohn's disease. Aliment Pharmacol Ther 2021. https://doi.org/10. 1111/apt.16551.

39. Plevris N, Jenkinson PW, Arnott ID, et al. Higher anti-tumor necrosis factor levels are associated with perianal fistula healing and fistula closure in Crohn's disease. Eur J Gastroenterol Hepatol 2020;32(1):32–7.

40. Strik AS, Löwenberg M, Buskens CJ, et al. Higher anti-TNF serum levels are associated with perianal fistula closure in Crohn's disease patients. Scand J Gastroenterol 2019;54(4):453–8.

41. Yarur AJ, Kanagala V, Stein DJ, et al. Higher infliximab trough levels are associated with perianal fistula healing in patients with Crohn's disease. Aliment Pharmacol Ther 2017;45(7):933–40.

42. El-Matary W, Walters TD, Huynh HQ, et al. Higher postinduction infliximab serum trough levels are associated with healing of fistulizing perianal Crohn's Disease in children. Inflamm Bowel Dis 2019;25(1):150–5.

43. Davidov Y, Ungar B, Bar-Yoseph H, et al. Association of induction infliximab levels with clinical response in perianal Crohn's Disease. J Crohns Colitis 2017;11(5): 549–55.

44. Colman RJ, Tsai Y-T, Jackson K, et al. Achieving target infliximab drug concentrations improves blood and fecal neutrophil biomarkers in Crohn's Disease. Inflamm Bowel Dis 2021;27(7):1045–51.

45. van Hoeve K, Dreesen E, Hoffman I, et al. Adequate infliximab exposure during induction predicts remission in paediatric patients with inflammatory bowel disease. J Pediatr Gastroenterol Nutr 2019;68(6):847–53.
46. Ungar B, Glidai Y, Yavzori M, et al. Association between infliximab drug and antibody levels and therapy outcome in pediatric inflammatory bowel diseases. J Pediatr Gastroenterol Nutr 2018;67(4):507–12.
47. Rinawi F, Ricciuto A, Church PC, et al. Association of early postinduction adalimumab exposure with subsequent clinical and biomarker remission in children with Crohn's Disease. Inflamm Bowel Dis 2021;27(7):1079–87.
48. Naviglio S, Lacorte D, Lucafò M, et al. Causes of treatment failure in children with inflammatory bowel disease treated with infliximab: a Pharmacokinetic Study. J Pediatr Gastroenterol Nutr 2019;68(1):37–44.
49. Clarkston K, Tsai Y-T, jackson k, et al. development of infliximab target concentrations during induction in pediatric Crohn's Disease Patients. J Pediatr Gastroenterol Nutr 2019;69(1):68–74.
50. Singh N, Rosenthal CJ, Melmed GY, et al. Early infliximab trough levels are associated with persistent remission in pediatric patients with inflammatory bowel disease. Inflamm Bowel Dis 2014;20(10):1708–13.
51. van Hoeve K, Dreesen E, Hoffman I, et al. Higher Infliximab trough levels are associated with better outcome in paediatric patients with inflammatory bowel disease. J Crohns Colitis 2018;12(11):1316–25.
52. Kang B, Choi SY, Choi YO, et al. Infliximab trough levels are associated with mucosal healing during maintenance treatment with infliximab in paediatric Crohn's Disease. J Crohns Colitis 2019;13(2):189–97.
53. Choi SY, Choi YO, Choe YH, et al. Potential utility of therapeutic drug monitoring of adalimumab in predicting short-term mucosal healing and histologic remission in pediatric Crohn's Disease Patients. J Korean Med Sci 2020;35(16):e114.
54. Lucafò M, Curci D, Bramuzzo M, et al. Serum Adalimumab levels after induction are associated with long-term remission in children with inflammatory bowel disease. Front Pediatr 2021;9:646671.
55. Choi SY, Kang B, Choe YH. Serum Infliximab Cutoff trough Level Values for Maintaining Hematological Remission in Pediatric Inflammatory Bowel Disease. Gut Liver 2019;13(5):541–8.
56. Stein R, Lee D, Leonard MB, et al. Serum Infliximab, Antidrug Antibodies, and Tumor Necrosis Factor Predict Sustained Response in Pediatric Crohn's Disease. Inflamm Bowel Dis 2016;22(6):1370–7.
57. Kang B, Choi SY, Choi YO, et al. Subtherapeutic Infliximab Trough Levels and Complete Mucosal Healing Are Associated With Sustained Clinical Remission After Infliximab Cessation in Paediatric-onset Crohn's Disease Patients Treated With Combined Immunosuppressive Therapy. J Crohns Colitis 2018;12(6):644–52.
58. Courbette O, Aupiais C, Viala J, et al. Trough Levels of Infliximab at Week 6 Are Predictive of Remission at Week 14 in Pediatric Crohn's Disease. J Pediatr Gastroenterol Nutr 2020;70(3):310–7.
59. Amil-Dias J, Kolacek S, Turner D, et al. Surgical Management of Crohn Disease in Children: Guidelines From the Paediatric IBD Porto Group of ESPGHAN. J Pediatr Gastroenterol Nutr 2017;64(5):818–35.
60. Nguyen GC, Loftus EV, Hirano I, et al. American Gastroenterological Association Institute Guideline on the Management of Crohn's Disease After Surgical Resection. Gastroenterology 2017;152(1):271–5.

61. Regueiro M, Feagan BG, Zou B, et al. Infliximab reduces endoscopic, but not clinical, recurrence of Crohn's Disease after ileocolonic resection. Gastroenterology 2016;150(7):1568–78.

62. Wright EK, Kamm MA, De Cruz P, et al. Anti-TNF therapeutic drug monitoring in postoperative Crohn's Disease. J Crohns Colitis 2018;12(6):653–61.

63. Bodini G, Savarino V, Peyrin-Biroulet L, et al. Low serum trough levels are associated with post-surgical recurrence in Crohn's disease patients undergoing prophylaxis with adalimumab. Dig Liver Dis 2014;46(11):1043–6.

64. Boivineau L, Guillon F, Altwegg R. Serum adalimumab concentration after surgery is correlated with postoperative endoscopic recurrence in Crohn's Disease Patients: one step before proactive therapeutic drug monitoring. J Crohns Colitis 2020;14(10):1500–1.

65. Kelsen JR, Grossman AB, Pauly-Hubbard H, et al. Infliximab therapy in pediatric patients 7 years of age and younger. J Pediatr Gastroenterol Nutr 2014;59(6):758–62.

66. Dotan I, Ron Y, Yanai H, et al. Patient factors that increase infliximab clearance and shorten half-life in inflammatory bowel disease: a population pharmacokinetic study. Inflamm Bowel Dis 2014;20(12):2247–59.

67. Jongsma MME, Winter DA, Huynh HQ, et al. Infliximab in young paediatric IBD patients: it is all about the dosing. Eur J Pediatr 2020;179(12):1935–44.

68. Winter DA, Joosse ME, de Wildt SN, et al. Pharmacokinetics, pharmacodynamics, and immunogenicity of infliximab in pediatric inflammatory bowel disease: a systematic review and revised dosing considerations. J Pediatr Gastroenterol Nutr 2020;70(6):763–76.

69. Cohen RZ, Schoen BT, Kugathasan S, et al. Management of anti-drug antibodies to biologic medications in children with inflammatory bowel disease. J Pediatr Gastroenterol Nutr 2019;69(5):551–6.

70. Hellmann J, Etter RK, Denson LA, et al. Quality improvement methodology optimizes infliximab levels in pediatric patients with inflammatory bowel disease. Pediatr Qual Saf 2021;6(3):e400.

71. Salvador-Martín S, Pujol-Muncunill G, Bossacoma F, et al. Pharmacogenetics of trough serum anti-TNF levels in paediatric inflammatory bowel disease. Br J Clin Pharmacol 2021;87(2):447–57.

72. Sazonovs A, Kennedy NA, Moutsianas L, et al. HLA-DQA1*05 carriage associated with development of anti-drug antibodies to infliximab and adalimumab in patients with Crohn's Disease. Gastroenterology 2020;158(1):189–99.

73. Wilson A, Peel C, Wang Q, et al. HLADQA1*05 genotype predicts anti-drug antibody formation and loss of response during infliximab therapy for inflammatory bowel disease. Aliment Pharmacol Ther 2020;51(3):356–63.

74. Rocha C, Lago P, Fernandes S, et al. Rapid test detection of anti-infliximab antibodies: performance comparison with three different immunoassays. Ther Adv Gastroenterol 2020;13. https://doi.org/10.1177/1756284820965790. 1756284820965790.

75. Facchin S, Buda A, Cardin R, et al. Rapid point-of-care anti-infliximab antibodies detection in clinical practice: comparison with ELISA and potential for improving therapeutic drug monitoring in IBD patients. Ther Adv Gastroenterol 2021;14. https://doi.org/10.1177/1756284821999902. 1756284821999902.

76. Dutzer D, Nasser Y, Berger AE, et al. Letter: new thresholds need to be defined when using point of care assays to monitor infliximab trough levels in IBD patients. Aliment Pharmacol Ther 2018;47(11):1571–3.

77. Berends SE, D'Haens GRAM, Schaap T, et al. Dried blood samples can support monitoring of infliximab concentrations in patients with inflammatory bowel disease: a clinical validation. Br J Clin Pharmacol 2019;85(7):1544–51.
78. Nasser Y, Labetoulle R, Harzallah I, et al. Comparison of Point-of-Care and Classical Immunoassays for the Monitoring Infliximab and Antibodies Against Infliximab in IBD. Dig Dis Sci 2018;63(10):2714–21.
79. Laserna-Mendieta EJ, Salvador-Martín S, Marín-Jiménez I, et al. Comparison of a new rapid method for determination of serum anti-adalimumab and anti-infliximab antibodies with two established ELISA kits. J Pharm Biomed Anal 2021;198: 114003.
80. Dubinsky MC, Phan BL, Singh N, et al. Pharmacokinetic dashboard-recommended dosing is different than standard of care dosing in infliximab-treated pediatric IBD Patients. AAPS J 2017;19(1):215–22.
81. Papamichael K, Cheifetz AS. Optimizing therapeutic drug monitoring in inflammatory bowel disease: a focus on therapeutic monoclonal antibodies. Expert Opin Drug Metab Toxicol 2022. https://doi.org/10.1080/17425255.2021. 2027367. In press.
82. Dubinsky MC, Mendiolaza ML, Phan BL, et al. Dashboard-Driven Accelerated Infliximab Induction Dosing Increases Infliximab Durability and Reduces Immunogenicity.. Inflamm Bowel Dis 2022. https://doi.org/10.1093/ibd/izab285. In press.

Diet in the Pathogenesis and Management of Crohn's Disease

Phillip Gu, MD[a], Linda A. Feagins, MD[b],*

KEYWORDS

- Diet • Inflammatory bowel disease • Crohn's disease • Ulcerative colitis

KEY POINTS

- Advice on the role of diet in Crohn's disease should be discussed with patients rountinely.
- The literature does not clearly identify any specific foods that cause or exacerbate Crohn's disease. However, various diet components may weaken or strengthen the gut barrier.
- A variety of diets have been studied for treating Crohn's disease, with exclusive enteral nutrition having the most supportive data to date.
- Additional research trials studiying diet are needed to help us better incorporate diet into the treatment regimen for Crohn's patients.

INTRODUCTION

With the increasing prevalence of Crohn's disease (CD), especially in newly industrialized countries such as Asia and South America, environmental exposures are amassing attention.[1–5] Diet, in particular, has gained significant interest with a high demand for more educational resources, especially among patients.[6,7] While 86% of patients say dietary knowledge is very important in their inflammatory bowel disease (IBD) care, 69% report receiving little to no information about diet from their provider.[6] Unfortunately, this may be a result of a limited amount of resources on diet in IBD for providers. One study found only 46% of gastrointestinal (GI) providers (n = 91) reported adequate access to nutritional resources to initiate and guide discussions with patients.[8] Unsurprisingly, this discrepancy in supply and demand leads patients to seek dietary advice from alternate sources such as the Internet. This can be risky, as Hou and colleagues illustrated in their review of online patient-targeted dietary

Funding: none.
[a] Division of Digestive and Liver Diseases, UT Southwestern Medical Center, 5323 Harry Hines Blvd, Dallas, TX 75390, USA; [b] Department of Medicine, Center for Inflammatory Bowel Diseases, University of Texas at Austin, Dell Medical School, Health Discovery Building, Z0900 1601 Trinity Street, Building B, Austin, TX 78712, USA
* Corresponding author.
E-mail address: Linda.Feagins@austin.utexas.edu

Gastroenterol Clin N Am 51 (2022) 319–335
https://doi.org/10.1016/j.gtc.2021.12.008
0889-8553/22/© 2021 Elsevier Inc. All rights reserved.

recommendations. They found online recommendations were highly restrictive and often conflicting.[9] The imbalance between supply and demand of information and unreliable recommendations found on other media outlets highlights the need for more research to better understand the role of diet in CD and underlines the need for more educational resources. This article discusses the role of diet in the pathogenesis, exacerbation, and treatment in CD.

Role of Diet in Pathogenesis of Crohn's Disease

As more countries industrialize and adopt a more Westernized diet, modern dietary patterns favor consuming more fats, sugars, and processed foods with additives and less fiber. Because these dietary trends coincide with the increasing incidence of CD worldwide, many suspect components of the Western diet contribute to the risk of developing CD. This section reviews major components of the Western diet that could contribute to CD pathogenesis: high meat, high fat, low fiber, and food additives.

High meat intake has been frequently proposed as a dietary risk factor for CD. Because meat contains sulfur amino acid, it yields hydrogen sulfide (H_2S) after gut bacterial fermentation. Subsequently, the hydrogen sulfide potentially promotes intestinal inflammation by inhibiting butyrate oxidation in colonocytes and/or impairing the intestinal barrier function by reducing the disulfide bonds of the mucus layer, which increases intestinal permeability to enteric pathogens.[10,11] Most studies characterizing meat's proinflammatory impact on the GI tract primarily describe its effect on the colon and in those with ulcerative colitis (UC).[12–14] The role of meat in the pathogenesis of CD is unclear, as its proinflammatory influence on the small intestine is less well described. In a systematic review, Hou, and colleagues noted only 1 out of 5 studies evaluating the association between meat and CD was significant (odds ratio [OR] 2.48 95% confidence interval [CI] [1.4–4.4]), specifically with consuming pork.[12] More studies are required to clarify the role of meat in CD pathogenesis and if it plays a larger role in UC.

Dietary fats have also been suggested as a risk factor in the development of CD, particularly polyunsaturated fatty acids (PUFAs). A Western diet typically contains a high n-6 PUFA to n-3 PUFA ratio. n-6 PUFAs, which include linoleic acid and arachidonic acid, are suggested to be proinflammatory, while n-3 PUFAs, especially eicosapentaenoic acid and docosahexaenoic acid (which are major component of omega 3 fish oil), are suggested to be anti-inflammatory. Although the proinflammatory effects of dietary fats on the intestine are not completely understood, 1 study observed mice that were fed a high fat and high sugar diet had a decrease in mucus layer thickness and increase barrier permeability.[15] This was associated with increased TNFα secretion and later allowed for invasive *Escherichia coli* to more readily colonize the gut mucosa and induce inflammation.

Currently, there have been few studies that have evaluated the role of dietary fats in the pathogenesis of CD, and the results are conflicting. In a large, prospective study of 170,000 women enrolled in the Nurses' Health Study (NHS), cumulative intake of total fat, saturated fats, n-6, and n-3 PUFAs were not associated with risk of developing CD or UC. Investigators found greater consumption of long-chain n-3 PUFA was only associated with lower risk of UC (hazard ratio (HR) 0.72, 95%CI 0.51–1.01).[16] Conversely, a nested case-control study found higher intake of docosahexaenoic acid was associated with lower risk of CD (OR 0.07, [95% CI 0.02–0.81] for highest vs lowest quintile; $P_{trend} =.04$).[17] Similar to meat, more studies are required to better understand the role of dietary fats in CD development and its proinflammatory effects on the intestines.

Contrary to meat and fat, fiber is suggested to be protective against developing CD. In a large prospective study of 170,000 women enrolled in the NHS, higher intake of fiber was associated with a 40% reduction in the risk of CD. Interestingly, the protective benefits of fiber appeared to be greatest in fiber derived from fruits.[18] Fiber from cereal, whole grain, or legumes did not modify risk. Fiber's anti-inflammatory properties are thought stem from its production of short chain fatty acids via metabolization by gut bacteria and aid in maintaining the intestinal barrier function. Fiber protects the intestinal barrier function by preserving the inner mucus layer, which contains antimicrobial peptides and immunoglobulins, and is essentially the first line of defense against intestinal bacteria.[19] Because fiber is a source of nutrition of gut bacteria, fiber depravation causes an imbalance of the gut microbiome to favor mucin-degrading bacteria and less fiber-degrading species. This microbiome shift results in thinning of the inner mucus layer.[17,18] In fact, the mucus layer in fiber-deprived mice is 5 to 6 times thinner than mice fed a fiber-rich diet.[20] The compromised mucus layer then allows for increased bacterial proximity to the intestinal epithelium, and, subsequently, higher risk for bacterial translocation and inflammation.

While the available data are limited, it is worth discussing the growing body of literature implicating food additives in the pathogenesis of CD including emulsifiers, inorganic microparticles, and food coloring agents. Emulsifiers, especially carrageenan, carboxymethylcellulose (CMC), and polysorbate-80 (P80), have been strongly implicated in promoting intestinal inflammation. Emulsifiers are food additives commonly used to give food products a smooth texture, prevent separation, and prolong shelf life. Common foods that contain emulsifiers include ice cream, nondairy milk alternatives, salad dressing, and pasta to name a few. Currently, majority of the research on emulsifiers and intestinal inflammation has been conducted on animal models. These studies have found emulsifiers most likely promote inflammation by altering the gut microbiome through decreasing diversity and promoting proinflammatory enteric bacteria.[21-23] Furthermore, animal studies have noted changes in emulsifier-exposed intestines that are associated with IBD pathogenesis such as decreased colonic butyrate levels,[24] thinner inner mucus layer,[21] increased intestinal permeability,[21,24,25] and increased gut bacterial translocation.[21,26] More relevant to CD, several studies have also noted colonic ulcerations and intestinal histopathologic changes such as villous architectural distortion and lymphoid hyperplasia with microgranulomas in animals exposed to emulsifiers.[27,28] One study found mice fed chow containing carrageenan developed small bowel lesions during the first 2 to 6 weeks followed by colonic lesions after 8 weeks.[29] These findings have important implications for the subphenotype of CD patients with disease extension during the course of their disease.

Similarly, inorganic microparticles, which are additives found in processed foods to prevent caking or preserve color, have been proposed as dietary risk factors in the pathogenesis of IBD.[30] Microparticles are bacteria-sized, non-biologic particles that are resistant to degradation, especially particulate oxides of titanium, aluminum, and silicon. However, the current data on the role of microparticles in IBD are controversial. Mice models have found microparticles promote colitis and visceral hypersensitivity.[31,32] However, a randomized-controlled trial (RCT) of 83 patients with active CD found a low microparticle diet did not improve clinical outcomes.[33] Finally, the most common food colorants Red 40 and Yellow 6 have been found to promote colitis in mice via increased interleukin-23 (IL-23) signaling.[34]

Overall, the literature does not identify any specific foods that cause CD. Instead, the role of diet in the pathogenesis of IBD is most likely an interplay of proinflammatory and anti-inflammatory dietary exposures interacting with the microbiome to strengthen or weaken our intestinal barrier function and resulting in varying degrees

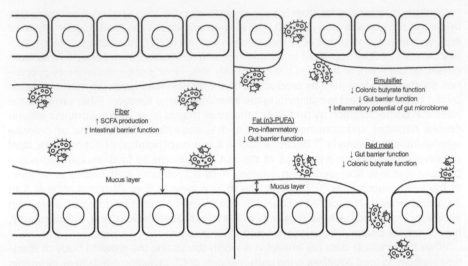

Fig. 1. Proposed mechanism behind diet and the pathogenesis of IBD: different dietary components interact with the gut microbiome to strengthen or weaken the gut barrier function that allows for varying degrees of enteric bacterial translocation, which may increase risk of developing IBD. (*From* Gu P, Feagins LA. Dining with inflammatory bowel disease: a review of the literature on diet in the pathogenesis and management of IBD. Inflamm Bowel Dis. 2020;26(2):181-191. https://doi.org/10.1093/ibd/izz268; with permission).

of bacterial translocation (**Fig. 1**). This hypothesis is supported by a recent study using the empirical dietary inflammatory pattern (EDIP) score to quantify an individual's dietary inflammatory potential and evaluate risk of developing IBD. From analyzing prospectively collected data from 208,834 subjects enrolled in NHS, NHS II, and Health Professionals Follow-up Study, the investigators found participants in the highest quartile score had a 51% higher risk of CD. Additionally, participants who shifted from a low to high inflammatory diet also had a greater risk of CD than those who maintained a low inflammatory diet (HR 2.05; 95% CI 1.10–3.79).[35]

Role of Diet in Exacerbation of Inflammation

IBD patients frequently make dietary modifications for various reasons, particularly for relapse prevention. Studies have reported 57% to 58% (total n = 407) of patients believe diet has a role in triggering symptoms, and 68% (n = 273) of patients self-impose dietary restrictions to prevent relapse.[7,36] These restrictive modifications often diminish quality of life, with 20% (n = 81) of patients refusing to dine out and 66% (n = 265) of patients depriving themselves of favorite foods to prevent relapse.[7]

Studies have not identified any specific dietary exposures that can increase inflammation and cause flares. To further complicate the picture, IBD patients with quiescent disease frequently have persistent GI symptoms, so it can be difficult to discriminate if dietary exacerbation of symptoms is related to inflammation or dietary intolerance. This predicament is highlighted by conflicting data on meat and relapse of IBD in 2 prospective studies.[13,37]

Regardless if there are data supporting whether certain foods exacerbate inflammation, IBD patients frequently impose dietary restrictions based on anecdotal evidence. Interestingly, there are common themes observed across several survey studies on dietary practices of IBD patients. Spicy foods, dairy products, fatty foods, and fibrous foods, particularly vegetables, are the most commonly identified trigger

Table 1
Quality of data on various dietary therapies for Crohn's disease

Diet	Case Series	Retrospective	Prospective	RCT
Exclusive enteral nutrition	X	X	X	X
Specific carbohydrate diet	X	X	X	
Low FODMAP		X	X	X
Mediterranean		X	X	
Paleo			X	
CD Anti-inflammatory diet	X			
Semivegetarian			X	X

foods.[7,36,38–40] Alcohol was also reported to exacerbate symptoms but was not consistently surveyed among studies.[7,38] Additionally, in a survey of 2300 IBD patients, Cohen and colleagues found that those with active disease were significantly more likely to avoid fruit, leafy and nonleafy vegetables, tomatoes, beans, and ice cream compared with those in remission.[38] Interestingly, IBD patients with active disease were more likely to consume soda than those without active disease. Finally, yogurt and rice were frequently reported to improve symptoms.

Although dietary exposures may not exactly exacerbate inflammation in IBD, dietary avoidance can help manage symptoms and should be tailored on an individual basis. Future studies are required to confirm the absence of inflammation in the setting of symptom exacerbation secondary to dietary exposures.

Dietary Therapeutics in Crohn's Disease

Multiple dietary therapies have been proposed for CD (**Table 1**) with variable quality of data to support their use. **Table 2** summarizes the rationale and recommendations for

Table 2
Dietary therapies that have been proposed to help treat Crohn's disease

Diet	Proposed Mechanism of Action	Typical Diet
EEN	• Possibly downregulates proinflammatory cytokines and alters the microbiome to decrease intestinal inflammation.	• Exclusive diet of formula (oral or via nasogastric tube) for 4–12 weeks • The CD-TREAT diet aims to mimic EEN with real foods[57] • The CD exclusion diet is a whole-food diet combined with partial enteral nutrition[58]
SCD	• Avoids foods that are thought to lead to intestinal injury caused by an overgrowth and imbalance toward proinflammatory gut microbes (ie, poorly absorbed carbohydrates, specifically di- and polysaccharide carbohydrates)	• Foods allowed include most fresh fruits and vegetables, meat, yogurt, nuts, seeds, hard cheeses, and certain legumes. • Avoid most grains such as wheat, barley, corn, rice, processed/canned foods, and milk.

(continued on next page)

Table 2
(continued)

Diet	Proposed Mechanism of Action	Typical Diet
Low FODMAP	• Avoids carbohydrates that are poorly absorbed, fermented by intestinal bacteria, and result in increased gas production and fluid load, thus causing GI distress. • Likely improves functional symptoms more than inflammatory symptoms	• 3-phase diet: 1. Elimination: avoid all high FODMAP food for 6 to 8 weeks 2. Reintroduction: Gradually reintroduce back high FODMAP foods to tolerance to identify trigger foods 3. Maintenance: follow an individualized diet that avoids problematic high FODMAP foods
Semivegetarian	• Avoids meat and high-fat foods that may impair intestinal barrier function and promote inflammation	• Low intake of animal proteins (fish once a week and meat once every 2 weeks)
Mediterranean	• Promotes diet high in omega-3s and low in omega-6s, which may reduce inflammation	• High in vegetables, fruits, whole grains, and healthy fat • Moderate in fish poultry, beans, and eggs • Limited red meat intake
Paleo	• Avoids foods and additives that may trigger intestinal inflammation, dysbiosis, and/or symptomatic food intolerance	• Encourages fruits, vegetables, nuts/seeds, lean meats, fish, and oils from nuts • Avoids grains, legumes, dairy, sugar, salt, potatoes, and highly processed foods • Autoimmune protocol diet is an extension of this diet and includes gluten avoidance[76]
CD Anti-inflammatory diet	• Aims to improve dysbiosis of the gut by modifying carbohydrates (reduced lactose and processed carbs), increased pre- and probiotics (soluble fiber, onions, fermented foods), increasing healthy fats • Minimize irritants to promote healing • Modifies textures of foods to improve absorption and minimize intact fiber	• Allows lean meat, poultry, fish, omega-3 eggs, select carbohydrates, select fruits and vegetables • Encourages prebiotics in the form of soluble fiber (bananas, oats, flax) • Limits dairy intake

each diet. This section highlights the 4 most studied diets and reviews their underlying pathophysiology, efficacy, and adherence rates.

Exclusive enteral nutrition

Of the different dietary therapies, EEN is the most well-studied with the strongest evidence to support its use in CD, especially in pediatric patients. In fact, in the 2014 European Society of Pediatric Gastroenterology, Hepatology, and Nutrition (ESPGHAN) and European Crohn's and Colitis Organization (ECCO) guidelines, 96% of experts agreed that EEN should be the recommended first-line induction therapy for children with active luminal CD over steroids.[41] Although the underlying pathophysiology behind EEN's therapeutic benefits in CD is unclear, many hypothesize that it downregulates proinflammatory cytokines and alters the microbiome to decrease intestinal inflammation.[42]

With EEN therapy, patients receive 100% of their nutrition through liquid formulations, either orally or via feeding tube, for 4 to 12 weeks. EEN comes in 3 major formulations: elemental, semielemental, and polymeric formulations. Elemental formulations contain only amino acids and are administered via tube feeds. Semielemental formulations contain peptides of varying lengths. Finally, polymeric formulations contain intact protein and can be ingested orally. Polymeric formulations are typically more palatable and, thankfully, are equally as efficacious as elemental and semielemental formulations.[43]

EEN has been extensively studied, with 9 meta-analyses to date evaluating the efficacy of EEN versus corticosteroids for inducing remission in CD (Table 3).[43–51] Although the overall consensus is mixed, studies evaluating EEN exclusively in pediatric patients have found it is at least noninferior to corticosteroids. One meta-analysis found EEN was 4.5 times more likely to achieve mucosal healing than corticosteroids (OR 4.50 [95% CI 1.64–12.32).[50] In contrast, studies that included adult patients found EEN was inferior to corticosteroids. An explanation behind this discrepancy between adults and pediatric patients undergoing EEN therapy has not been identified but is most likely related to adherence and tolerability. However, there are data suggesting EEN has beneficial effects in adults with complex CD. In a prospective, observational study of 41 adult CD patients with fistulas, strictures, and abscesses, 80.5% achieved clinical remission, and 75% of subjects with enterocutaneous fistulas achieved fistula

Table 3
Summary of 9 meta-analyses on exclusive enteral nutrition in Crohn's disease

Study	# Of studies	Total n	Population	Outcome: EEN vs Corticosteroid
Fernandez-Banareset al,[44] 1995	9	419	Adult	Inferior (0.35, [95% CI 0.23–0.53])
Griffithset al,[45] 1995	8	143	Adult	Inferior (OR 0.35, [95% CI 0.23–0.53])
Messori et al,[46] 1996	7	N/A	Adult	Inferior (RTF 0.35, [(95% CI 0.23–0.53])
Heuschkel et al,[47] 2000	5	147	Pediatric	Noninferior (RR = 0.95, [95% CI 0.67–1.34])
Zachos et al,[48] 2001	4	153	Adult and pediatric	Inferior (OR 0.30, [95% CI 0.17–0.52])
Zachos et al,[43] 2007	6	352	Adult and pediatric	Inferior (OR 0.33, [95% CI 0.23–0.56])
Dziechciarz et al,[49] 2007	4	144	Pediatric	Noninferior (RR = 0.97, [95% CI 0.7–1.4])
Swaminath et al,[50] 2017	8	451	Pediatric	Noninferior (OR1.26, [95% CI 0.77–2.05])
Narula et al,[51] 2018	8	223	Adult and Pediatric	Adult: Inferior (RR: 0.65, [95% CI 0.52–0.82]) Pediatric: noninferior (RR 1.35, [95% CI 0.92–1.97])

Abbreviations: OR, odds ratio; RR, relative risk; RTF, risk of treatment failure.

closure.[52] Another prospective study of 59 CD patients reported a 331% increase in luminal cross-sectional area of inflammatory strictures on imaging after 12 weeks of EEN.[53] EEN may also be an effective adjunct therapy with biologic agents. In a meta-analysis comparing patients on infliximab (IFX) and EEN versus IFX monotherapy, 74.5% of patients on IFX and EEN therapy versus 49.2% of patients on IFX monotherapy sustained remission after 1 year (OR 2.93; 95% CI: 1.66–5.17, $P<.01$). Finally, prior studies have suggested EEN may not be effective in colonic CD.[54,55] However, a more recent study found disease location did not influence likelihood of clinical remission in children with CD treated with EEN.[56]

Because palatability is a major barrier to EEN therapy adherence, there have been a couple of studies dedicated to identifying strategies to circumnavigate this barrier. In the CD-TREAT trial, investigators designed a diet using regular foods with similar composition to EEN and found that it had better adherence than traditional EEN in adults.[57] As part of the study, investigators also conducted a small open-label trial in 5 children with active CD (n = 5) and found 60% achieved clinical remission after 8 weeks. There was also a 55% decrease in fecal calprotectin compared with baseline. Likewise, in an RCT, investigators evaluated the tolerability and efficacy of inducing remission using of a combination diet of the CD exclusion diet (CDED), a whole food diet, with partial enteral nutrition (PEN) versus EEN in pediatric patients with mild-to-moderate CD.[58] The investigators found CDED + PEN was significantly better tolerated than EEN ($P=.002$; OR for tolerance of CDED + PEN 13.92 [95%CI 1.68–115.14]) while equally efficacious for inducing steroid-free remission at 6 weeks (75% (n = 30) on CDED + PEN versus 59% (n = 20) on EEN, $P=.38$). These studies offer promising dietary alternatives for EEN to improve adherence while maintaining efficacy. They also offer insight into strategies to apply EEN in the adult IBD population as well as help further clarify dietary factors that may contribute to the development and exacerbation of IBD.

In conclusion, EEN is a well-studied dietary intervention for treating CD and is recommended as the first-line agent for inducing remission in pediatric patients in Europe. In adults, the adoption of EEN has not been as widespread. Currently, only Japan has adopted EEN as a first-line agent in adult CD patients.[59] This highlights the need for RCTs to better understand its efficacy in adult CD patients.

Specific carbohydrate diet

Specific carbohydrate diet (SCD) was first described in 1924 by Sidney Haas for the treatment of celiac disease in children. It was initially termed the banana diet, because it required patients to eat numerous bananas daily along with milk, cottage cheese, meats, and vegetables while eliminating starches. SCD garnered attention for treating IBD after Elaine Gottschall, a biochemist, described how her daughter was cured of UC after following SCD in the book *Breaking the Vicious Cycle*.

The underlying concept behind SCD hypothesizes intestinal disorders such as IBD, IBS, and CD are due to intestinal injury caused by an overgrowth and imbalance of proinflammatory gut microbes from consuming poorly absorbed carbohydrates, specifically di- and polysaccharide carbohydrates. As such, SCD recommends avoiding most grains such as wheat, barley, corn, rice, processed/canned foods, and milk. Patients can eat monosaccharide carbohydrates such as glucose, fructose, and galactose, which are easily absorbed, in order to prevent further expansion of proinflammatory gut microbes. SCD allows most fresh fruits and vegetables, meat, yogurt, nuts, and hard cheeses just to name a few. While seemingly restrictive, SCD appears to have a high adherence rate. In a case series of 50 patients, mean adherence rate was 95%, with the mean duration of following SCD 35 months.[60] Likewise,

Table 4
Summary of available studies on specific carbohydrate diet and Crohn's disease

Study	Study Design	Total n	Cohort	Results
Obih et al,[66] 2016	Retrospective observational	26	Pediatric IBD patients	• Mean PCDAI decreased from 32.8 ± 13.2–8.8 ± 8.5 after 6 months • Mean PUCAI decreased from 28.3 ± 10.3–18.3 ± 31.7 after 6 months
Suskind,[68] 2014	Retrospective observational	7	Pediatric CD patients	• All patients' PCDAI decreased to 0 after 3 months on SCD • Improvement to normalization of albumin, CRP, and Hct
Burgis et al,[69] 2016	Retrospective observational	11	Pediatric CD patients	• Significant improvement of hct, albumin, and ESR on strict SCD (P=.006, .002, 0.002, respectively) • Laboratory values were stable on liberalized SCD • 90% (n = 10) gained weight percentile, and 82% (n = 9) had stable or increased height percentiles on strict SCD
Cohen et al,[71] 2014	Prospective observational	9	Pediatric CD patients	• Decrease in Harvey-Bradshaw Index (3.3 ± 2.0–0.6 ± 1.3; P=.007) and PCDAI (21.1 ± 5.9–7.8 ± 7.1, P=.011) at 12 wk • Capsule endoscopy evaluation for mucosal healing showed decline in mean Lewis score (2153 ± 732–732 ± 433, P=.012) at 12 weeks
Lewis et al,[62] 2021	RCT	194	Adult CD patients	• Similar rates of symptomatic remission (CDAI<150) at week 6 for patients on SCD (46.5%, n = 46) and Mediterranean diet (43.5%, n = 40; P=.77) • CRP normalization not common in either diets (SCD 5.4%, Mediterranean diet 3.6%)
Kaplan et al,[63] 2021	N-of-1 trial	54	Pediatric IBD patients	• High probability strict SCD (sSCD) and modified SCD (mSCD) improved GI symptoms and pain intereference measures • High probability sSCD and mSCD reduced fecal calprotectin compared with baseline • Low probability sSCD more effective than mSCD

Abbreviations: PCDAI, Pediatric Crohn's disease activity index; PUCAI, Pediatric ulcerative colitis activity index.

in a survey of 417 patients, 96% of patients were able to continue SCD, with only 7 patients citing difficulty to maintain as the reason for discontinuing the diet.[61]

Most evidence supporting SCD in CD is limited by retrospective or case series study designs and primarily involve pediatric patients (**Table 4**). However, in the recently completed the DINE-CD trial, investigators conducted an RCT in 194 adult CD patients with mild-to-moderate symptoms (defined as short Crohn's Disease Activity Index (sCDAI) 176–399) to compare the efficacy of the Mediterranean diet (MD) versus SCD in inducing symptomatic remission at 6 weeks (defined as sCDAI <150 in the absence of initiation or increase in any CD medication).[62] The investigators found similar efficacy in achieving symptomatic remission at 6 weeks with MD (43.5%, n = 40) and SCD (46.5%, n = 46, P = .77). Interestingly, C-reactive protein normalization was not common in either diets (MD 3.6%; SCD 5.4%). The study also provided reassuring data that both diets were well tolerated despite increased consumption of fruits and vegetables. In a similar study, investigators of the PRODUCE trial evaluated the effectiveness of strict SCD (sSCD) versus modified SCD (mSCD) versus usual diet in reducing symptoms and inflammation in pediatric IBD patients with elevated inflammatory markers.[63] The study implemented a unique n-of-1 study design where the patient serves as his or her own control, and treatment is systematically varied over time. The investigators enrolled 54 patients and found sSCD and mSCD had high probability of improving in GI symptoms and pain inter-reference measures. They also found both diets resulted in a reduction of fecal calprotectin compared with baseline for both diets. However, there was low probability that sSCD was more effective than mSCD.

Although the current evidence does not demonstrate SCD is more effective than other dietary therapies, there are now RCT data demonstrating that SCD is an effective dietary intervention to at least improve GI symptoms. Moreover, the finding that SCD and MD are equally efficacious suggests that it is more important to avoid certain dietary elements such as processed foods and to increase intake of whole foods like fruits and vegetables rather than adhere to a specific, restrictive dietary regimen. This is welcome news for CD patients, as many risk malnutrition from following restrictive diets.

Low FODMAP

A low FODMAP diet, which stands for fermentable oligosaccharides, disaccharides, monosaccharides, and polyols, is traditionally prescribed for patients suffering from IBS and other functional GI disorders. The underlying concept behind the diet states that high FODMAP foods are typically poorly absorbed carbohydrates that, when fermented by intestinal bacteria, result in increased gas production, fluid load, and ultimately GI distress in certain individuals. The diet involves 3 phases: elimination, reintroduction, and maintenance. The elimination phase is notoriously difficult, because patients are given an extensive list of foods to avoid. Given its highly restrictive nature, especially during the elimination phase, there are concerns for developing nutritional deficiencies with long-term use. For instance, short-term exclusion of high FODMAP foods are associated with lower carbohydrate and calcium intake.[64] Dedicated evidence for nutritional deficiencies associated with long-term use of low FODMAP diet is lacking. However, it is still important to remember that the elimination phase is intended to be short term, and, once a patient's GI symptoms have improved, he or she should progress to the reintroduction phase.

Currently, the data on the effectiveness of low FODMAP in IBD are uncertain (**Table 5**). There have been 3 RCTs, but these trials were designed to evaluate the efficacy of low FODMAP diet in treating IBS-like symptoms in IBD patients who were predominantly in remission.[65–67] Among the 3 trials, there was consensus that low FODMAP diet improved GI symptoms and quality of life compared with a control diet. Additionally, the studies found that changes in inflammatory markers did not differ between low FODMAP and control diet. Based on these studies, the role of a low FODMAP diet in IBD patients is best for addressing concomitant IBS-like symptoms rather than active inflammation. The data also reiterate the fact that IBD patients frequently suffer from functional GI symptoms despite quiescent disease and require a unique set of strategies to manage.[68]

Table 5
Summary of available studies on low FODMAP diet and inflammatory bowel disease

Study	Study Design	Total n	Cohort	Results
Pedersen et al,[74] 2017	Randomized controlled open-label trial	89	Adult IBD patients with quiescent to mild/moderate disease and coexisting IBS symptoms	• Significantly larger proportion of responders (at least 50-point reduction in IBS symptom severity system) in low FODMAP (LF) group (81%) vs normal diet group (46%, OR:5.30 [95% CI 1.81–15.55]). • LF group had significantly greater increase than normal diet group in short IBD quality-of-life questionnaire score at week 6 (median 60, IQR51–65 vs median 50, IQR 39–60, $P<.01$).
Gearry et al,[75] 2009	Survey study	52	Adult IBD patients who received instruction on low FODMAP diet	• Approximately 50% of patients had improvement in at least 5 out of 10 overall symptoms on LF • Significant improvement in abdominal symptoms, abdominal pain, bloating, wind, and diarrhea on LF ($P<.02$)
Prince et al,[76] 2016	Retrospective observational	88	Adult IBD patients with functional GI symptoms independent of degree of inflammation	• Significant increase in proportion of patients reporting satisfactory relief of functional-like GI symptoms after LF (16% at baseline vs 78% at follow-up, $P<.001$) • Improvement in proportion of patients reporting normal stool frequency (once every 3 d to 3 times/d) (60% at baseline vs 81% at follow-up, $P<.001$) after LF
Halmos et al,[66] 2016	Randomized controlled cross-over trial	9	Adult CD patients in clinical remission	• GI symptom severity of GI symptoms was 50% lower on the LF compared with typical diet ($P<.001$). • Neither diet had an effect on fecal calprotectin

(continued on next page)

		Total		
Study	Study Design	n	Cohort	Results
Cox,[65] 2020	RCT	52	Adult CD patients in remission	• Higher proportion of patients reported improvement in GI symptoms on LF diet (52%, n = 14) compared with control diet (16%, n = 4; P=.007) • Neither diet had effect on inflammatory markers

Table 5 (continued)

Semivegetarian diet

Because of data implicating high intake of meats and fats and the protective effect of fiber in the pathogenesis of CD, investigators have suggested a semivegetarian diet may have a beneficial role. However, evidence supporting this diet is weak. Currently, the use of a semivegetarian diet in CD is supported by 2 small prospective studies that included 22 to 40 patients. One study based in Japan found consuming a semivegetarian diet, where only fish was allowed once a week, and meat was allowed once every 2 weeks, was associated with remission in 94% (15/16) compared with 33% of patients (2/6) in the omnivorous diet group.[69] The adherence rate of was high, with 73% (n = 16) of patients maintaining the study diet. The second study used an immunoglobulin 4 (IgG4)-guided exclusion diet, where animal proteins were most commonly eliminated. Investigators reported symptomatic improvement in 90% of patients (n = 26) who followed the dietary interventions.[70] Only 5 of 40 subjects failed to adhere to the diet throughout the study. In contrast to these 2 small studies, a large RCT of 213 CD patients found reduced meat intake (consuming no more than 1 serving of red or processed meat per month) did not reduce the risk of CD flare compared to those with high meat intake (consuming at least 2 servings of red or processed meat per week).[37] The average adherence rate was 57%. Based on these studies, the role of reducing meat consumption is muddy and likely inconsequential in treating CD. Interestingly, these studies do not address dietary fiber intake. Based on prior studies suggesting that increased fiber intake reduces risk of developing CD while the role of high meat intake is less clear, one may gain more benefit from efforts focusing on increasing plant fiber intake rather than reducing meat consumption. This may help explain the discrepancies between the studies as Asian versus Western dietary patterns vary in terms of vegetable and fruit intake independent of quantity of meat consumption. Further studies are needed to better understand if increasing plant fiber intake from has a role in treating IBD when following a semivegetarian diet.

It is also worth mentioning that curcumin, which is a naturally occurring substance found in turmeric, is a promising dietary agent for treating IBD via its action on NF-κB.[71–73] One RCT in 30 patients with mild-to-moderate CD found 360 mg/d of a highly bioavailable curcumin derivative achieved clinical remission in 40% (n = 8) compared with 0 patients in the placebo arm (P=.020). Additionally, compared with baseline, there was a significant decrease in simple endoscopic score for CD (SESCD) at 12 weeks in the curcumin group (12.4–8.0, P=.032) but not the placebo group (15.0–10.3, P=.220). In UC, 2 to 3 g daily in combination with 5-ASA is effective in inducing and maintaining remission in mild-to-moderate disease.[74,75] Although more prospective studies are needed to confirm its efficacy, curcumin may be a promising dietary adjunct therapy to conventional IBD therapies in select patients.

Finally, there are a couple of notable trials exploring dietary interventions in CD in the pipeline. The COmbinAtion therapy of diet with biologicalS for CD (OATS) study will investigate the safety and efficacy of the Food influence on the Intestinal microbiota (FIT) diet. The FIT diet consists of a semivegetarian diet that is high in fiber and low in saturated fat and sulfites. It also excludes added sugars, processed foods, and food emulsifiers (carrageenan and polysorbate-80). Specifically, the investigators will evaluate the FIT diet as an add-on therapy during the induction and maintenance phases of biologic therapy in CD. The Inflammatory Bowel Disease Mediterranean Diet (IBDMED) study will investigate the effect a Mediterranean diet in newly diagnosed CD patients in India and compare the effects with CD patients who receive the same intervention in Israel. With the influx of dietary intervention trials, dietary therapies will hopefully be commonly prescribed for patients in the near future.

SUMMARY

For most patients, diet is a fundamental component in the management of their CD. Unfortunately, 50% to 69% of patients do not receive any information about it.[6,7] With the increasing prevalence of CD, it is important for providers to have the knowledge and resources to educate patients about the dietary aspects of CD.

This review article summarized the available literature on the role of diet in the pathogenesis, exacerbation, and treatment of CD. Although the data do not identify any certain foods in the pathogenesis of CD, the interplay of dietary exposures on the intestinal microbiome and barrier function may increase certain individuals' susceptibility to CD. Similarly, there is no evidence that certain foods exacerbate inflammation in CD in people, but studies have found certain foods are more prone to exacerbate GI symptoms. This may be a consequence of a sensitized gut from chronic inflammation. Finally, there has been tremendous growth in the number of studies evaluating dietary therapies in CD. Currently, EEN has the strongest evidence for its use, especially in pediatric patients, but emerging trials in the pipeline may identify new effective dietary interventions in CD. Overall, the future of incorporating diet into the treatment CD is bright, and dietary therapies may soon be part of the standard of care.

CLINICS CARE POINTS

- Patients with Crohn's disease want to discuss their diet and how it may help manage their disease with their physicians.- Informing patients that diet has no role in treating their Crohn's disease should be avoided.
- Embedding a GI-trained dietitian in the clinic is an invaluable resource for patients.

CONFLICTS OF INTEREST

L.A. Feagins has previously received research support from Arena Pharmaceuticals, Corevitas, LLC, Janssen Pharmaceuticals, and Takeda Pharmaceuticals. P. Gu has nothing to disclose.

REFERENCES

1. Molodecky NA, Soon IS, Rabi DM, et al. Increasing incidence and prevalence of the inflammatory bowel diseases with time, based on systematic review. Gastroenterology 2012;142(1):46–54, e42; quiz e30.

2. Sood A, Midha V, Sood N, et al. Incidence and prevalence of ulcerative colitis in Punjab, North India. Gut 2003;52(11):1587–90.

3. Ng SC, Tang W, Ching JY, et al. Incidence and phenotype of inflammatory bowel disease based on results from the Asia-pacific Crohn's and colitis epidemiology study. Gastroenterology 2013;145(1):158–165 e152.

4. Ng SC. Emerging leadership lecture: Inflammatory bowel disease in Asia: emergence of a "Western" disease. J Gastroenterol Hepatol 2015;30(3):440–5.

5. Thia KT, Loftus EV Jr, Sandborn WJ, et al. An update on the epidemiology of inflammatory bowel disease in Asia. Am J Gastroenterol 2008;103(12):3167–82.

6. Bernstein KI, Promislow S, Carr R, et al. Information needs and preferences of recently diagnosed patients with inflammatory bowel disease. Inflamm Bowel Dis 2011;17(2):590–8.

7. Limdi JK, Aggarwal D, McLaughlin JT. Dietary practices and beliefs in patients with inflammatory bowel disease. Inflamm Bowel Dis 2016;22(1):164–70.

8. Tinsley A, Ehrlich OG, Hwang C, et al. Knowledge, attitudes, and beliefs regarding the role of nutrition in IBD among patients and providers. Inflamm Bowel Dis 2016;22(10):2474–81.

9. Hou JK, Lee D, Lewis J. Diet and inflammatory bowel disease: review of patient-targeted recommendations. Clin Gastroenterol Hepatol 2014;12(10):1592–600.

10. Roediger WE, Duncan A, Kapaniris O, et al. Reducing sulfur compounds of the colon impair colonocyte nutrition: implications for ulcerative colitis. Gastroenterology 1993;104(3):802–9.

11. Ijssennagger N, Belzer C, Hooiveld GJ, et al. Gut microbiota facilitates dietary heme-induced epithelial hyperproliferation by opening the mucus barrier in colon. Proc Natl Acad Sci U S A 2015;112(32):10038–43.

12. Hou JK, Abraham B, El-Serag H. Dietary intake and risk of developing inflammatory bowel disease: a systematic review of the literature. Am J Gastroenterol 2011;106(4):563–73.

13. Jowett SL, Seal CJ, Pearce MS, et al. Influence of dietary factors on the clinical course of ulcerative colitis: a prospective cohort study. Gut 2004;53(10):1479–84.

14. Llewellyn SR, Britton GJ, Contijoch EJ, et al. Interactions between diet and the intestinal microbiota alter intestinal permeability and colitis severity in mice. Gastroenterology 2018;154(4):1037–1046 e1032.

15. Martinez-Medina M, Denizot J, Dreux N, et al. Western diet induces dysbiosis with increased E coli in CEABAC10 mice, alters host barrier function favouring AIEC colonisation. Gut 2014;63(1):116–24.

16. Ananthakrishnan AN, Khalili H, Konijeti GG, et al. Long-term intake of dietary fat and risk of ulcerative colitis and Crohn's disease. Gut 2014;63(5):776–84.

17. Chan SS, Luben R, Olsen A, et al. Association between high dietary intake of the n-3 polyunsaturated fatty acid docosahexaenoic acid and reduced risk of Crohn's disease. Aliment Pharmacol Ther 2014;39(8):834–42.

18. Ananthakrishnan AN, Khalili H, Konijeti GG, et al. A prospective study of long-term intake of dietary fiber and risk of Crohn's disease and ulcerative colitis. Gastroenterology 2013;145(5):970–7.

19. McGuckin MA, Linden SK, Sutton P, et al. Mucin dynamics and enteric pathogens. Nat Rev Microbiol 2011;9(4):265–78.

20. Desai MS, Seekatz AM, Koropatkin NM, et al. A dietary fiber-deprived gut microbiota degrades the colonic mucus barrier and enhances pathogen susceptibility. Cell 2016;167(5):1339–1353 e1321.

21. Chassaing B, Koren O, Goodrich JK, et al. Dietary emulsifiers impact the mouse gut microbiota promoting colitis and metabolic syndrome. Nature 2015; 519(7541):92–6.
22. Shang Q, Sun W, Shan X, et al. Carrageenan-induced colitis is associated with decreased population of anti-inflammatory bacterium, *Akkermansia muciniphila*, in the gut microbiota of C57BL/6J mice. Toxicol Lett 2017;279:87–95.
23. Viennois E, Merlin D, Gewirtz AT, et al. Dietary emulsifier-induced low-grade inflammation promotes colon carcinogenesis. Cancer Res 2017;77(1):27–40.
24. Singh RK, Wheildon N, Ishikawa S. Food additive P-80 impacts mouse gut microbiota promoting intestinal inflammation, obesity and liver dysfunction. SOJ Microbiol Infect Dis 2016;4(1).
25. Fahoum L, Moscovici A, David S, et al. Digestive fate of dietary carrageenan: evidence of interference with digestive proteolysis and disruption of gut epithelial function. Mol Nutr Food Res 2017;61(3).
26. Swidsinski A, Ung V, Sydora BC, et al. Bacterial overgrowth and inflammation of small intestine after carboxymethylcellulose ingestion in genetically susceptible mice. Inflamm Bowel Dis 2009;15(3):359–64.
27. Moyana TN, Lalonde JM. Carrageenan-induced intestinal injury in the rat–a model for inflammatory bowel disease. Ann Clin Lab Sci 1990;20(6):420–6.
28. Watt J, Marcus R. Carrageenan-induced ulceration of the large intestine in the guinea pig. Gut 1971;12(2):164–71.
29. Pricolo VE, Madhere SM, Finkelstein SD, et al. Effects of lambda-carrageenan induced experimental enterocolitis on splenocyte function and nitric oxide production. J Surg Res 1996;66(1):6–11.
30. Lomer MC, Thompson RP, Powell JJ. Fine and ultrafine particles of the diet: influence on the mucosal immune response and association with Crohn's disease. Proc Nutr Soc 2002;61(1):123–30.
31. Pineton de Chambrun G, Body-Malapel M, Frey-Wagner I, et al. Aluminum enhances inflammation and decreases mucosal healing in experimental colitis in mice. Mucosal Immunol 2014;7(3):589–601.
32. Esquerre N, Basso L, Dubuquoy C, et al. Aluminum ingestion promotes colorectal hypersensitivity in rodents. Cell Mol Gastroenterol Hepatol 2019;7(1):185–96.
33. Lomer MC, Grainger SL, Ede R, et al. Lack of efficacy of a reduced microparticle diet in a multi-centred trial of patients with active Crohn's disease. Eur J Gastroenterol Hepatol 2005;17(3):377–84.
34. He Z, Chen L, Catalan-Dibene J, et al. Food colorants metabolized by commensal bacteria promote colitis in mice with dysregulated expression of interleukin-23. Cell Metab 2021;33(7):1358–71.e5.
35. Lo CH, Lochhead P, Khalili H, et al. Dietary inflammatory potential and risk of Crohn's disease and ulcerative colitis. Gastroenterology 2020;159(3):873–883 e871.
36. Zallot C, Quilliot D, Chevaux JB, et al. Dietary beliefs and behavior among inflammatory bowel disease patients. Inflamm Bowel Dis 2013;19(1):66–72.
37. Albenberg L, Brensinger CM, Wu Q, et al. A diet low in red and processed meat does not reduce rate of Crohn's disease flares. Gastroenterology 2019;157(1): 128–136 e125.
38. Cohen AB, Lee D, Long MD, et al. Dietary patterns and self-reported associations of diet with symptoms of inflammatory bowel disease. Dig Dis Sci 2013;58(5): 1322–8.
39. de Vries JHM, Dijkhuizen M, Tap P, et al. Patient's dietary beliefs and behaviours in inflammatory bowel disease. Dig Dis 2019;37(2):131–9.

40. Jowett SL, Seal CJ, Phillips E, et al. Dietary beliefs of people with ulcerative colitis and their effect on relapse and nutrient intake. Clin Nutr 2004;23(2):161–70.
41. Ruemmele FM, Veres G, Kolho KL, et al. Consensus guidelines of ECCO/ES-PGHAN on the medical management of pediatric Crohn's disease. J Crohns Colitis 2014;8(10):1179–207.
42. Hansen T, Duerksen DR. Enteral nutrition in the management of pediatric and adult Crohn's disease. Nutrients 2018;10(5).
43. Zachos M, Tondeur M, Griffiths AM. Enteral nutritional therapy for induction of remission in Crohn's disease. Cochrane Database Syst Rev 2007;1:CD000542.
44. Fernandez-Banares F, Cabre E, Esteve-Comas M, et al. How effective is enteral nutrition in inducing clinical remission in active Crohn's disease? A meta-analysis of the randomized clinical trials. JPEN J Parenter Enteral Nutr 1995; 19(5):356–64.
45. Griffiths AM, Ohlsson A, Sherman PM, et al. Meta-analysis of enteral nutrition as a primary treatment of active Crohn's disease. Gastroenterology 1995;108(4): 1056–67.
46. Messori A, Trallori G, D'Albasio G, et al. Defined-formula diets versus steroids in the treatment of active Crohn's disease: a meta-analysis. Scand J Gastroenterol 1996;31(3):267–72.
47. Heuschkel RB, Menache CC, Megerian JT, et al. Enteral nutrition and corticosteroids in the treatment of acute Crohn's disease in children. J Pediatr Gastroenterol Nutr 2000;31(1):8–15.
48. Zachos M, Tondeur M, Griffiths AM. Enteral nutritional therapy for inducing remission of Crohn's disease. Cochrane Database Syst Rev 2001;3:CD000542.
49. Dziechciarz P, Horvath A, Shamir R, et al. Meta-analysis: enteral nutrition in active Crohn's disease in children. Aliment Pharmacol Ther 2007;26(6):795–806.
50. Swaminath A, Feathers A, Ananthakrishnan AN, et al. Systematic review with meta-analysis: enteral nutrition therapy for the induction of remission in paediatric Crohn's disease. Aliment Pharmacol Ther 2017;46(7):645–56.
51. Narula N, Dhillon A, Zhang D, et al. Enteral nutritional therapy for induction of remission in Crohn's disease. Cochrane Database Syst Rev 2018;4:CD000542.
52. Yang Q, Gao X, Chen H, et al. Efficacy of exclusive enteral nutrition in complicated Crohn's disease. Scand J Gastroenterol 2017;52(9):995–1001.
53. Hu D, Ren J, Wang G, et al. Exclusive enteral nutritional therapy can relieve inflammatory bowel stricture in Crohn's disease. J Clin Gastroenterol 2014;48(9): 790–5.
54. Seidman EG. Nutritional management of inflammatory bowel disease. Gastroenterol Clin North Am 1989;18(1):129–55.
55. Afzal NA, Davies S, Paintin M, et al. Colonic Crohn's disease in children does not respond well to treatment with enteral nutrition if the ileum is not involved. Dig Dis Sci 2005;50(8):1471–5.
56. Buchanan E, Gaunt WW, Cardigan T, et al. The use of exclusive enteral nutrition for induction of remission in children with Crohn's disease demonstrates that disease phenotype does not influence clinical remission. Aliment Pharmacol Ther 2009;30(5):501–7.
57. Svolos V, Hansen R, Nichols B, et al. Treatment of active Crohn's disease with an ordinary food-based diet that replicates exclusive enteral nutrition. Gastroenterology 2019;156(5):1354–1367 e1356.
58. Levine A, Wine E, Assa A, et al. Crohn's disease exclusion diet plus partial enteral nutrition induces sustained remission in a randomized controlled trial. Gastroenterology 2019;157(2):440–450 e448.

59. Day A, Wood J, Melton S, et al. Exclusive enteral nutrition: An optimal care pathway for use in adult patients with active Crohn's disease. JGH Open 2020; 4(2):260–6.

60. Kakodkar S, Farooqui AJ, Mikolaitis SL, et al. The specific carbohydrate diet for inflammatory bowel disease: a case series. J Acad Nutr Diet 2015;115(8): 1226–32.

61. Suskind DL, Wahbeh G, Cohen SA, et al. Patients perceive clinical benefit with the specific carbohydrate diet for inflammatory bowel disease. Dig Dis Sci 2016;61(11):3255–60.

62. Lewis J. Trial of specific carbohydrate and Mediterranean diets to induce remission of Crohn's disease (DINE-CD). DDW Virtual, 2021.

63. Kaplan HC. Personalized research on diet in ulcerative colitis and Crohn's disease (PRODUCE). Crohn's and Colitis Congress Virtual, 2021.

64. Staudacher HM. Nutritional, microbiological and psychosocial implications of the low FODMAP diet. J Gastroenterol Hepatol 2017;32(Suppl 1):16–9.

65. Cox SR, Lindsay JO, Fromentin S, et al. Effects of low FODMAP diet on symptoms, fecal microbiome, and markers of inflammation in patients with quiescent inflammatory bowel disease in a randomized trial. Gastroenterolog 2020;158(1):176–188 e177.

66. Halmos EP, Christophersen CT, Bird AR, et al. Consistent prebiotic effect on gut microbiota with altered FODMAP intake in patients with Crohn's disease: a randomised, controlled cross-over trial of well-defined diets. Clin Transl Gastroenterol 2016;7:e164.

67. Pedersen N, Ankersen DV, Felding M, et al. Low-FODMAP diet reduces irritable bowel symptoms in patients with inflammatory bowel disease. World J Gastroenterol 2017;23(18):3356–66.

68. Halpin SJ, Ford AC. Prevalence of symptoms meeting criteria for irritable bowel syndrome in inflammatory bowel disease: systematic review and meta-analysis. Am J Gastroenterol 2012;107(10):1474–82.

69. Chiba M, Abe T, Tsuda H, et al. Lifestyle-related disease in Crohn's disease: relapse prevention by a semi-vegetarian diet. World J Gastroenterol 2010; 16(20):2484–95.

70. Rajendran N, Kumar D. Food-specific IgG4-guided exclusion diets improve symptoms in Crohn's disease: a pilot study. Colorectal Dis 2011;13(9):1009–13.

71. Singh S, Aggarwal BB. Activation of transcription factor NF-kappa B is suppressed by curcumin (diferuloylmethane) [corrected]. J Biol Chem 1995; 270(42):24995–5000.

72. Kumar A, Dhawan S, Hardegen NJ, et al. Curcumin (Diferuloylmethane) inhibition of tumor necrosis factor (TNF)-mediated adhesion of monocytes to endothelial cells by suppression of cell surface expression of adhesion molecules and of nuclear factor-kappaB activation. Biochem Pharmacol 1998;55(6):775–83.

73. Jobin C, Bradham CA, Russo MP, et al. Curcumin blocks cytokine-mediated NF-kappa B activation and proinflammatory gene expression by inhibiting inhibitory factor I-kappa B kinase activity. J Immunol 1999;163(6):3474–83.

74. Hanai H, Iida T, Takeuchi K, et al. Curcumin maintenance therapy for ulcerative colitis: randomized, multicenter, double-blind, placebo-controlled trial. Clin Gastroenterol Hepatol 2006;4(12):1502–6.

75. Lang A, Salomon N, Wu JC, et al. Curcumin in combination with mesalamine induces remission in patients with mild-to-moderate ulcerative colitis in a randomized controlled trial. Clin Gastroenterol Hepatol 2015;13(8):1444–1449 e1441.

76. Konijeti GG, Kim N, Lewis JD, et al. Efficacy of the autoimmune protocol diet for inflammatory bowel disease. Inflamm Bowel Dis 2017;23(11):2054–60.

Complementary and Alternative Medicine in Crohn's Disease

Jennifer Seminerio, MD

KEYWORDS

- Complementary and alternative medicine • Crohn's disease
- Inflammatory bowel disease

KEY POINTS

- Complementary and alternative medicine is an ever-growing part of inflammatory bowel disease with data suggesting more than half of patients have or are using it as part of their overall care
- There are a variety of options available for patients that include mind-based therapies, body-based therapies, supplements, and probiotics.
- There is a lack of well-designed clinical trials to assess the efficacy and safety of these therapies within inflammatory bowel disease
- There is a lack of education among health care providers, which includes gaps in knowledge, understanding, and ability to discuss these therapies with patients.

INTRODUCTION

Complementary and alternative medicine (CAM) is the use of a combined alternative medicine and conventional therapeutic approach to treatment. Alternative medicine is defined as practices that encompass herbal and dietary supplements, probiotics, traditional Chinese medicines, mind-body techniques and is considered nonconventional and nonmedically evidence-based.

CAM is increasing within IBD. Literature supports the use of prebiotics, probiotics, and supplements for gut dysbiosis, mental wellbeing, and quality of life (QoL). Patients turn to CAM for a variety of reasons that include a desire for a holistic approach to supplement conventional therapy and a perception that herbal therapies are less toxic and harmless because they are "natural." Specifically, patients feel a sense of control as these therapies are often accessible and taken without the involvement of health care providers, industry leaders, and insurance authorization. They also may turn to alternative medicine and or CAM when they have had a lack of response to conventional therapy.[1–3]

University of South Florida, The Carol and Frank Morsani Center, 13330 USF Laurel Drive, 6th Floor, Tampa, FL 33612, USA
E-mail address: jenniferlsem@usf.edu

Gastroenterol Clin N Am 51 (2022) 337–351
https://doi.org/10.1016/j.gtc.2021.12.009
0889-8553/22/© 2022 Elsevier Inc. All rights reserved.

Predictors of CAM use include a history of psychiatric comorbidities, dissatisfaction with the patient–doctor relationship, and a history of side effects from conventional treatment. Interestingly, patients with higher utilization of corticosteroids also tend to have higher rates of CAM use.[3,4] Other factors include a history of friends and family using CAM, disease duration, female gender, a higher income, degree of education, or higher socioeconomic status, vegetarianism, and geographic location. Specifically, the Mountain, Pacific, and Midwest regions have the highest usage of CAM.[4-6]

Inflammatory bowel disease (IBD) is a chronic inflammatory state seen within the gastrointestinal tract. Clinical symptoms range from abdominal pain, diarrhea, gastro-intestinal bleeding, tenesmus, urgency, frequency, incontinence, weight loss, fatigue, and arthralgia and are related to an inflammatory cascade of neutrophils and macro-phages producing a range of cytokines, proteolytic enzymes, and free radicals.[7]

Crohn's disease is a lifelong condition that occurs in both males and females with prevalence increasing in newly industrialized countries, and incidence highest in North America and Europe.[8] The precise cause of Crohn's disease remains unknown although evidence points toward a spectrum of genetic susceptibility, environmental triggers and an aberrant immunologic response.[7] The QoL is of immense importance when it comes to this disease as there is no cure and exceedingly high costs from ther-apies, clinical care, and diagnostic modalities. Furthermore, potential adverse thera-peutic effects exist in addition to misconceptions regarding the safety, efficacy, and cost-effectiveness of both conventional and alternative therapies.

CAM use over the past decade has increased up to 60% in some studies.[3] Howev-er, well-conducted clinical trials are lacking with regards to CAM use and IBD. The tri-als that do exist typically favor CAM in mild IBD. In real-world clinical practice, it is difficult to assess improvement with alternative therapies as up to 75% of patients fail to discuss use with their provider.[6,9] Reasons include a perceived lack of knowl-edge by their health care provider, lack of appointment time, and fear. That being said, the most commonly used alternative therapy in the United States is herbal supplements.

Ultimately, it is important to better understand that CAM uses both as a tool to help patients gain and maintain remission, as well as to ensure that compliance with con-ventional therapies is not lost.[5] Below is the comprehensive review of the literature on current CAM modalities used within patients with IBD, specifically Crohn's disease.

METHODS

A systematic literature review was performed on CAM therapies and included specific treatment trials, systematic reviews, and meta-analysis on specific treatments as well as review articles tackling the topic of CAM therapy with relevant articles referenced throughout this review.

Mind-Based Therapies

It has been published that patients with IBD have higher rates of depression, anxi-ety.[10-12] The European Crohn's and Colitis Organization (ECCO) states anxiety and depression are seen at higher rates preceding a diagnosis of IBD.[13] A systemic review from 2016 found 768 abstracts were evaluated with only one trial on anxiety treatment and IBD, and no well-designed studies on depression and IBD.[14,15] Therapies including stress management, relaxation, mindfulness, hypnosis, yoga, exercise, cognitive-behavioral therapy (CBT), and biofeedback have all been used in IBD.

Biofeedback is a form of relaxation therapy used to assess how your body responds to and controls pain. It is associated with significant improvement in QoL in a variety of conditions. A study looking at patient's subjective outcomes specifically relating to incontinence and evacuatory disorders in the setting of ileoanal pouch anastomosis found an improved QoL after biofeedback.[16] Biofeedback may also be successful for fecal incontinence in quiescent IBD per a retrospective analysis.[17]

Cognitive-behavioral therapy (CBT) is based on the core principle that psychological problems are in part based on ineffective ways of thinking stemming from learned behavior that can be changed. The idea is to teach better coping strategies that will lead to a decrease in symptoms and an improvement in QoL. The idea that this could be used advantageously in IBD has been studied with mixed data. A randomized controlled trial (RCT) of patients with IBD showed improvement in QoL scores and a decrease in depression and anxiety.[18] However, another RCT among patients with IBD revealed no difference in Crohn's Disease Activity Index (CDAI) scores when CBT was added to standard therapy after 24 months.[19] A meta-analysis of the available data show small, short-term benefits of CBT on QoL and depression.[20] Finally, a single-center RCT evaluated the efficacy of CBT for the management of IBD-related fatigue. Although small in scale barriers to CBT included time, finance, and training constraints. Initial results showed a reduction in fatigue and improved QoL scores.[21] ECCO has stated that CBT can have short-term benefits on QoL and coping with early reports showing promise.[13] It should be noted that although CBT may improve QoL there has been a lack of data to suggest an effect on disease activity, anxiety, depression, and stress.[22]

Mindfulness is conscious awareness used as a form of psychological treatment. When combined with cognitive therapy mindfulness-based cognitive therapy (MBCT) forms.[23] Multiple approaches such as meditation are used with the goal of creating an overall attitude devoid of judgment. Studies are limited in IBD but an RCT found improved QoL scores and lowered anxiety and depression at 6 months in the treatment group who underwent mental body scan, meditation, yoga, group discussions, and sharing of experiences.[23] Another study revealed improvement in psychological and physical symptoms of IBD with reduced CRP levels.[24] In contrast, an RCT looking at complimentary mindfulness, found no change in fecal calprotectin or CRP in patients already in remission.[25] A review of literature found no role for relaxation techniques in unselected patients with IBD.[26]

Gut-directed hypnosis aims to link disconnect between the brain and gut. Therapists are trained to guide an individual into a relaxed state of altered awareness at which point guided suggestions, imagery, and relaxation techniques lead to a therapeutic effect.[27] A literature review from 2014 found 6 studies and 1 abstract with improved QoL scores and reductions in GI symptoms.[27] Despite the success of gut-directed hypnosis in IBS, sufficient data are still lacking in IBD.

Holistic or Comprehensive Health Wellness programs are increasing both via live events and or streamed teleconferences. The goals of these retreats are to target individuals with chronic disease and expose them to relaxation, stress reduction, and mind–body therapies.[3] They may make therapies more obtainable but are limited due to cost, misinformation, misguidance, scams, sham therapies, and exposure risk. Little data exist on overall benefit but a non-IBD trial on a 1 week wellness retreat revealed that experiences may lead to improvement in health and well-being over a 6-week follow-up. The area demands further research.[28] A systematic review of residential retreats found a total of 23 studies, 8 of which were RCTs. Participants and outcome measures varied but all studies reported positive outcomes that ranged from 0 to 5 years poststudy inclusion. These studies varied widely with small sample sizes, poor methodology, lack of follow-up data, and adverse effects making conclusions difficult to translate.[29]

Body-Based Interventions

Yoga is grounded within the Hindu spiritual and ascetic discipline and involves breath control, meditation, and bodily posture. It is widely practiced and is felt to be a health-amplifying technique. Another RCT in both types of IBD in remission found improvements in patient-reported outcomes (PRO), anxiety, and abdominal pain. No differences were noted in inflammatory markers.[30] ECCO recommendations state that yoga can improve QoL but there is not enough evidence on IBD symptom effects.[13]

Exercise is considered any activity that requires physical effort performed with the intention to improve health and fitness.[31] Exercise in IBD is linked to improved QoL scores, decreased rates of disease flare and improved bone density.[32,33] In animal models of colitis exercise led to a decreased expression of proinflammatory cytokines TNF-α and IL-1, and increased expression of IL-6 and IL-10.[33] Previous publications have acknowledged that exercise in IBD can be limited by fatigue, joint pain, abdominal pain, diarrhea, or urgency, tenesmus, and depression.[33] Sedentary occupations increased incidence of IBD.[34] In prospective female cohorts, physically active women had a 44% reduction in the risk of developing CD compared with sedentary women[35] and this was also seen as a relative risk reduction in a case-control study.[36] Meta-analysis on physical activity and IBD revealed a protective effect against developing CD.[37] Another prospective trial found exercise decreased the likelihood of flare in patients already in remission from CD at 6 months.[38]

Chronic vagal nerve stimulation involves delivering electrical impulses to the vagus nerve. It has been studied in epilepsy and treatment-resistant depression.[39] It can have side effects including coughing and shortness of breath.[39] In animal models with intestinal inflammation data revealed that stimulated rats had improved stool quality and decreases in rectal bleeding, CRP, and inflammatory cells within the intestine. Conclusions hypothesize a possible effective IBD treatment in humans.[40] A pilot study on vagus nerve stimulation that was well tolerated revealed that after 1 year 5 patients were in clinical remission and 6 endoscopic remissions in CD.[41] The therapy is difficult to access but certainly opens up the need for additional research.

Acupuncture is an integrative medicine that involves pricking skin tissue with needles. It is used to alleviate pain and treat various physical, mental, and emotional conditions. The art originated in ancient China but is widely practiced. Moxibustion is a form of heat therapy wherein dried plant materials called "moxa" are burned on or near the skin to increase Qi in the body and dispel pathogenic mechanisms.[3] They can be used in combination or as standalone treatments. ECCO states that given limited evidence alone or in combination they cannot be recommended for the treatment of IBD.[13] A combination study of acupuncture and moxibustion performed in quiescent CD concluded both therapies decreased CDAI, but differed in potential outcomes and long-term efficacy.[42] Within CD, patients not on conventional therapies saw a decrease in CDAI, CRP, and histopathologic abnormalities.[43] Patients with CD were evaluated with acupuncture alone versus placebo and CDAI score decreased in another study.[44] A systematic review and meta-analysis from 2010 found 5 RCTs all of the low methodologic quality comparing moxibustion with conventional drug therapy. Moxibustion response was favored in 3 trials comparing it to sulfasalazine and 2 comparing sulfasalazine plus other medications.[45] Another systemic review and meta-analysis from 2013 revealed within 43 RCT, 10 trials found moxibustion and/or acupuncture superior to sulfasalazine. The analysis noted heterogeneity and low methodologic quality.[46]

Supplements

Curcumin is derived from the rhizomatous plant (Curcuma longa) and is a part of the ginger family. It is the active ingredient of turmeric.[3] Curcumin belongs to a family of natural compounds called curcuminoids and is thought to possess antioxidant, anti-inflammatory, anticancer, and neuroprotective properties.[47] It's a frequently studied herbal therapy and was shown to reduce histologic inflammation in colitis mouse models through the inhibition of the NF-κB pathway and reduction of the proinflammatory cytokine response.[47-50] Several human RCTs have been performed and benefit for both induction and maintenance has been seen. In CD, a systemic review of the literature showed that curcumin reduced IL-1, a possible mechanism for loss of response to Remicade.[51] Patients using curcumin had lower CDAI scores.[51] Ultimately, use dates back to the 1700s for a multitude of clinical conditions. That being said, formulation and brands vary, and side effects include bloating, nausea, and lose stools.[3,52] ECCO recommends curcumin as a complementary therapy and positioned it as a therapy to induce remission in mild-to-moderate UC.[13]

Fish oil comes naturally from tuna, salmon, mackerel, sardines among others, and is known to increase omega-3 fatty acids (FA), DHA, and EPA Omega-3. It decreases the production of IL-1, IL-6, and tumor necrosis factor [TNF].[3,53] Thus, research examining the effects of both natural and commercially produced fish oils on disease outcomes in IBD has been warranted. In CD one study showed an advantage of omega-3 FA in comparison to omega-6 FA with regards to the inhibition of proinflammatory cytokines.[54] In another CD study, CRP decreased after 9 weeks in the omega 3 FA group.[55] Systemic reviews and meta-analysis found that in 6 studies a marginal benefit in CD remission was seen with omega 3 FA.[56,57] There was high heterogeneity and small sample size. Two large studies EPIC1 and EPIC2 evaluated the use of 4g daily of omega 3 FA versus placebo for 58 weeks and found no significant difference in outcome measures regarding the prevention of relapse in CD.[58] Alternative preparations for omega 3 FA have also been studied, specifically seal oil, which is high in omega-3 FA comparing it to the cod liver. In this study, a tendency toward joint pain improvement in both groups was seen.[59] Yet another study compared seal oil to soy oil, which is rich in omega-6 FA and found that seal oil significantly reduced IBD-related joint pains in the short term.[60] ECCO states that omega-3 fatty acids might be beneficial in maintaining remission in CD but that high-quality data are limited and necessary.[13]

Traditional Chinese medicine (TCM) is based on the principles of yin and yang, which is the belief in balance and harmony within one's body. When this balance is off, Qi is blocked and we are at risk of disease. Various herbal agents fall within the TCM realm. In IBD, studies are limited but a retention enema composed of Chinese herbals found that there was improvement in symptoms, endoscopic and histologic disease in patients with IBD. This was hypothesized as a modality for disease treatment.[61] An opinion statement publication on TCM noted it to be popular among patients.[62] There are different herbs within the umbrella of TCM and several have been evaluated.

Boswellia serrata is a traditional Ayurvedic remedy with anti-inflammatory properties and data that show a positive correlation between the antioxidant activity and maintenance of the integrity and function of the intestinal epithelium.[63] In a RCT patients with underlying CD in remission were randomized to Boswelan or placebo for 52 weeks; unfortunately, the trial was terminated due to lack of efficacy. There was no advantage seen but overall Boswellia serrata extract was noted to be tolerable.[64]

Tripterygium wilfordii (GTW) is another TCM with anti-inflammatory and immunomodulatory effects. It can inhibit cytokines IL-1, IL-2, IL-6, and reduce TNF-alpha and NF-κB. Full understanding is unknown.[65] In a postoperative CD single-blinded study, GTW versus 5-ASA was evaluated over 52 weeks. Clinical and endoscopic recurrence was seen less commonly in the GTW group without serious adverse events and was thought to be superior to 5-ASA.[66] A similar study in CD over 52 weeks comparing GTW to 5-ASA found similar results in high-dose GTW, but no difference with low-dose GTW and placebo. It should be noted that more adverse effects were seen in the high-dose GTW. These did not lead to study withdrawal.[67] Finally, GTW versus azathioprine was studied for recurrence of postoperative CD. In this study, GTW was inferior to azathioprine at 52 weeks with higher rates of endoscopic recurrence and similar rates of clinical recurrence.[68]

Artemisia absinthium is commonly known as wormwood. It is used throughout the world for both its leaves and stems. It is thought to reduce inflammation and carcinogens.[69] An RCT study looked at patients with CD on steroids who received wormwood versus placebo. There was an improvement in steroid tapering among patients given wormwood. Patients given wormwood also had higher rates of clinical remission that extended to week 20. Findings suggest a steroid-tapering effect for wormwood.[70] In another study, the TNF-alpha suppression effect of wormwood was tested in a small subgroup of patients with CD and CDAI score of at least 200. All meds were continued and TNF-alpha levels were recorded with a greater score decrease in the wormwood group. Additionally, a positive mood effect was seen in the wormwood group compared with placebo.[71] These studies are small but give insight into a beneficial effect.

Daikenchuto (DKT) is a traditional Japanese Kampo medicine that has been used for postoperative ileus with clinical efficacy and ability to decrease CRP.[72] In a postoperative CD study, DKT was studied to prevent recurrent surgical need over 3 years in comparison to 5-ASA and azathioprine. There was a significantly lower reoperation rate in the DKT group and additional studies are necessary.[72]

Cannabis has also become increasingly popular within IBD in the form of medical marijuana. It is derived from Cannabis sativa with 2 major active compounds known as cannabidiol and θ-9-tetrahydrocannabinol (THC). This is a U.S. Schedule I substance and per federal law is illegal but individual states may allow it. It represents the most widely used recreational drug in the world and epidemiologic studies suggest up to 15% of patients with IBD use cannabis but studies are small and data are limited.[73] Previous authors have noted a lack of quality data discussing optimal dosing, mode of administration as well as questions regarding long-term side effects. Despite this public opinion regards cannabis as a harmless drug and more importantly one with medical efficacy. Data are necessary to better understand cannabis and its use in IBD.[73] ECCO currently states that the use of cannabis may be associated with a reduction of some symptoms in IBD but that there is no good evidence to show that it positively affects the course of disease.[13] The initial cannabis study was a retrospective observational study in CD and found improvement in PRO and need for additional medications. It was hypothesized as having a potentially positive effect but prospective studies were needed.[74] There are animal studies that have demonstrated an anti-inflammatory effect but without conversion into human patients with IBD. It was noted as of 2020 that there remain only 3 small placebo-controlled studies regarding the use of cannabis in active Crohn's disease.[75] Within these studies clinical improvement was seen without corresponding laboratory improvement. The expert opinion is: "Cannabis seems to have a therapeutic potential in IBD. This potential must not be neglected; however, cannabis research is still at a very early stage. The complexity of the plant and the diversity of different cannabis chemovars create an inherent difficulty in cannabis research. We need more studies investigating the effect of the various cannabis compounds. These effects can then be investigated in randomized placebo-controled clinical trials to fully explore the potential of cannabis treatment in IBD."[75]

Parasites

Whipworm is a parasite with a possible role in IBD treatment. It is understood that environmental factors which include helminths play a role in the development of IBD.[76] Whipworm or Trichuris suis ova is a nonpathogenic parasite. It has been studied in IBD in small clinical trials that have shown promise in inducing clinical remission[77] and possible prevention of the immune dysregulation that leads to ongoing disease.[78] That being said, harmful effects may limit use. A more recent RCT looked at the safety and tolerability of whipworm ova. Patients were given a single dose and followed over 14 days. The patients were followed over 6 months with no dose-dependent relationship seen and a single dose did not result in treatment-related side effects.[79]

Bovine colostrum (BC) is milk produced by female mammals for the first 3 days after parturition. Commercially produced colostrum is available in the form of powder, concentrate, lozenges, supplemented milk, beverages, yogurts, butter, and even chewing gums. That being said there are differences in quality, quantity, and bioavailability and the majority of the U.S. farms did not meet minimum immunologic and bacteriologic criteria.[80] BC use in IBD has been of interest but there is limited data. There is currently no data on supplement BC in the CD patient population although a small study was conducted looking at BC enemas in UC.[81]

Vitamins and Minerals

Vitamin D is a well-studied and often coprescribed vitamin in IBD-related care. Considerable evidence exists that associates low vitamin D levels with degrees of inflammation. Deficiency in IBD ranges from 10% to 75% of patients[82] and cause has been associated with reduced physical activity, decreases in diet, malabsorption, and impairments in conversion.[82] There are significantly higher rates of low serum levels of the major circulating form of vitamin D, 25-hydroxyvitamin D (25-OH-D) in IBD with some seasonal association seen.[83] It is thought that supplementation with vitamin D may prevent the onset of IBD although once the diagnosis is made it may help to decrease disease severity.[83] In one pilot study, patients with active UC and low vitamin D were given oral liquid supplementation over 12 weeks and results found that clinical disease activity consistently declined, but inflammatory markers were not changed..[84] A pilot study in CD looked at the dose of vitamin D necessary to raise levels above 40 ng/mL. The study found that when low levels were increased to the desired level, CDAI scores reduced and QoL scores improved significantly but no significant lab changes were seen suggesting that vitamin D restoration may be useful in CD.[85] A systematic review and meta-analysis looked at 14 eligible studies of both IBD cases and controls. In IBD there were 64% higher odds of vitamin D deficiency when compared with controls. Additionally, it was noted that latitude did not influence results.[86] A study evaluating vitamin and zinc deficiency found that serum 25(OH)D levels may be useful to characterize disease status.[87] Ongoing RCTs are necessary to explore deficiency and its role in disease.

Vitamins B12 and folate represent another significant deficiency seen in IBD, especially given the location in the terminal ileum for which these nutrients are absorbed. A systematic review and meta-analysis found that folate concentration was lower in control patients but no difference was seen with serum B12. Ultimately it was concluded that folate deficiency may be linked to IBD but causation was not proven.[88]

Vitamin K deficiency has been seen in IBD but its role remains unclear. In a recent cross-sectional study vitamin K deficiency was assessed for a correlation to disease activity in pediatric patients with IBD. Results found that vitamin K deficiency was more common with higher disease activity in CD and less common in infliximab-treated patients but further research is necessary.[89] It is also noted that in vitro data suggest a protective role for vitamin K and participants in the Framingham Offspring Study found that levels of vitamin K were inversely associated with inflammatory markers. This suggests a protective role for vitamin K that requires further study.[90]

Zinc is a mineral that has been shown to play a role in wound repair, tissue regeneration, and altered immune response. It is also proposed that increased proinflammatory cytokines and reactive oxygen species which are found in higher amounts in IBD are associated with underlying zinc deficiency. Thus, zinc supplementation can benefit patients with IBD. An IBD data registry looked at patients with a minimum of 2 zinc measurements and found that zinc deficiency was associated with increased risk of hospitalizations, surgeries, and disease-related complications, whereas zinc normalization resulted in improvement in the aforementioned outcomes.[91]

Probiotics

There is enormous commercial and patient-centric interest in the gut microbiome especially when it comes to IBD. Within this, prebiotics and probiotics are wide-accepted by patients without large degrees of evidence regarding specific species and formulations. The current literature has demonstrated alterations in gut microbiota in patients with IBD as well as in colitic animal models. There has also been promising on gut microbiota-based therapeutic approaches among animal models when it comes to therapeutic potential. Insufficient data and confusing results from previous studies have led to failures in our ability to clearly define the microbiome necessary to ameliorate disease and recommend a specific probiotic or prebiotic approach.[92] The American College of Gastroenterology (AGA) Clinical Practice Guidelines addressed the role of probiotics, specifically in the management of gastrointestinal disorders and ultimately did not recommend their use outside of a clinical trial as a result of knowledge gaps caused by low sample sizes, as well as study design and treatment heterogeneity.[93] Furthermore, ECCO states insufficient evidence to support the use of prebiotics, probiotics or both in patients with CD, either in the induction or the maintenance of remission.[13] Within CD there was no benefit of probiotics in inducing remission of active CD, preventing relapse of quiescent CD, or in preventing relapse of CD after surgically induced remission.[94] Within the CD studies lactobacillus has been studied but with nonfavorable outcomes. In one study of postop patients with CD those given placebo had less endoscopic recurrence with higher rates of clinical recurrence in the lactobacillus-treated group.[95] In another trial lactobacillus was given as adjunct treatment in pediatric cases whereby the disease was in remission and found no differences between groups.[96] In one additional study looking at postoperative recurrence in CD found a slight nonsignificant difference in the probiotic-treated group but overall recurrence did not differ.[97] Ultimately, more data are necessary to fully understand the utilization of probiotics in CD but initial studies were not promising.

Diet

Diet is an emerging area of research within the CD arena and with a plethora of options available for patients and little data to back it up its important that ongoing data evolve. The Diet to INducE Remission in Crohn's disease (DINE-CD) study was an RCT that looked at 2 different diets. These included the Specific Carbohydrate Diet (SCD) and the Mediterranean style diet. The goal was to see if these diets acted as a method to improve QoL and CD symptoms. The results of this study revealed that study participants on both diets had improvement and resolution of symptoms with 43.5% of

Mediterranean-style diet followers and 46.5% of SCD diet followers achieving symptomatic remission. Additional findings included improvement in fatigue, pain, sleep disturbance, and social isolation.

These diets were well tolerated but given the ease of the Mediterranean style diet this may be preferred for patients.[98]

SUMMARY

CAM therapy encompasses an enormous variety of treatment options and needs to be taken seriously given their overall patient-centric use and availability. There are limited data with large heterogeneity in what is available, which restricts our diagnostic and therapeutic understanding of their role in IBD and specifically within patients with CD. Furthermore, knowledge gaps exist with regard to overall safety and interactions with conventional therapies. The use of CAM therapies has been increasing with reports of more than half of all patients with IBD having tried some form of CAM therapy. The biggest conclusion we can currently gain with regards to CAM therapy is that this is a part of IBD culture now and into the future. Without well-designed and funded clinical studies to rely on, we leave ourselves vulnerable to the limitations of these therapies and the inability to regulate and give appropriate recommendations. Additionally, further research will allow health care providers the ability to educate and direct patients and families about the potential benefits and adverse effects of these therapies.

CLINICS CARE POINTS

- Mind-based therapy data show an overall improvement in QoL scores with the lack of corresponding evidence of improvement in inflammation and endoscopic appearance as well as limitations on availability.

- Body-based therapy data show improvement in QoL as well as improvement in inflammatory markers, disease state, and overall lifetime risk but may be limited due to patient capabilities and overall availability.

- Supplements are plentiful with large heterogeneity within trials and some safety concerns although some supplements, specifically curcumin, may induce maintain remission.

- Probiotics vary with regards to type and data are limited by the conflicting studies and altering formulations with more comprehensive data necessary

DISCLOSURE

The authors have nothing to disclose.

REFERENCES

1. Cheifetz AS, Gianotti R, Luber R, et al. Complementary and Alternative Medicines Used by Patients With Inflammatory Bowel Diseases. Gastroenterology 2017; 152(2):415–29.e15.
2. Fabian A, Rutka M, Ferenci T, et al. The use of complementary and alternative medicine is less frequent in patients with inflammatory bowel disease than in patients with other chronic gastrointestinal disorders. Gastroenterol Res Pract 2018; 2018:9137805.
3. Lin SC, Cheifetz AS. The Use of Complementary and Alternative Medicine in Patients With Inflammatory Bowel Disease. Gastroenterol Hepatol (N Y) 2018;14(7): 415–25.

4. Koning M, Ailabouni R, Gearry RB, et al. Use and Predictors of Oral Complementary and Alternative Medicine by Patients With Inflammatory Bowel Disease: A Population-Based, Case-Control Study. Inflamm Bowel Dis 2013;19(4):767–78.

5. Bertomoro P, Renna S, Cottone M, et al. Regional variations in the use of complementary and alternative medicines (CAM) for inflammatory bowel disease patients in Italy: an IG-IBD study. J Crohns Colitis 2010;4(3):291–300.

6. Mountifield R, Andrews JM, Mikocka-Walus A, et al. Doctor communication quality and Friends' attitudes influence complementary medicine use in inflammatory bowel disease. World J Gastroenterol 2015;21(12):3663–70.

7. Guan QD. A Comprehensive Review and Update on the Pathogenesis of Inflammatory Bowel Disease. J Immunol Res 2019;2019:7247238.

8. Ng SC, Shi HY, Hamidi N. Worldwide incidence and prevalence of inflammatory bowel disease in the 21st century: a systematic review of population-based studies (vol 390, pg 2769, 2018). Lancet 2020;396(10256):E56.

9. Park DI, Cha JM, Kim HS, et al. Predictive factors of complementary and alternative medicine use for patients with inflammatory bowel disease in Korea. Complement Ther Med 2014;22(1):87–93.

10. Mizrahi MC, Reicher-Atir R, Levy S, et al. Effects of guided imagery with relaxation training on anxiety and quality of life among patients with inflammatory bowel disease. Psychol Health 2012;27(12):1463–79.

11. Bernstein CN, Singh S, Graff LA, et al. A Prospective Population-Based Study of Triggers of Symptomatic Flares in IBD. Am J Gastroenterol 2010;105(9):1994–2002.

12. Peppas S, Pansieri C, Piovani D, et al. The Brain-Gut Axis: Psychological Functioning and Inflammatory Bowel Diseases. J Clin Med 2021;10(3).

13. Torres J, Ellul P, Langhorst J, et al. European Crohn's and Colitis Organisation Topical Review on Complementary Medicine and Psychotherapy in Inflammatory Bowel Disease. J Crohns Colitis 2019;13(6):673–685e.

14. Fiest KM, Hitchon CA, Bernstein CN, et al. Systematic review and meta-analysis of interventions for depression and anxiety in persons with rheumatoid arthritis. J Clin Rheumatol 2017;23(8):425–34.

15. Fiest KM, Bernstein CN, Walker JR, et al. Systematic review of interventions for depression and anxiety in persons with inflammatory bowel disease. BMC Res Notes 2016;9(1):404.

16. Segal JP, Chan H, Collins B, et al. Biofeedback in patients with ileoanal pouch dysfunction: a specialist centre experience. Scand J Gastroenterol 2018;53(6):665–9.

17. Vasant DH, Limdi JK, Solanki K, et al. Anorectal Dysfunction in Quiescent Inflammatory Bowel Disease: is there a role for biofeedback therapy? Gut 2016;65:A116.

18. Bennebroek Evertsz F, Bockting CL, Stokkers PC, et al. The effectiveness of cognitive behavioral therapy on the quality of life of patients with inflammatory bowel disease: multi-center design and study protocol (KL!C- study). BMC Psychiatry 2012;12:227.

19. Mikocka-Walus A, Bampton P, Hetzel D, et al. Cognitive-Behavioural Therapy for Inflammatory Bowel Disease: 24-Month data from a randomised controlled trial. Int J Behav Med 2017;24(1):127–35.

20. Gracie DJ, Irvine AJ, Sood R, et al. Effect of psychological therapy on disease activity, psychological comorbidity, and quality of life in inflammatory bowel disease: a systematic review and meta-analysis. Lancet Gastroenterol Hepatol 2017;2(3):189–99.

21. Artom M, Czuber-Dochan W, Sturt J, et al. Cognitive-behavioural therapy for the management of inflammatory bowel disease-fatigue: a feasibility randomised controlled trial. Pilot Feasibility Stud 2019;5:145.
22. Knowles SR, Monshat K, Castle DJ. The efficacy and methodological challenges of psychotherapy for adults with inflammatory bowel disease: a review. Inflamm Bowel Dis 2013;19(12):2704–15.
23. Neilson K, Ftanou M, Monshat K, et al. A Controlled Study of a Group Mindfulness Intervention for Individuals Living With Inflammatory Bowel Disease. Inflamm Bowel Dis 2016;22(3):694–701.
24. Gerbarg PL, Jacob VE, Stevens L, et al. The Effect of Breathing, Movement, and Meditation on Psychological and Physical Symptoms and Inflammatory Biomarkers in Inflammatory Bowel Disease: a randomized controlled trial. Inflamm Bowel Dis 2015;21(12):2886–96.
25. Jedel S, Hoffman A, Merriman P, et al. A randomized controlled trial of mindfulness-based stress reduction to prevent flare-up in patients with inactive ulcerative colitis. Digestion 2014;89(2):142–55.
26. Timmer A, Preiss JC, Motschall E, et al. Psychological interventions for treatment of inflammatory bowel disease. Cochrane Database Syst Rev 2011;(2): CD006913.
27. Moser G. The role of hypnotherapy for the treatment of inflammatory bowel diseases. Expert Rev Gastroenterol Hepatol 2014;8(6):601–6.
28. Cohen MM, Elliott F, Oates L, et al. Do wellness tourists get well? An Observational Study of Multiple Dimensions of Health and Well-Being After a Week-Long Retreat. J Altern Complement Med 2017;23(2):140–8.
29. Naidoo D, Schembri A, Cohen M. The health impact of residential retreats: a systematic review. BMC Complement Altern Med 2018;18(1):8.
30. Sharma P, Poojary G, Dwivedi SN, et al. Effect of Yoga-Based Intervention in Patients with Inflammatory Bowel Disease. Int J Yoga Therap 2015;25(1):101–12.
31. Gleeson M, Bishop NC, Stensel DJ, et al. The anti-inflammatory effects of exercise: mechanisms and implications for the prevention and treatment of disease. Nat Rev Immunol 2011;11(9):607–15.
32. Robinson RJ, Krzywicki T, Almond L, et al. Effect of a low-impact exercise program on bone mineral density in Crohn's disease: a randomized controlled trial. Gastroenterology 1998;115(1):36–41.
33. Engels M, Cross RK, Long MD. Exercise in patients with inflammatory bowel diseases: current perspectives. Clin Exp Gastroenterol 2018;11:1–11.
34. Bernstein CN, Kraut A, Blanchard JF, et al. The relationship between inflammatory bowel disease and socioeconomic variables. Am J Gastroenterol 2001;96(7): 2117–25.
35. Khalili H, Ananthakrishnan AN, Konijeti GG, et al. Physical activity and risk of inflammatory bowel disease: prospective study from the Nurses' Health Study cohorts. BMJ 2013;347:f6633.
36. Persson PG, Leijonmarck CE, Bernell O, et al. Risk indicators for inflammatory bowel disease. Int J Epidemiol 1993;22(2):268–72.
37. Wang Q, Xu KQ, Qin XR, et al. Association between physical activity and inflammatory bowel disease risk: A meta-analysis. Dig Liver Dis 2016;48(12):1425–31.
38. Jones PD, Kappelman MD, Martin CF, et al. Exercise decreases risk of future active disease in patients with inflammatory bowel disease in remission. Inflamm Bowel Dis 2015;21(5):1063–71.

39. O'Reardon JP, Cristancho P, Peshek AD. Vagus nerve stimulation (VNS) and treatment of depression: to the brainstem and beyond. Psychiatry (Edgmont) 2006; 3(5):54–63.
40. Payne SC, Furness JB, Burns O, et al. Anti-inflammatory effects of abdominal vagus nerve stimulation on experimental intestinal inflammation. Front Neurosci 2019;13:418.
41. Sinniger V, Pellissier S, Fauvelle F, et al. A 12-month pilot study outcomes of vagus nerve stimulation in Crohn's disease. Neurogastroenterol Motil 2020;32(10): e13911.
42. Bao C, Wang D, Liu P, et al. Effect of Electro-Acupuncture and Moxibustion on Brain Connectivity in Patients with Crohn's Disease: A Resting-State fMRI Study. Front Hum Neurosci 2017;11:559.
43. Bao CH, Zhao JM, Liu HR, et al. Randomized controlled trial: Moxibustion and acupuncture for the treatment of Crohn's disease. World J Gastroenterol 2014; 20(31):11000–11.
44. Joos S, Brinkhaus B, Maluche C, et al. Acupuncture and moxibustion in the treatment of active Crohn's disease: a randomized controlled study. Digestion 2004; 69(3):131–9.
45. Lee DH, Kim JI, Lee MS, et al. Moxibustion for ulcerative colitis: a systematic review and meta-analysis. BMC Gastroenterol 2010;10:36.
46. Ji J, Lu Y, Liu H, et al. Acupuncture and moxibustion for inflammatory bowel diseases: a systematic review and meta-analysis of randomized controlled trials. Evid Based Complement Alternat Med 2013;2013:158352.
47. Vecchi Brumatti L, Marcuzzi A, Tricarico PM, et al. Curcumin and inflammatory bowel disease: potential and limits of innovative treatments. Molecules 2014; 19(12):21127–53.
48. Salh B, Assi K, Templeman V, et al. Curcumin attenuates DNB-induced murine colitis. Am J Physiol Gastrointest Liver Physiol 2003;285(1):G235–43.
49. Ukil A, Maity S, Karmakar S, et al. Curcumin, the major component of food flavour turmeric, reduces mucosal injury in trinitrobenzene sulphonic acid-induced colitis. Br J Pharmacol 2003;139(2):209–18.
50. Sugimoto K, Hanai H, Tozawa K, et al. Curcumin prevents and ameliorates trinitrobenzene sulfonic acid-induced colitis in mice. Gastroenterology 2002;123(6): 1912–22.
51. Schneider A, Hossain I, VanderMolen J, et al. Comparison of remicade to curcumin for the treatment of Crohn's disease: a systematic review. Complement Ther Med 2017;33:32–8.
52. Gupta SC, Patchva S, Aggarwal BB. Therapeutic roles of curcumin: lessons learned from clinical trials. AAPS J 2013;15(1):195–218.
53. Cabre E, Manosa M, Gassull MA. Omega-3 fatty acids and inflammatory bowel diseases - a systematic review. Br J Nutr 2012;107 Suppl 2:S240–52.
54. Nielsen AA, Jørgensen LG, Nielsen JN, et al. Omega-3 fatty acids inhibit an increase of proinflammatory cytokines in patients with active Crohn's disease compared with omega-6 fatty acids. Aliment Pharmacol Ther 2005;22(11–12): 1121–8.
55. Eivindson M, Grønbaek H, Nielsen JN, et al. Insulin-like growth factors (IGFs) and IGF binding proteins in active Crohn's disease treated with omega-3 or omega-6 fatty acids and corticosteroids. Scand J Gastroenterol 2005;40(10):1214–21.
56. Lev-Tzion R, Griffiths AM, Leder O, et al. Omega 3 fatty acids (fish oil) for maintenance of remission in Crohn's disease. Cochrane Database Syst Rev 2014;(2): CD006320.

57. Turner D, Shah PS, Steinhart AH, et al. Maintenance of remission in inflammatory bowel disease using omega-3 fatty acids (fish oil): a systematic review and meta-analyses. Inflamm Bowel Dis 2011;17(1):336–45.
58. Feagan BG, Sandborn WJ, Mittmann U, et al. Omega-3 free fatty acids for the maintenance of remission in Crohn disease: the EPIC Randomized Controlled Trials. JAMA 2008;299(14):1690–7.
59. Brunborg LA, Madland TM, Lind RA, et al. Effects of short-term oral administration of dietary marine oils in patients with inflammatory bowel disease and joint pain: a pilot study comparing seal oil and cod liver oil. Clin Nutr 2008;27(4):614–22.
60. Bjorkkjaer T, Brunborg LA, Arslan G, et al. Reduced joint pain after short-term duodenal administration of seal oil in patients with inflammatory bowel disease: comparison with soy oil. Scand J Gastroenterol 2004;39(11):1088–94.
61. Ling XH, Yu X, Kong DJ, et al. Treatment of inflammatory bowel disease with Chinese drugs administered by both oral intake and retention enema. Chin J Integr Med 2010;16(3):222–8.
62. Salaga M, Zatorski H, Sobczak M, et al. Chinese herbal medicines in the treatment of IBD and colorectal cancer: a review. Curr Treat Options Oncol 2014;15(3):405–20.
63. Catanzaro D, Rancan S, Orso G, et al. Boswellia serrata preserves intestinal epithelial barrier from oxidative and inflammatory damage. PLoS One 2015;10(5):e0125375.
64. Holtmeier W, Zeuzem S, Preiss J, et al. Randomized, placebo-controlled, double-blind trial of Boswellia serrata in maintaining remission of Crohn's disease: good safety profile but lack of efficacy. Inflamm Bowel Dis 2011;17(2):573–82.
65. Fangxiao M, Yifan K, Jihong Z, et al. Effect of Tripterygium wilfordii Polycoride on the NOXs-ROS-NLRP3 Inflammasome Signaling Pathway in Mice with Ulcerative Colitis. Evid Based Complement Alternat Med 2019;2019:9306283.
66. Ren J, Wu X, Liao N, et al. Prevention of postoperative recurrence of Crohn's disease: tripterygium wilfordii polyglycoside versus mesalazine. J Int Med Res 2013;41(1):176–87.
67. Sun J, Shen X, Dong J, et al. Tripterygium wilfordii Hook F as Maintenance Treatment for Crohn's Disease. Am J Med Sci 2015;350(5):345–51.
68. Zhu W, Li Y, Gong J, et al. Tripterygium wilfordii Hook. f. versus azathioprine for prevention of postoperative recurrence in patients with Crohn's disease: a randomized clinical trial. Dig Liver Dis 2015;47(1):14–9.
69. Algieri F, Rodriguez-Nogales A, Rodriguez-Cabezas ME, et al. Botanical Drugs as an Emerging Strategy in Inflammatory Bowel Disease: a review. Mediators Inflamm 2015;2015:179616.
70. Omer B, Krebs S, Omer H, et al. Steroid-sparing effect of wormwood (Artemisia absinthium) in Crohn's disease: a double-blind placebo-controlled study. Phytomedicine 2007;14(2–3):87–95.
71. Krebs S, Omer TN, Omer B. Wormwood (Artemisia absinthium) suppresses tumour necrosis factor alpha and accelerates healing in patients with Crohn's disease - A controlled clinical trial. Phytomedicine 2010;17(5):305–9.
72. Kanazawa A, Sako M, Takazoe M, et al. Daikenchuto, a traditional Japanese herbal medicine, for the maintenance of surgically induced remission in patients with Crohn's disease: a retrospective analysis of 258 patients. Surg Today 2014;44(8):1506–12.
73. Naftali T, Dor M. Cannabis for the Treatment of Inflammatory Bowel Disease: a true medicine or a false promise? Rambam Maimonides Med J 2020;11(1).

74. Naftali T, Lev LB, Yablecovitch D, et al. Treatment of Crohn's disease with cannabis: an observational study. Isr Med Assoc J 2011;13(8):455–8.
75. Naftali T. An overview of cannabis based treatment in Crohn's disease. Expert Rev Gastroenterol Hepatol 2020;14(4):253–7.
76. Huang X, Zeng LR, Chen FS, et al. Trichuris suis ova therapy in inflammatory bowel disease: a meta-analysis. Medicine (Baltimore) 2018;97(34):e12087.
77. Summers RW, Elliott DE, Qadir K, et al. Trichuris suis seems to be safe and possibly effective in the treatment of inflammatory bowel disease. Am J Gastroenterol 2003;98(9):2034–41.
78. Yazdanbakhsh M, Kremsner PG, van Ree R. Allergy, parasites, and the hygiene hypothesis. Science 2002;296(5567):490–4.
79. Sandborn WJ, Elliott DE, Weinstock J, et al. Randomised clinical trial: the safety and tolerability of Trichuris suis ova in patients with Crohn's disease. Aliment Pharmacol Ther 2013;38(3):255–63.
80. Sienkiewicz M, Szymańska P, Fichna J. Supplementation of Bovine Colostrum in Inflammatory Bowel Disease: Benefits and Contraindications. Adv Nutr 2021; 12(2):533–45.
81. Khan Z, Macdonald C, Wicks AC, et al. Use of the 'nutriceutical', bovine colostrum, for the treatment of distal colitis: results from an initial study. Aliment Pharmacol Ther 2002;16(11):1917–22.
82. Holick MF. Vitamin D deficiency. N Engl J Med 2007;357(3):266–81.
83. Fletcher J, Cooper SC, Ghosh S, et al. The Role of Vitamin D in Inflammatory Bowel Disease: mechanism to management. Nutrients 2019;11(5).
84. Garg M, Rosella O, Rosella G, et al. Evaluation of a 12-week targeted vitamin D supplementation regimen in patients with active inflammatory bowel disease. Clin Nutr 2018;37(4):1375–82.
85. Yang L, Weaver V, Smith JP, et al. Therapeutic effect of vitamin d supplementation in a pilot study of Crohn's patients. Clin Transl Gastroenterol 2013;4:e33.
86. Del Pinto R, Pietropaoli D, Chandar AK, et al. Association between inflammatory bowel disease and vitamin d deficiency: a systematic review and meta-analysis. Inflamm Bowel Dis 2015;21(11):2708–17.
87. Mechie NC, Mavropoulou E, Ellenrieder V, et al. Serum vitamin D but not zinc levels are associated with different disease activity status in patients with inflammatory bowel disease. Medicine (Baltimore) 2019;98(15):e15172.
88. Pan Y, Liu Y, Guo H, et al. Associations between Folate and Vitamin B12 Levels and inflammatory bowel disease: a meta-analysis. Nutrients 2017;9(4).
89. Nowak JK, Grzybowska-Chlebowczyk U, Landowski P, et al. Prevalence and correlates of vitamin K deficiency in children with inflammatory bowel disease. Sci Rep 2014;4:4768.
90. Shea MK, Booth SL, Massaro JM, et al. Vitamin K and vitamin D status: associations with inflammatory markers in the Framingham Offspring Study. Am J Epidemiol 2008;167(3):313–20.
91. Siva S, Rubin DT, Gulotta G, et al. Zinc Deficiency is Associated with Poor Clinical Outcomes in Patients with Inflammatory Bowel Disease. Inflamm Bowel Dis 2017; 23(1):152–7.
92. Khan I, Ullah N, Zha L, et al. Alteration of Gut Microbiota in Inflammatory Bowel Disease (IBD): Cause or Consequence? IBD Treatment Targeting the Gut Microbiome. Pathogens 2019;8(3):126.
93. Su GL, Ko CW, Bercik P, et al. AGA clinical practice guidelines on the role of probiotics in the management of gastrointestinal disorders. Gastroenterology 2020; 159(2):697–705.

94. Derwa Y, Gracie DJ, Hamlin PJ, et al. Systematic review with meta-analysis: the efficacy of probiotics in inflammatory bowel disease. Aliment Pharmacol Ther 2017;46(4):389–400.
95. Prantera C, Scribano ML, Falasco G, et al. Ineffectiveness of probiotics in preventing recurrence after curative resection for Crohn's disease: a randomised controlled trial with Lactobacillus GG. Gut 2002;51(3):405–9.
96. Bousvaros A, Guandalini S, Baldassano RN, et al. A randomized, double-blind trial of Lactobacillus GG versus placebo in addition to standard maintenance therapy for children with Crohn's disease. Inflamm Bowel Dis 2005;11(9):833–9.
97. Marteau P, Lémann M, Seksik P, et al. Ineffectiveness of Lactobacillus johnsonii LA1 for prophylaxis of postoperative recurrence in Crohn's disease: a randomised, double blind, placebo controlled GETAID trial. Gut 2006;55(6):842–7.
98. Lewis JD, Sandler RS, Brotherton C, et al. A randomized trial comparing the specific carbohydrate diet to a mediterranean diet in adults with Crohn's Disease. Gastroenterology 2021;161(3):837.e9.

Surgical Management of Crohn's Disease

Valery Vilchez, MD[a], Amy L. Lightner, MD[a,b,c,d,e],*

KEYWORDS

- Crohn's disease • Resection • Strictureplasty • Bowel conservation

KEY POINTS

- Surgery for Crohn's disease is directed at symptom relief and is an adjunct to maximal medical therapy.
- Bowel preservation is a key in Crohn's disease surgery.
- Patients are arriving to the operating room with more advanced disease activity and a longer duration of immunosuppression.
- A multidisciplinary approach is imperative for patients with medically refractory Crohn's disease because of the increasing complexity of patient and medical management.

Progression of transmural inflammation through the bowel wall, a defining characteristic feature of Crohn's disease (CD), results in intra-abdominal abscess formation, enteroentero or enterocutaneous fistula, and intestinal perforation, whereas recurrent episodes of focal inflammations leads to stricture formation. Most operations are performed to address the bowel wall damage created by one of these complications. Often, the surgeon may need to address all these manifestations during a single operation. An important principle to remember is that surgery is not curative but is rather an adjunct to maximal medical therapy. It is important to always try to minimize the amount of bowel resected assuming that the patient may require a subsequent bowel resection in the future.

INDICATIONS FOR SURGERY

Despite making significant advances in medical therapy, up to 70% of patients eventually require an operation.[1,2] The leading indication for surgery is disease that is

---

[a] Department of Colorectal Surgery, Digestive Disease Surgical Institute, Cleveland Clinic, Cleveland, OH, USA; [b] Center for Regenerative Medicine and Surgery, Cleveland Clinic, 9500 Euclid Avenue, Cleveland, OH, USA; [c] Digestive Disease and Surgery Institute, Cleveland Clinic, 9500 Euclid Avenue, Cleveland, OH, USA; [d] Lerner Research Institute, Cleveland Clinic, 9500 Euclid Avenue, Cleveland, OH, USA; [e] Center for Immunotherapy, Cleveland Clinic, 9500 Euclid Avenue, Cleveland, OH, USA
* Corresponding author. Cleveland Clinic, 9500 Euclid Avenue, Cleveland, OH 44195.
E-mail address: Lightna@ccf.org

Gastroenterol Clin N Am 51 (2022) 353–367
https://doi.org/10.1016/j.gtc.2021.12.010
0889-8553/22/© 2021 Elsevier Inc. All rights reserved.

refractory to medical management. The end result presents as obstruction, fistulae, abscesses, bleeding, or perforation.[3] It is important to remember that a multidisciplinary approach is central to the management of this patient population. The patient, gastroenterologist, and surgeon should be in close communication as the patient's disease severity increases and surgery becomes a potential solution. Before exhausting all medical options, a patient should at least have had a surgical consultation to understand the risks and benefits of an operation versus increased medical management with associated parenteral nutrition to optimize the management. Ideally, a consensus is reached by all parties involved before the patient is taken to the operating room. Once the decision is made to proceed with an operation, careful preoperative planning should ensure to optimize patients' perioperative outcomes.

PREOPERATIVE CONSIDERATIONS

The decision to operate is made in the context of the patient's preoperative nutritional status, immunosuppressive regimen, and controlled source of infection. The patient's nutritional status is often compromised by severe disease and long-standing poor nutrition. Total parenteral nutrition may be indicated if the patient is severely malnourished to achieve improvement in wound healing and prevention of anastomotic leaks.[4]

Evidence regarding the impact of preoperative exposure to biologics on surgical outcomes remains controversial and difficult to completely discern. Several studies have now reported an increased risk and no increased risk of infectious and general complications with preoperative exposure to an anti–tumor necrosis factor-α.[5–12] Overall, it seems that biologics may not mechanistically result in postoperative morbidity, but that rather they are a marker of disease severity and are an additional factor to consider when considering the optimal timing of surgery or need for diversion. Although necessary for treatment, these medications can impair wound healing and increase the rate of postoperative infectious complications.[8–12] Preoperative steroids are known to increase perioperative complications[10]; therefore, an attempt should be done to taper the steroids to the lowest possible dose without exacerbating the patient's symptoms and hold biologics agents 1 month before surgery.

Patients with abscesses should be drained percutaneously before going to the operating room, unless contraindicated because of need for emergent surgery. For intra-abdominal abscesses, adequate drainage may obviate surgery altogether; if not, it at least minimizes the degree of intra-abdominal inflammation allowing for a more limited bowel resection.[13,14] If infection or abscesses are present at the time of the operation, the surgeon should consider postoperative antibiotic therapy and delayed closure of open operative incisions.

Once it is decided that the patient will proceed with surgery the surgical plan should incorporate detailed information from imaging, endoscopy, and prior operative reports. Cross-sectional imaging with computed tomography or magnetic resonance enterography provides important information about the distribution of disease, undrained collections, preoperative anatomy including localization of fistulizing disease, and an estimate of remaining small bowel length.[15]

A final important step before taking a patient to the operating room is a discussion regarding the potential need of diversion. Because anxiety around stoma formation is common among patients with CD, early comprehensive education and support from an enterostomal therapist is important. It is also important to consider preoperative stoma marking if the patient has any suspicion of requiring a stoma, especially in complex reoperative CD where unexpected intraoperative findings or technical difficulties may mandate stoma creation.

OPERATIVE CONSIDERATIONS

Once patient optimization and preoperative planning are completed, the initial operation for CD should focus on bowel preservation, careful measurement and description of remaining bowel, how to maximize a minimally invasive approach, and prepare for subsequent operations after the index operation.

Laparoscopic surgery is ideal for patients with CD, a young cohort with high lifetime potential need for reoperation. Both randomized and nonrandomized studies have demonstrated safety and decreased morbidity and mortality with laparoscopic versus open resection in patients with CD.[16–21] Laparoscopic surgery has shown decreased length of stay, shorter time to return of bowel function, decreased cost, improved postoperative complication rate, and decreased small bowel obstructions (35% vs 11%) for small bowel and ileocolonic CD.[16–24] Patient selection is again important. A thickened mesentery, fistulizing disease, and phlegmon surrounding abscess cavities present challenges to safely performing a case laparoscopically. Thus, again, patient selection and intraoperative decision making becomes key.

Margin status used to be a more controversial topic in CD surgery. Retrospective reviews had showed disease-free margins of 4 cm or "radical" disease-free margins of 10 cm compared with placebo had a lower recurrence rates. However, later larger studies[25] and prospective studies[26] showed no difference in recurrence rate. Fazio and colleagues[26] evaluated recurrence in 131 ileocolectomy patients randomized to undergo resections with proximal margins either 2 or 12 cm from the macroscopically diseased tissue followed up for median of 56 months. Clinical recurrence was demonstrated in 33% versus 29% of those with limited and extended resections, respectively, and no relationship was found between microscopic CD found at the resection margin and disease recurrence. The standard practice today is to resect all gross macroscopically involved bowel without any particular gross margin length to preserve as much bowel length as possible. Following bowel resection, careful measurement and description of remaining bowel should be performed for any potential future intervention.

The concept of extended mesenteric excision is currently being evaluated in two randomized controlled trials given the promising retrospective findings that performing an extended mesenteric excision reduces postoperative recurrence rates.[27,28] Coffey and colleagues[27] evaluated the role of the mesentery in ileocolic CD. Surgical recurrence rates were compared between two cohorts: Cohort A underwent conventional ileocolic resection where the mesentery was divided flush with the intestine, whereas Cohort B underwent resection that included excision of the mesentery. Surgical technique was an independent determinant of outcome ($P = .007$). The authors demonstrated that advanced mesenteric disease predicted increased surgical recurrence (hazard ratio, 4.7; 95% confidence interval, 1.71–13.01; $P = .003$).[27]

Considerations in Stricturing Phenotype

Indications for an operation in the setting of stricturing CD include persistent obstructive symptoms that do not resolve with maximal escalation of medical therapy, chronic steroid use, weight loss, or the need for chronic pain medications.[1,2,10] Repeated episodes of inflammation, remodeling, and scarring of the bowel wall occur more often in small bowel than the colon. Regardless of the location, the normal pliable tissue is replaced with thickened nondistensible segments that narrow the lumen. On initial exploration in the setting of known obstructive disease, the entire bowel should be examined for any evidence of disease. Obvious strictures should be marked with sutures. If there are any questionable areas of narrowing during visual and tactile examination of the bowel, a sizing device is run through the small bowel to assess diameter and distensibility. The length of the stricture, number of strictures, number of prior operations, and remaining small bowel length all contribute to the intraoperative decision making of bowel resection versus strictureplasty. At an initial operation, a long segment stricture may be resected if the remaining small bowel looks healthy. However, if there are multiple segments or the remaining small bowel has areas of narrowing, strictureplasty should be considered because of the concern for short bowel as an outcome.

Considerations in Fistulizing Phenotype

Ongoing transmural inflammation can result in fistula formation between loops of bowel, bowel to bladder, bowel to abdominal wall, or bowel to any other structure or organ in the abdomen and pelvis. Historically, intra-abdominal CD fistulas were treated with bowel rest, intravenous nutrition, proximal diversion, and occasional resection. The introduction of infliximab in 1998 changed the paradigm of operative indication given its efficacy in closing abdominal wall and perianal fistulas.[29] The initial multicenter, double-blind, randomized, placebo-controlled trial to look at the efficacy of infliximab in treating CD fistulas included 94 patients with draining abdominal or perineal fistulas. The authors reported nearly 55% of all patients had closure of all fistulas and nearly 70% had a significant reduction in the number of draining fistulas.[29] In the follow-up trial of long-term outcomes (54 weeks of follow-up), 36% of patients had complete absence of fistulas at 1 year compared with 19% in the placebo group.[30] In another more recent study including 48 patients with CD with enterocutaneous fistulas alone, the authors found a third of patients achieved closure within 3 months of infliximab initiation.[31] Therefore, for fistulizing disease patients now undergo a 3-month trial of infliximab in hopes of achieving remission and avoiding surgical intervention.

The type of operation performed depends on the anatomic location of the fistula and degree of associated sepsis. For enterocutaneous fistula, the goal is to resect the bowel and skin communicating via the fistula. This should only be attempted once the patient has exhausted maximal medical therapy, the skin surrounding the fistula is soft and pliable, sepsis has been controlled, and the patient is nutritionally optimized. Preoperative planning for potential mesh placement with loss of abdominal domain is necessary. When resecting the small bowel, the consistent principles of bowel preservation should be kept in mind. The bowel is resected often with a primary anastomosis, and the skin and abdominal wall are excised back to healthy tissue. If the abdominal wall cannot be closed, mesh is inserted. Prosthetic material, such as Prolene or Gortex, is contraindicated because of infection risk, but biologic meshes, now abundantly available, are used. The mesh should be placed as an underlay with normal surrounding tissue, and drains placed under any flaps to prevent seroma formation. Enteroentero fistulas may not be clinically significant unless a large segment of bowel is bypassed. If found preoperatively, preoperative planning should include imaging to best delineate the anatomy before an operation. When an operation is undertaken, often only one segment of bowel is actively involved with CD, whereas the other is a bystander. When this is seen, the actively inflamed segment with fistula should be resected, whereas the other is repaired primarily following fistula take down. This allows for increased bowel preservation with minimal morbidity and mortality.[32]

Considerations in Inflammatory Phenotype

In the setting of segmental medically refractory colitis, patients should also be approached with the same bowel-preserving perspective unless there is multifocal dysplasia or malignancy, in which case subtotal colectomy (STC) or total proctocolectomy should be considered. No studies have shown the need to resect to histologically negative margins.[33,34] Thus, in the setting of segmental colonic colitis, it is recommended to perform excision and primary anastomosis of the grossly affected segment. At the time of surgery, a flexible sigmoidoscope or colonoscope should be available in case the extent of mucosal disease should be evaluated before making a primary anastomosis. Following surgery, resumption of CD medications remains nonstandardized. If, at the time of resection, a significant burden of disease was noted, biologics may be resumed 2 to 4 weeks following surgery.[10,12]

In the case of rectal-sparing Crohn's colitis, two options are available: STC with ileorectal anastomosis (IRA), or total proctocolectomy with end ileostomy.[35,36] In the case of rectal-sparing Crohn's colitis, STC with IRA is safely performed with nearly 70% still functioning at 5 years. When the rectum is not spared, and medical management has been exhausted, total proctocolectomy and end ileostomy are performed.[37] In patients with known preoperative CD, who are motivated to maintain intestinal continuity with a clear understanding of the potential increased risk of recurrent disease, ileal pouch–anal anastomosis construction is feasible and may have functional outcomes equivalent to the outcomes of patients with ulcerative colitis (UC). Even in highly selected patients with CD, pouch failure rates remain higher than in patients with UC, but lower than patients who develop CD in the years after ileal pouch–anal anastomosis.[38]

In patients with isolated proctitis, two options remain. Either the patient may be diverted with a loop ileostomy and medical therapy maximized, or the patient may be offered a proctectomy. In the patient with significant perianal disease, in which an abdominal perineal resection would leave a significant perianal defect, a combination of these surgical approaches may be used. A diversion may first be performed to quiet and minimize the perianal fistulizing disease, followed by a proctectomy with closure of the anus and ability to retain the sphincter complex in the anal canal. Unfortunately, for patients diverted for severe perianal disease with associated proctitis, the stomal reversal rate is only 22%, even in the era of biologic therapy; for proctitis alone the stomal reversal rate is slightly improved at 50%. The most important factors associated with stoma reversal are the presence of proctitis and number of prior setons placed, reflecting the severity of perianal disease.[39] Although diversion may be attempted, in most patients with severe proctitis, proctectomy is eventually required. Without colonic involvement or neoplasia, the colon may be preserved in this patient population. A retrospective outcome analysis of 10 consecutive patients who underwent intersphincteric proctectomy with end-colostomy for refractory distal and perianal CD with normal proximal colon was recently performed. The authors showed that intersphincteric proctectomy with colostomy seems to be an ineffective surgery for perianal CD with coexisting proctitis and results in a high risk of recurrence of the disease in the remaining colon.[40]

Type of Anastomosis

Basic principles of bowel anastomosis should be maintained when performing any anastomosis in CD. The anastomosis should be free of tension, with adequate blood flow, and lack of contamination of the field. The type of anastomosis, handsewn versus stapled, and configuration of a side-to-side versus end-to-end have been widely studied without definitive preference in terms of leak or recurrence rate in patients with CD.[41,42]

Although no anastomotic type has been found to be superior to another in patients with CD,[41–44] some principles should still be applied individually to each case. The first is bowel size discrepancy. In the setting of significant size discrepancy, an end-to-end anastomosis may be more challenging to perform than a side-to-side. Early postoperative outcomes are comparable with regard to anastomotic leak rate and surgical site infection.[44] The second is staple height. There are two staple sizes: 3.6 mm and 4.8 mm. When the bowel wall is thickened, a 4.8-mm staple height may be best for the bowel wall, but at the expense of decreased hemostasis achieved compared with the 3.6-mm stapler. Bowel wall thickness and hemostasis must be weighed intraoperatively. Third, the evaluation of disease recurrence associated with the type of anastomosis performed becomes important.[45] A multicenter randomized study of end-to-end versus side-to-side found equivalent endoscopic recurrence (42.5% vs 37.9%; $P = .55$) and a symptomatic recurrence rate (21.9% vs 22.7%; $P = .92$) in the end-to-end compared with side-to-side group 12 months postresection.[41] To date, none of the commonly performed anastomotic techniques are favored with regard to recurrence of CD at the anastomotic site.

The Kono-S anastomosis was developed to potentially minimize risk of recurrence (**Fig. 1**). This technique uses a linear stapler-cutter to transversely divide the tissue for resection. The corners of the two stapled lines are sutured together and antimesenteric longitudinal enterotomies are created on both sides. The enterotomies are then closed transversely in two layers resulting in an antimesenteric functional end-to-end anastomosis. This technique has shown promise in a small cohort of 18 patients, 43% of whom have undergone follow-up endoscopic surveillance with an average Rutgeerts score of 0.7 (0–3) at a mean of 6.8 months.[46] More recently, the first randomized controlled trial comparing Kono-S anastomosis and standard anastomosis in 79 patients with CD was completed. The authors demonstrated a significant reduction in postoperative endoscopic and clinical recurrence rate for patients who underwent Kono-S anastomosis at 24 months.[47]

The nature of the stricture and the amount of the remaining bowel are key factors in determining whether a strictureplasty is appropriate. Strictureplasty may be performed at any place along the length of the bowel including the duodenum, jejunum, ileum, and rarely even the colon. Strictureplasty is not appropriate if the segment involves a bowel perforation or an extensive inflammatory phlegmon.

The first reported strictureplasty for the treatment of CD was by Lee and Papaioannou in 1982.[48] Since then, many techniques for strictureplasty have been described, each dependent on the length of the stricture, bowel diameter, and multifocality of

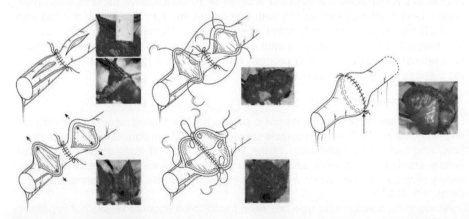

Fig. 1. Kono-S anastomosis.

the disease process. More surgeons are advocating the use of strictureplasty in place of resection for first time ileocolic disease.[49,50]

For strictures less than 4 to 5 cm in length, a Heineke-Mikulicz technique is used, opening the stricture longitudinally and the closing transversely (**Fig. 2**). Two sutures (3–0 either nonabsorbable or absorbable) are placed at the midpoint of the stricture, to be used as stay sutures to open the strictureplasty. An antimesenteric longitudinal incision is made over the stricture using electrocautery, and extended onto normal bowel of equal distance proximally and distally. Frozen section biopsies from all strictures should be sent to rule out the presence of dysplasia. The enterotomy is then closed in a transverse, two-layered handsewn fashion, so the bowel lumen is not narrowed.

For longer strictures, a Finney strictureplasty is used to prevent narrowing at the inlet or tension on the transverse closure (**Fig. 3**). This technique resembles a side-to-side anastomosis, and is useful in the setting of a single long stricture or multiple short segment strictures in close proximity. This form of strictureplasty requires the bowel to be folded on itself such that the two ends of the enterotomy are opposed. The bowel is usually closed in a two-layer manner using running suture. The outer layer of the back wall begins at the middle of the enterotomy, incorporates the seromuscular layers of the bowel wall, and stops at the end of the enterotomy. The inner layer begins at the same site as the outer layer, but includes all layers of the bowel. After this, the inner layer is continued onto the front wall in a Connell fashion. Lastly, the back outer layer is carried onto the front wall while incorporating only the seromuscular layers.

In a much less common scenario when there is significant size discrepancy between the proximal and distal bowel, a Moskel-Walske-Neumayer strictureplasty is performed. The stricture is opened along the antimesenteric border as a Y-shaped enterotomy with the "Y" portion in the dilated bowel just proximal to the stricture. The strictured segment is then pulled apart and the antimesenteric segment of the proximal bowel is advanced into the strictured area and closed in a transverse fashion

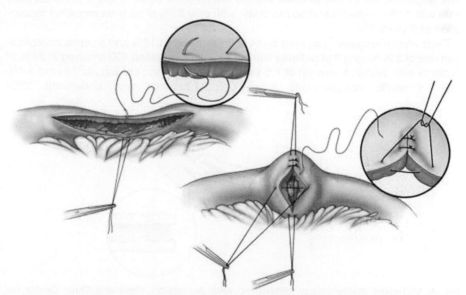

Fig. 2. Heineke-Mikulicz strictureplasty. (*Reprinted with permission,* Cleveland Clinic Center for Medical Art & Photography ©2022. All Rights Reserved.).

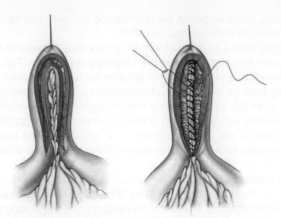

Fig. 3. Finney strictureplasty. (*Reprinted with permission*, Cleveland Clinic Center for Medical Art & Photography ©2022. All Rights Reserved.).

with one side of the closure being normal bowel along the entire length and the other being the two strictured bowel edges.

The most difficult type of stricture to address is the long, greater than 20 cm, stricture or series of strictures in close proximity. Given the amount of compromised bowel, resection is not recommended. Michelassi[51] developed a unique technique to address this anatomic challenge. A side-to-side isoperistaltic strictureplasty is made by first completely dividing the bowel transversely in the middle of the strictured segment. The mesentery is then divided perpendicular to the long axis of the bowel to permit the now two segments of strictured bowel to lay side by side along the entire length of strictured bowel (**Fig. 4**). Both strictured segments are then opened along the antimesenteric border and sewn to one another in an isoperistaltic fashion. The advantage of this technique is that it avoids to bypass the segment of the stricture. The largest series of 184 patients across six different centers found the technique safe with 11% morbidity and no mortality, with only 23% of patients requiring reoperation at 5 years.[49]

Dietz and colleagues[50] reported an overall morbidity of 18% and a septic complication rate of 5% among 314 patients with 1124 strictureplasties. CD recurred in 34% of patients with median follow-up of 7.5 years. Yamamoto and colleagues[52] found a 4% rate of septic complications among 1112 patients who underwent 3259

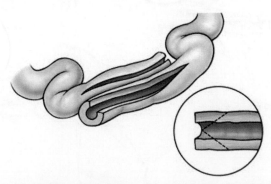

Fig. 4. Michelassi strictureplasty. (*Reprinted with permission*, Cleveland Clinic Center for Medical Art & Photography ©2022. All Rights Reserved.).

strictureplasties, and a site-specific recurrence rate of only 3% (5-year recurrence rate, 28%). Campbell and colleagues[53] compared the type of strictureplasty performed and found no difference in immediate and long-term complication rates between the conventional (Heineke-Mikulicz and Finney) and nonconventional (Michelassi) technique among 1516 patients with 4538 strictureplasties.

DISEASE-SPECIFIC SCENARIOS
Surgical Management of Perianal Disease

Perianal disease is a particularly morbid manifestation of CD affecting up to 20% of patients, with a lifetime risk of 20% to 40%.[54] Fistulas can tract from the rectum to the perianal skin, vagina, or sphincter complex. Initially, drainage of any active infection or abscess is undertaken, and placement of a seton (vessel loop or suture) through the fistula tract can promote ongoing source control while more aggressive medical and surgical managements are being placed. Unfortunately, there are no available data concerning the ideal time to remove the seton, and this is performed on empirical basis, reported to range between 3 and 58 months by some authors.[55]

Definitive treatment of perianal disease is notoriously difficult. Infliximab heals only half of perianal fistulas at 1 year; adalimumab and certolizumab have even worse results and are not recommended in place of infliximab. Seton placement can be permanent, and additional surgical options carry a risk of incontinence because of sphincter impairment. A more invasive option of diversion with a temporary loop ileostomy does work to quiet perianal disease when combined with medical therapy. However, once reversed and intestinal continuity is restored, 70% to 80% of patients have recurrence of symptoms despite biologic therapy, making this treatment option temporary and limited.[56–58] Newer treatment modalities including adipose-derived mesenchymal stem cells have improved clinical and radiographic healing rates, but widespread adoption of these treatment modalities has yet to occur.[57]

Duodenal Crohn's Disease

Gastroduodenal CD is rare, occurring in only 0.5% to 4% of all patients with CD.[59] Similar to any other location in the gastrointestinal tract, treatment is a combination of medical, endoscopic, and surgical intervention. Most of the patients with duodenal CD have concurrent involvement of the terminal ileum or large intestine at presentation. Given the challenging anatomic location and increased major surgical morbidity medical therapy should be exhausted before proceeding with surgery. The most common phenotype of duodenal CD is stricturing disease, and typically presents with short-segment strictures, often surrounded by ulcerated mucosa. The most common indication for surgery therefore is the presence of refractory obstructive symptoms despite maximal medical therapy or failed endoscopic therapy. Patients may also present with pancreatitis caused by local invasion into the pancreas or duodenoenteric fistulas resulting from distal obstruction. In the setting of obstructive-like symptoms, total parenteral nutrition should be considered before an operation in the case of long-standing obstruction and weight loss of greater than 10%. Additionally, iron supplementation should be given, and vitamin D and calcium considered. In cases where there is a short stricture length of less than 2 cm, endoscopic balloon dilation is a viable alternative to surgery.

Up to 40% of patients with duodenal CD eventually become medically refractory and ultimately require surgery.[60] Before surgery, patients should be evaluated for synchronous small bowel and/or colonic involvement, or even perianal disease, to document the extent of disease and surgical planning. The surgical management of duodenal compromise is performed in three ways: bypass, strictureplasty, or resection. Given the anatomic challenges associated with duodenectomy, bypass and strictureplasty are more widely favored when feasible. When patients have duodenal narrowing or obstruction, bypass procedures, such as gastrojejunostomy and Roux-en-Y duodenojejunostomy, are undertaken. However, morbidity need for reoperation because of marginal ulceration, obstruction of the afferent limb, and duodenal fistula approaches one-third of patients.[61,62] Therefore, strictureplasty should be used when feasible as a safe option to preserve bowel.[63] When patients present with fistulizing disease from adjacent organs, the involved bowel (eg, ileum or colon) should be resected, and the duodenum repaired primarily. Before primary repair, the duodenal edges should be cleaned.

Rectovaginal Fistulas

Rectovaginal fistulas are a particularly distressing complication of CD that affects 2% of women with CD.[64] Surgical intervention is reserved for patients who have failed medical management and continue to experience symptoms with an unacceptable quality of life. For patients who undergo surgical repair, the disease should be quiescent and the rectum distensible. Proximal diversion before surgical repair may be required to achieve these goals. In general, for distal rectovaginal fistulas where less than 15% of the internal sphincter is involved, a simple fistulotomy may be performed. Alternatives include an endorectal advancement flap or noncutting seton placement in patients who do not have active rectal inflammation. Some series of experts in the area have shown good results with advancement flaps. Joo and colleagues[65] reported sustained closure in 74% of 26 patients with fistulizing CD treated with an endorectal advancement flap, and Hull and Fazio[66] reported 68% ultimate healing.

Dysplasia or Cancer

All patients with CD longer than 8 years should undergo annual surveillance colonoscopy because of an increased risk of colorectal cancer over the general population.[67] Exceptions are made for patients with primary sclerosing cholangitis who should typically begin screening at the time of diagnosis and then undergo surveillance annually. Patients with a strong family history of colorectal cancer (age <50, first-degree relative) should typically also undergo more frequent surveillance. The recommendation for dysplasia detection in patients with CD is based largely on the experience with patients with UC and typically involves high-definition white light colonoscopy with random four-quadrant biopsies (taken at 10-cm intervals with a total of ≥32 biopsies) or chromoendoscopy with targeted biopsies.[67–70] When dysplasia is found on endoscopy, the histology should always be confirmed by a second pathologist before discussion of surgical intervention. The management of patients with CD with dysplasia continues to evolve over time and currently depends on whether or not the dysplasia is invisible or visible or is unifocal or multifocal and if complete endoscopic excision of a visible lesion is achieved.[67,68] Patients with unifocal low-grade dysplasia can continue surveillance. Patients with multifocal low-grade dysplasia or high-grade dysplasia should undergo surgical intervention. If patients have rectal-sparing disease and are reliable for ongoing endoscopic surveillance, an STC with IRA is reasonable to perform. If there is rectal dysplasia, long-standing chronic inflammation in the setting of colonic dysplasia, or an unreliable patient who will likely be lost from ongoing surveillance, total proctocolectomy and end ileostomy is the operation of choice. In the setting of a colon or rectal cancer, a total proctocolectomy and end ileostomy is also the operation of choice, and the surgeon should be mindful of high vessel ligation and adequate lymph node sampling in this setting.

Disease Recurrence and Reoperative Crohn's Disease

Within 1 year of surgery, subclinical endoscopic recurrence occurs at the anastomosis in 90% of patients with CD, symptomatic clinical recurrence occurs in 30%, and 5% of patients require another operation.[71,72] Over time, approximately 70% of patients who have had operations need further surgery.[73] Smoking, perforating disease, and previous resection have been identified individually from retrospective studies as risk factors for earlier postoperative recurrence, but these factors have not been used to tailor postoperative initiation of medical therapy.[74,75] Recurrent mucosal disease after an operation typically precedes any clinical symptoms, and its severity predicts the subsequent clinical disease.[72] Therefore, early endoscopy might be useful in earlier initial and more aggressive use of postoperative medical therapy.[76]

The most common indication for reoperative CD is recurrent inflammatory or stricturing disease and less often, fistulizing disease. A few preoperative strategies are used to assist with the conduct of the case. First, selective placement of ureteral stents to assist in the identification of the ureters during the operation is helpful in the setting of retroperitoneal inflammation or alteration of the course of the ureters. Second, if the operation has the potential of involving the rectum or left colon, the patient should be placed in the combined for access to the pelvis and perineum. Third, a flexible endoscope should be available in the room to allow for intraoperative mucosal or anastomotic evaluation.

CLINICS CARE POINTS

- Bowel preservation is of importance when operating on Crohn's disease.
- Preoperative imaging and endosocpy is needed to 'stage' a Crohn's patient and understand the extent of disease.
- Drainage of sepsis is critical prior to surgical intervention.

REFERENCES

1. Bernell O, Lapidus A, Hellers G. Risk factors for surgery and postoperative recurrence in Crohn's disease. Ann Surg 2000;231(1):38–45.
2. Peyrin-Biroulet L, Harmsen WS, Tremaine WJ, et al. Surgery in a population-based cohort of Crohn's disease from Olmsted County, Minnesota (1970-2004). Am J Gastroenterol 2012;107(11):1693–701.
3. Andrews HA, Keighley MR, Alexander-Williams J, et al. Strategy for management of distal ileal Crohn's disease. Br J Surg 1991;78(6):679–82.
4. Semrad CE. Use of parenteral nutrition in patients with inflammatory bowel disease. Gastroenterol Hepatol (N Y) 2012;8(6):393–5.
5. Brouquet A, Maggiori L, Zerbib P, et al. Anti-TNF therapy is associated with an increased risk of postoperative morbidity after surgery for ileocolonic Crohn's disease: results of a prospective nationwide cohort. Ann Surg 2018;267(2):221–8.
6. Appau KA, Fazio VW, Shen B, et al. Use of infliximab within 3 months of ileocolonic resection is associated with adverse postoperative outcomes in Crohn's patients. J Gastrointest Surg 2008;12(10):1738–44.

7. Billioud V, Ford AC, Tedesco ED, et al. Preoperative use of anti-TNF therapy and postoperative complications in inflammatory bowel diseases: a meta-analysis. J Crohn's Colitis 2013;7(11):853–67.

8. Colombel JF, Loftus EV Jr, Tremaine WJ, et al. The safety profile of infliximab in patients with Crohn's disease: the Mayo Clinic experience in 500 patients. Gastroenterology 2004;126(1):19–31.

9. Fumery M, Seksik P, Auzolle C, et al. Postoperative complications after ileocecal resection in Crohn's disease: a prospective study from the REMIND Group. Am J Gastroenterol 2017;112(2):337–45.

10. Indar AA, Young-Fadok TM, Heppell J, et al. Effect of perioperative immunosuppressive medication on early outcome in Crohn's disease patients. World J Surg 2009;33(5):1049–52.

11. Cohen BLFP, Kane SV, Herfarth HH, et al. Prospective cohort of ulcerative colitis and Crohn's disease patients undergoing surgery to identify risk factors for postoperative injection. San Diego (CA): Digestive Disease Week; 2019.

12. Lightner AL, Mathis KL, Tse CS, et al. Postoperative outcomes in vedolizumab-treated patients undergoing major abdominal operations for inflammatory bowel disease: retrospective multicenter cohort study. Inflamm Bowel Dis 2018;24(4):871–6.

13. Gutierrez A, Lee H, Sands BE. Outcome of surgical versus percutaneous drainage of abdominal and pelvic abscesses in Crohn's disease. Am J Gastroenterol 2006;101(10):2283–9.

14. Sahai A, Belair M, Gianfelice D, et al. Percutaneous drainage of intra-abdominal abscesses in Crohn's disease: short and long-term outcome. Am J Gastroenterol 1997;92(2):275–8.

15. Allen BC, Leyendecker JR. MR enterography for assessment and management of small bowel Crohn's disease. Radiol Clin North Am 2014;52(4):799–810.

16. Bergamaschi R, Pessaux P, Arnaud JP. Comparison of conventional and laparoscopic ileocolic resection for Crohn's disease. Dis Colon Rectum 2003;46(8):1129–33.

17. Duepree HJ, Senagore AJ, Delaney CP, et al. Advantages of laparoscopic resection for ileocecal Crohn's disease. Dis Colon Rectum 2002;45(5):605–10.

18. Larson DW, Pemberton JH. Current concepts and controversies in surgery for IBD. Gastroenterology 2004;126(6):1611–9.

19. Lesperance K, Martin MJ, Lehmann R, et al. National trends and outcomes for the surgical therapy of ileocolonic Crohn's disease: a population-based analysis of laparoscopic vs. open approaches. J Gastrointest Surg 2009;13(7):1251–9.

20. Milsom JW, Hammerhofer KA, Bohm B, et al. Prospective, randomized trial comparing laparoscopic vs. conventional surgery for refractory ileocolic Crohn's disease. Dis Colon Rectum 2001;44(1):1–8 [discussion: 8-9].

21. Nguyen SQ, Teitelbaum E, Sabnis AA, et al. Laparoscopic resection for Crohn's disease: an experience with 335 cases. Surg Endosc 2009;23(10):2380–4.

22. Reissman P, Salky BA, Pfeifer J, et al. Laparoscopic surgery in the management of inflammatory bowel disease. Am J Surg 1996;171(1):47–50 [discussion: 50-41].

23. Soop M, Larson DW, Malireddy K, et al. Safety, feasibility, and short-term outcomes of laparoscopically assisted primary ileocolic resection for Crohn's disease. Surg Endosc 2009;23(8):1876–81.

24. Holubar SD, Dozois EJ, Privitera A, et al. Laparoscopic surgery for recurrent ileocolic Crohn's disease. Inflamm Bowel Dis 2010;16(8):1382–6.

25. Raab Y, Bergstrom R, Ejerblad S, et al. Factors influencing recurrence in Crohn's disease. An analysis of a consecutive series of 353 patients treated with primary surgery. Dis Colon Rectum 1996;39(8):918–25.
26. Fazio VW, Marchetti F, Church M, et al. Effect of resection margins on the recurrence of Crohn's disease in the small bowel. A randomized controlled trial. Ann Surg 1996;224(4):563–71 [discussion: 571-563].
27. Coffey CJ, Kiernan MG, Sahebally SM, et al. Inclusion of the mesentery in ileocolic resection for Crohn's disease is associated with reduced surgical recurrence. J Crohn's Colitis 2018;12(10):1139–50.
28. Li Y, Mohan H, Lan N, et al. Mesenteric excision surgery or conservative limited resection in Crohn's disease: study protocol for an international, multicenter, randomized controlled trial. Trials 2020;21(1):210.
29. Present DH, Rutgeerts P, Targan S, et al. Infliximab for the treatment of fistulas in patients with Crohn's disease. N Engl J Med 1999;340(18):1398–405.
30. Sands BE, Anderson FH, Bernstein CN, et al. Infliximab maintenance therapy for fistulizing Crohn's disease. N Engl J Med 2004;350(9):876–85.
31. Amiot A, Setakhr V, Seksik P, et al. Long-term outcome of enterocutaneous fistula in patients with Crohn's disease treated with anti-TNF therapy: a cohort study from the GETAID. Am J Gastroenterol 2014;109(9):1443–9.
32. Michelassi F, Stella M, Balestracci T, et al. Incidence, diagnosis, and treatment of enteric and colorectal fistulae in patients with Crohn's disease. Ann Surg 1993; 218(5):660–6.
33. Bordeianou L, Stein SL, Ho VP, et al. Immediate versus tailored prophylaxis to prevent symptomatic recurrences after surgery for ileocecal Crohn's disease? Surgery 2011;149(1):72–7.
34. Malireddy K, Larson DW, Sandborn WJ, et al. Recurrence and impact of postoperative prophylaxis in laparoscopically treated primary ileocolic Crohn's disease. Arch Surg 2010;145(1):42.
35. Nuij VJ, Zelinkova Z, Rijk MC, et al. Dutch Delta IBD Group. Phenotype of inflammatory bowel disease at diagnosis in the Netherlands: a population-based inception cohort study (the Delta Cohort). Inflamm Bowel Dis 2013;19:2215–22.
36. Thia KT, Sandborn WJ, Harmsen WS, et al. Risk factors associated with progression to intestinal complications of Crohn's disease in a population-based cohort. Gastroenterology 2010;139(4):1147–55.
37. Angriman I, Pirozzolo G, Bardini R, et al. A systematic review of segmental vs subtotal colectomy and subtotal colectomy vs total proctocolectomy for colonic Crohn's disease. Colorectal Dis 2017;19(8):e279–87.
38. Lightner AL, Jia X, Zaghiyan K, et al. IPAA in known preoperative Crohn's disease. Dis Colon Rectum 2021;64(3):355–64.
39. Gu J, Valente MA, Remzi FH, et al. Factors affecting the fate of faecal diversion in patients with perianal Crohn's disease. Colorectal Dis 2015;17(1):66–72.
40. De Buck van Overstraeten A, Wolthuis AM, Vermeire S, et al. Intersphincteric proctectomy with end-colostomy for anorectal Crohn's disease results in early and severe proximal colonic recurrence. J Crohn's Colitis 2013;7(6):e227–31.
41. McLeod RS, Wolff BG, Ross S, et al. Investigators of the CT. Recurrence of Crohn's disease after ileocolic resection is not affected by anastomotic type: results of a multicenter, randomized, controlled trial. Dis Colon Rectum 2009;52(5): 919–27.
42. Neutzling CB, Lustosa SA, Proenca IM, et al. Stapled versus handsewn methods for colorectal anastomosis surgery. Cochrane Database Syst Rev 2012;2: CD003144.

43. Scarpa M, Angriman I, Barollo M, et al. Role of stapled and hand-sewn anastomoses in recurrence of Crohn's disease. Hepatogastroenterology 2004;51(58): 1053–7.

44. Zurbuchen U, Kroesen AJ, Knebel P, et al. Complications after end-to-end vs. side-to-side anastomosis in ileocecal Crohn's disease: early postoperative results from a randomized controlled multi-center trial (ISRCTN-45665492). Langenbecks Arch Surg 2013;398(3):467–74.

45. Yamamoto T. Factors affecting recurrence after surgery for Crohn's disease. World J Gastroenterol 2005;11(26):3971–9.

46. Fichera A, Zoccali M, Kono T. Antimesenteric functional end-to-end handsewn (Kono-S) anastomosis. J Gastrointest Surg 2012;16(7):1412–6.

47. Luglio G, Rispo A, Imperatore N, et al. Surgical prevention of anastomotic recurrence by excluding mesentery in Crohn's disease: the SuPREMe-CD Study - a randomized clinical trial. Ann Surg 2020;272(2):210–7.

48. Lee EC, Papaioannou N. Minimal surgery for chronic obstruction in patients with extensive or universal Crohn's disease. Ann R Coll Surg Engl 1982;64(4):229–33.

49. Michelassi F, Taschieri A, Tonelli F, et al. An international, multicenter, prospective, observational study of the side-to-side isoperistaltic strictureplasty in Crohn's disease. Dis Colon Rectum 2007;50(3):277–84.

50. Dietz DW, Remzi FH, Fazio VW. Strictureplasty for obstructing small-bowel lesions in diffuse radiation enteritis: successful outcome in five patients. Dis Colon Rectum 2001;44(12):1772–7.

51. Michelassi F. Side-to-side isoperistaltic strictureplasty for multiple Crohn's strictures. Dis Colon Rectum 1996;39(3):345–9.

52. Yamamoto T, Fazio VW, Tekkis PP. Safety and efficacy of strictureplasty for Crohn's disease: a systematic review and meta-analysis. Dis Colon Rectum 2007;50(11):1968–86.

53. Campbell L, Ambe R, Weaver J, et al. Comparison of conventional and nonconventional strictureplasties in Crohn's disease: a systematic review and meta-analysis. Dis Colon Rectum 2012;55(6):714–26.

54. Schwartz DA, Loftus EV Jr, Tremaine WJ, et al. The natural history of fistulizing Crohn's disease in Olmsted County, Minnesota. Gastroenterology 2002;122(4): 875–80.

55. Buchanan GN, Owen HA, Torkington J, et al. Long-term outcome following loose-seton technique for external sphincter preservation in complex anal fistula. Br J Surg 2004;91(4):476–80.

56. Hong MK, Craig Lynch A, Bell S, et al. Faecal diversion in the management of perianal Crohn's disease. Colorectal Dis 2011;13(2):171–6.

57. Mennigen R, Heptner B, Senninger N, et al. Temporary fecal diversion in the management of colorectal and perianal Crohn's disease. Gastroenterol Res Pract 2015;2015:286315.

58. Garcia-Olmo D, Herreros D, Pascual I, et al. Expanded adipose-derived stem cells for the treatment of complex perianal fistula: a phase II clinical trial. Dis Colon Rectum 2009;52(1):79–86.

59. Reynolds HL Jr, Stellato TA. Crohn's disease of the foregut. Surg Clin North Am 2001;81(1):117–35, viii.

60. Nugent FW, Roy MA. Duodenal Crohn's disease: an analysis of 89 cases. Am J Gastroenterol 1989;84(3):249–54.

61. Murray JJ, Schoetz DJ Jr, Nugent FW, et al. Surgical management of Crohn's disease involving the duodenum. Am J Surg 1984;147(1):58–65.

62. Ross TM, Fazio VW, Farmer RG. Long-term results of surgical treatment for Crohn's disease of the duodenum. Ann Surg 1983;197(4):399–406.

63. Worsey MJ, Hull T, Ryland L, et al. Strictureplasty is an effective option in the operative management of duodenal Crohn's disease. Dis Colon Rectum 1999; 42(5):596–600.

64. Makowiec F, Jehle EC, Starlinger M. Clinical course of perianal fistulas in Crohn's disease. Gut 1995;37(5):696–701.

65. Joo JS, Weiss EG, Nogueras JJ, et al. Endorectal advancement flap in perianal Crohn's disease. Am Surg 1998;64(2):147–50.

66. Hull TL, Fazio VW. Surgical approaches to low anovaginal fistula in Crohn's disease. Am J Surg 1997;173(2):95–8.

67. Lightner AL, Vogel JD, Carmichael JC, et al. The American Society of Colon and Rectal Surgeons clinical practice guidelines for the surgical management of Crohn's disease. Dis Colon Rectum 2020;63(8):1028–52.

68. Farraye FA, Odze RD, Eaden J, et al. AGA technical review on the diagnosis and management of colorectal neoplasia in inflammatory bowel disease. 74.e1-774. Gastroenterology 2010;138:746–74 [quiz: e12-3].

69. Shah SC, Ten Hove JR, Castaneda D, et al. High risk of advanced colorectal neoplasia in patients with primary sclerosing cholangitis associated with inflammatory bowel disease. Clin Gastroenterol Hepatol 2018;16:1106–11013 e3.

70. American Society for Gastrointestinal Endoscopy Standards of Practice Committee, Shergill AK, Lightdale JR, Bruining DH, et al. The role of endoscopy in inflammatory bowel disease. Gastrointest Endosc 2015;81:1101–11021.e1-13.

71. Olaison G, Smedh K, Sjodahl R. Natural course of Crohn's disease after ileocolic resection: endoscopically visualised ileal ulcers preceding symptoms. Gut 1992; 33(3):331–5.

72. Rutgeerts P, Geboes K, Vantrappen G, et al. Predictability of the postoperative course of Crohn's disease. Gastroenterology 1990;99(4):956–63.

73. Landsend E, Johnson E, Johannessen HO, et al. Long-term outcome after intestinal resection for Crohn's disease. Scand J Gastroenterol 2006;41(10):1204–8.

74. Reese GE, Nanidis T, Borysiewicz C, et al. The effect of smoking after surgery for Crohn's disease: a meta-analysis of observational studies. Int J Colorectal Dis 2008;23(12):1213–21.

75. Simillis C, Yamamoto T, Reese GE, et al. A meta-analysis comparing incidence of recurrence and indication for reoperation after surgery for perforating versus non-perforating Crohn's disease. Am J Gastroenterol 2008;103(1):196–205.

76. Rutgeerts P, Van Assche G. What is the role of endoscopy in the postoperative management of Crohn's disease? Inflamm Bowel Dis 2008;14(Suppl 2):S179–80.

Intestinal Cancer and Dysplasia in Crohn's Disease

Scott Friedberg, MD, David T. Rubin, MD*

KEY POINTS

- Crohn's disease of the colon has a significantly increased risk of dysplasia and CRC development after 8 years of disease.
- Prevention of CRC in Crohn's disease is focused on risk stratification and secondary prevention with screening and surveillance colonoscopic examinations.
- Dysplasia management should be guided by the visibility of lesions, focality, resectability, and shared decision making.
- Adenocarcinoma of the small bowel in areas affected by Crohn's disease is rare, but is important to consider in patients with long-standing unresected disease and when there are obstructive symptoms.

INTRODUCTION

Since the mid-twentieth century, there has been evidence that ulcerative colitis (UC) increases the risk of colorectal cancer (CRC), which is likely due to multiple factors, but most directly linked to longstanding unchecked inflammation.[1–4] Crohn's disease (CD) was initially not part of this paradigm. However, this has changed with studies of CD of the colon, in which it is now recognized that CD may carry a similar association of adenocarcinoma.[5,6] Today, it is established that CD is associated with an increased risk of dysplasia and CRC, as well as potentially with other malignancies. As a result, the prevention of cancer is a critically important goal in the management of CD. This review provides an overview of the current understandings of the link between CD and CRC and dysplasia, with a particular focus on clinical management.

COLORECTAL DYSPLASIA/CANCER
Background

The etiology of dysplasia and cancer development in CD is not known. The pathogenesis seems to be via a different pathway than sporadic CRC development and does not typically follow the adenoma-carcinoma sequence, but rather may progress without the clear development of polypoid dysplasia in transition from dysplasia to

University of Chicago Medicine Inflammatory Bowel Disease Center
* Corresponding author. University of Chicago Medicine Inflammatory Bowel Disease Center, Section of Gastroenterology, Hepatology, and Nutrition, University of Chicago Medical Center, 5841 S. Maryland Avenue, MC 4076, Chicago, IL 60637.
E-mail address: drubin@medicine.bsd.uchicago.edu

Gastroenterol Clin N Am 51 (2022) 369–379
https://doi.org/10.1016/j.gtc.2021.12.011
0889-8553/22/© 2022 Elsevier Inc. All rights reserved.

adenocarcinoma.[7] Both of these pathways seem to be driven in part by genomic alterations; however, they have distinct molecular fingerprints; specifically, p53 overexpression and decreased rate of APC and KRAS mutations have been observed in IBD-associated neoplasia.[8] Additionally, IBD-associated neoplasia is more likely to have mucinous differentiation and signet ring cell differentiation, both of which are significantly associated with the presence of c-MYC amplification.[9] It is likely that various immune pathways, oxidative stress, and the microbiota changes all play intertwined roles that have yet to be fully characterized.[10]

Colonic and rectal involvement of CD is a predictor of CRC risk in these patients. In particular, there is an increased risk of colorectal dysplasia and cancer when CD involves at least one-third of the large intestine.[11] The overall relative risk has been found to be 1.6 to 2.5, which is driven mostly by those with Crohn's colitis, who have a relative risk as high as 4.5 to 5.6.[1,12] The cumulative risk of dysplasia or cancer has been reported to be as high as 22% after 4 surveillance examinations.[13] In contrast, CD of the ileum alone has not been shown to be a risk factor of increased CRC development (relative risk: 1.1).[12,14]

Not only are patients with Crohn's colitis more likely to develop CRC but also they have a higher rate of CRC-related death (hazard ratio (HR): 1.74 [1.54–1.96]). Additionally, a diagnosis of CRC in CD is associated with an increased mortality rate (HR: 1.42 [1.16–1.75]).[15]

In addition to disease extent, disease duration of 8 or more years after diagnosis is a significant risk factor for cancer development (**Fig. 1**).[11,16–18] This duration-related risk is similar between patients with UC and CD. Some evidence suggests that the duration-related increased risk of cancer in both UC and CD may be increased earlier than 8 years following diagnosis[11,18]. Earlier age of diagnosis, irrespective of duration, has also been associated with increased cancer risk.

Cumulative inflammation is an increasingly recognized driver of cancer risk in UC, and presumably CD.[19–23] More recently, longitudinal inflammation in UC has been expressed as a cumulative inflammatory burden (CIB), calculated by the microscopic severity of inflammation (rated 0–3) multiplied by the length of surveillance interval in years.[19,20] Cumulative inflammation has not been studied in CD, and this is likely due to both the inherent patchiness of disease, that is also often more difficult to access endoscopically, as well as its less well-established grading scales for histology. Despite the lack of studies in CD, however, the principle behind cumulative

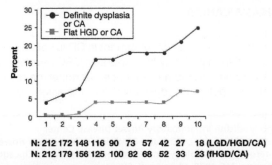

Fig. 1. Cumulative probability of an initial finding of dysplasia or cancer on surveillance examinations over years. (*From* Friedman S, Rubin PH, Bodian C, Harpaz N, Present DH. Screening and surveillance colonoscopy in chronic Crohn's colitis: results of a surveillance program spanning 25 years. Clin Gastroenterol Hepatol. 2008;6(9):993-954. https://doi.org/10.1016/j.cgh.2008.03.019; with permission).

inflammation can likely be extrapolated to CD in unresected segments of bowel and neoplastic risk as well.

There are a number of additional factors that are associated with an increased risk of the development of neoplasia in CD (**Fig. 2**). The presence of concomitant primary sclerosing cholangitis (PSC) increases the risk of dysplasia and CRC in UC and may possibly in CD as well, although studies have not demonstrated consistent results.[21,24,25] The presence of dysplasia in patients with CD is associated with an increased risk for CRC, and at a similar rate to what is observed in patients with UC.[26] Presuming the effectiveness of secondary prevention with colonoscopic surveillance, any barrier limiting the ability to perform or to provide surveillance to patients with CD also increases the risk of dysplasia and CRC development. This may include mechanical barriers such as nontraversable strictures, but may also include social determinants of health (SDOH) barriers (eg, financial barriers or poor health literacy).[27] Lastly, while not studied particularly in the CD population, it is presumed that the risk of neoplasia development in CD is also increased by a family history of CRC and personal history of adenomatous polyps.

Prevention

Prevention begins with risk stratification to identify those patients who are at increased risk and therefore, eligible for the prevention of CRC. Risk stratification is performed by taking into consideration the risks described above (phenotype, extent of rectal and colonic involvement, cumulative inflammation, presence of PSC, and so forth). It is presumed that these risk factors may be cumulative or even synergistic but a validated model for combining them has not been developed. Despite progress in the development of prognostic tests for CD, there are not yet specific biomarkers that predict neoplasia.

It is presumed that objective control of the chronic inflammation in CD may reduce the risk of subsequent neoplasia, but this is unproven (**Table 1**). Nonetheless, with the movement toward earlier aggressive therapy and treat-to-target strategies, it is hoped that the subsequent risk of neoplasia will be reduced. Close monitoring ensures that steps can be taken to reduce cumulative inflammation (**Fig. 3**). The utility of such approaches and incorporation of such tests as the Endoscopic Healing Index[28] in the prevention of cancer is unproven and should be included in future research priorities.

Environment also likely serves a role in oncogenesis. Although the relationship remains speculative, it likely includes diet and may include exposure to ionizing radiation from diagnostic imaging. Patients with CD may accumulate exposure to ionizing

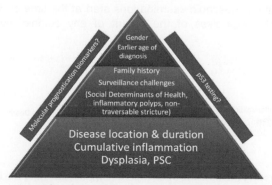

Fig. 2. A model to assist with colorectal cancer risk stratification in Crohn's disease.

Table 1
Known and unknown risks and facts about crohn's disease and intestinal adenocarcinoma

What is Known/Proven?	What is Presumed/Unproven?
Crohn's disease of the large and small bowel is associated with the development of intestinal adenocarcinoma and dysplasia	Degree and cumulative inflammation is associated with the development of dysplasia and intestinal adenocarcinoma
Specific risk factors have been identified: • Longer duration of Crohn's disease • The presence of concomitant primary sclerosing cholangitis • Family history of CRC	Control of inflammation will reduce the risk of neoplasia of the bowel
Colorectal cancer carries higher mortality in Crohn's disease than without Crohn's disease	Sureveillance colonoscopies in Crohn's disease prevent CRC and death from CRC

radiation from repeated barium or computed tomography (CT) scans, with a significant proportion of patients accumulating greater than CED 50 millisieverts (mSv), which is a level considered potentially harmful, although a direct link to CRC has not been demonstrated.[29]

Primary prevention

It is of interest to identify agents which may prevent the development of dysplasia or CRC in CD, but to date, there are none. Even in UC, whereby there has been much written about the potential chemoprotective properties of 5-ASA, this has now been minimized with newer, more controlled studies.[30] In fact, in the studies of UC-associated neoplasia, when controlling for degree of inflammation, the benefits previously ascribed to 5-ASA are significantly reduced or eliminated entirely.[21] As mentioned, it is presumed that control of inflammation may result in less neoplasia over time, but this has not been studied in CD. Nonetheless in UC, there is growing evidence that deep remission is associated with lower risks of subsequent neoplasia.[31,32]

Secondary prevention

The main approach to CRC prevention in CD is colonoscopic screening and surveillance to identify precancerous dysplasia or early-stage CRC. The current recommendations suggest interval colonoscopic surveillance for patients with CD of 8 or more year's duration and in those individuals with greater than one-third colonic involvement.[11,17] As in UC, the exception is for patients with concurrent PSC, in whom it is recommended that colonoscopic examinations start at the time of diagnosis and be performed annually, regardless of the extent of any colonic involvement. Each

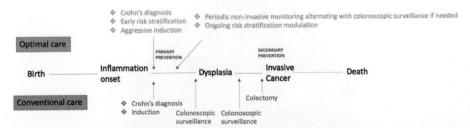

Fig. 3. Model illustrating the timeline of oncogenesis in IBD, stressing the importance of primary prevention.

surveillance plan should be individualized. Surveillance should still be considered in those stratified into other higher risk categories, even if there is less than one-third colonic involvement or 8 years of the diagnosis.

There is not yet a validated nonendoscopic modality to screen or survey for CRC in UC or CD. Endoscopic methods are classified as either standard definition (SD) or high-definition (HD), as well as either white-light (WL), narrow-band imaging (NBI), or dye-spray chromoendoscopy (CE). These modalities have been compared in the UC population and it has been demonstrated that with modern HD technology most dysplasia is visible with WL. There is generally minimal difference when NBI or CE is added.[33–35] The data and findings in UC studies may be extrapolated to CD of the colon and rectum, but this has not been proven and may be more difficult given the more frequent nodularity of the mucosa in CD than that which is seen in UC. The role of artificial intelligence (AI) enhanced endoscopic surveillance in the diagnosis of neoplasia in CD is not established.

There has been an evolution in understanding the relative yield of nontargeted (four quadrant) biopsies compared with targeted biopsies alone. Conventional thought was that nontargeted biopsies provided increased yield to identify invisible dysplastic lesions; however, recent data suggest that most lesions are visible and that nontargeted biopsies may have a yield only on the order of 0.1% to 0.2%.[29] An updated approach would be to combine targeted and nontargeted biopsies with separation by the segment of the bowel and clear labeling of specimens. Nontargeted biopsies would be favorable if the endoscopist is less comfortable identifying dysplasia, if there is inflammation obscuring clear views, and also in areas that may seem endoscopically normal to clarify the true extent of colorectal involvement. Any suspicious lesion, whether polypoid or nonpolypoid based on the modified Paris classification, should be targeted or removed during these examinations.[36,37] These lesions should also be described in relation to the patients' colitis.[30,38]

Expert-based consensus and guidelines based on limited or low-quality evidence have generally recommended that after an initial negative screening examination, surveillance should be repeated every one to 3 years, based on the findings from the prior examination (including the amount of active inflammation) and combined risk factors for neoplasia.[17] For example, the presence of inflammatory polyps poses difficulty with surveillance and thus should require more frequent surveillance and additional nontargeted biopsies. If dysplasia is found in such an area of polyposis, surgery is an appropriate consideration. More recently, guidelines have proposed that surveillance intervals can be extended to 5 years in certain populations with quiescent disease and repeatedly negative examinations for dysplasia (Table 2).[38]

The frequency of endoscopic surveillance following dysplasia, similarly to surveillance without dysplasia, should be individualized. Intervals generally span between 3 months and 12 months, depending on the type of resection (EMR, ESD) and other previously mentioned factors, such as the presence of inflammatory polyps, ability to survey closely, and so forth. More recently, data in UC suggest that after 2 consecutive negative examinations, the surveillance interval can be lengthened.[39] The AGA practice update suggests that interval for surveillance take into consideration the individual patient risks, the inflammation on the prior examination, and any history of prior dysplasia in choosing intervals.[38]

Management of Crohn's-associated dysplasia is generally considered the same as that for UC-associated dysplasia. Management is dictated by the focality, grade, and resectability of the lesion (Fig. 4). If the lesion is resectable and resected, patients must subsequently be risk stratified into an ongoing, more frequent surveillance program.

Table 2
Timing of next colonoscopy when no dysplasia detected at present colonoscopy

Physicians should err toward the more frequent surveillance category if at least one higher risk factor exists. Timing based on past and ongoing CRC risk factors and mucosal features that may obscure dysplasia.

1 y	2 or 3 y	5 y
• Moderate or severe inflammation (and extent) • PSC • Family history of CRC in first-degree relative (FDR) age < 50 • Dense pseudopolyposis • History of invisible dysplasia or higher risk visible dysplasia < 5 y ago	• Mild inflammation (any extent) • Strong family history of CRC (but no FDR < age 50) • Features of prior severe colitis (moderate pseudopolyps, extensive mucosal scarring) • History of invisible dysplasia or higher risk visible dysplasia >5 y ago • History of lower risk visible dysplasia < 5 y ago	• Continuous disease remission since the last colonoscopy with mucosal healing on current examination, plus either of: • ≥ 2 consecutive examinations without dysplasia • Minimal historical colitis extent (ulcerative proctitis or < 1/3 of colon in CD)

From Murthy SK, Feuerstein JD, Nguyen GC, Velayos FS. AGA Clinical Practice Update on Endoscopic Surveillance and Management of Colorectal Dysplasia in Inflammatory Bowel Diseases: Expert Review. Gastroenterology. 2021;161(3):1043-1051.e4. https://doi.org/10.1053/j.gastro.2021.05.063; with permission.

Details on specific methods of endoscopic resection are outside the scope of this review.

When a lesion is unresectable or multifocal, surgery is generally recommended. Conventionally, surgical considerations for IBD-associated neoplasia have been limited to total proctocolectomy with end ileostomy; however, there is emerging evidence that subtotal colectomy with ileorectal anastomosis or segmental colectomy, followed by active surveillance, can be appropriate, as the risk for metachronous lesions is low.[40–43] This is particularly relevant in patients with CD who may have a patchy or segmental disease that is amenable to this approach and who, unlike patients with UC, are usually not candidates for ileal pouch-anal anastomosis (IPAA). Notably, management must be guided by shared decision making, as certain patients will prefer a preemptive or "prophylactic" colectomy and others will value a colonic preservation strategy.

Invisible dysplastic lesions are believed to be rare when nontargeted biopsies are taken; however, when discovered, we recommend repeating endoscopy at a center whereby CE expertise is available to better characterize the extent of dysplasia. Depending on the extent and grade, it can be decided with the patient whether to continue frequent endoscopic surveillance alone or proceed with a colectomy.

Additional considerations exist when medically managing patients with active Crohn's-associated CRC. There has been some concern of a link between specific biologic therapies, such as anti-TNF therapy, and progression of active cancer. While studies generally have not revealed any clear link, there remains some uncertainty. Treatment of IBD during active cancer should thus be a multidisciplinary effort between the gastroenterology, oncology, and surgical teams. In contrast with active cancer, a personal history of cancer has not been shown to be contraindicative to using any immunosuppressive therapy for CD.[44]

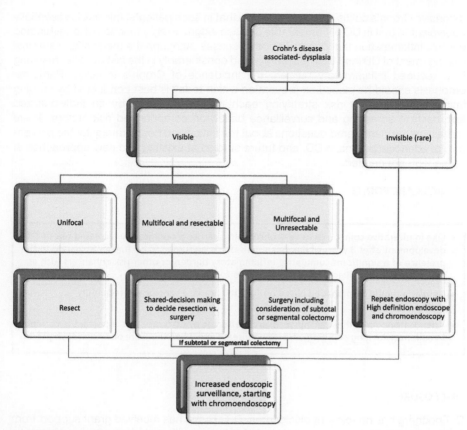

Fig. 4. Management of Crohn's-associated dysplasia.

SMALL BOWEL ADENOCARCINOMA

The ileum is the most common site of Crohn's involvement and those who have ileal or any small intestinal involvement are at a significantly increased risk of developing small bowel adenocarcinoma, with a relative risk of 18 to 33.2 and a standardized incidence ratio (SIR) of 22.[14,45,46] As compared with sporadic small bowel adenocarcinoma which occurs evenly distributed throughout the small bowel, small bowel adenocarcinoma in CD is primarily found in the ileum.[47] Despite this increased risk of small bowel adenocarcinoma in CD, however, the absolute risk remains quite low at 0.3 cases per 1000 patient-years, and thus screening is not currently recommended. There are no prospective studies to inform the value of surveillance, but the case series and reports of small bowel adenocarcinoma are usually in patients who have not had a prior resection, have long duration disease, and often present with new obstructive symptoms.[48,49] In the absence of other recommendations, having a low threshold for the surgical resection of such lesions is prudent.[50]

SUMMARY

CD is associated with an increased risk of adenocarcinoma of the involved portions of the bowel. Most notable is the risk of colorectal dysplasia and cancer that is seen in extensive Crohn's colitis. Today it is known that in such patients, this risk is essentially equivalent to that in UC of comparable disease extent, likely a function of longstanding chronic inflammation that occurs in both diseases. Although the medical and surgical management of CD (and UC) has progressed considerably in the last decade, resulting in a reduced inflammatory burden, the incidence of Crohn's is rising. Particular emphasis should be placed on prevention which today is best conducted by curbing inflammation and by risk stratifying each patient, followed by an individualized approach to screening and surveillance based on compounded risk factors. There remain many unanswered questions about the cause and best strategy for the prevention of adenocarcinoma in CD, and future studies of existing and new approaches at prevention are needed.

CLINICS CARE POINTS

- Like in ulcerative colitis, extensive Crohn's colitis carries a significantly increased risk of CRC development after 8 years of diagnosis. This risk is presumed to be further increased in the presence of a significant cumulative inflammatory burden or other risk enhancers such as PSC, dysplasia, surveillance challenges, and so forth.
- Dysplasia should be managed based on focality, grade, endoscopic resectability, and shared decision making.
- Adenocarcinoma of the small bowel in areas affected by CD is rare, but important to consider in patients with long-standing unresected disease and when there are obstructive symptoms.

DISCLOSURE

S. Friedberg has no relevant disclosures. D.T. Rubin has received grant support from Takeda; and has served as a consultant for Abbvie, Altrubio, Arena Pharmaceuticals, Bristol-Myers Squibb, Genentech/Roche, Gilead Sciences, Iterative Scopes, Janssen Pharmaceuticals, Lilly, Pfizer, Prometheus Biosciences, Takeda, and Techlab Inc.

REFERENCES

1. Herrinton LJ, Liu L, Levin TR, et al. Incidence and mortality of colorectal adenocarcinoma in persons with inflammatory bowel disease From 1998 to 2010. Gastroenterology 2012;143(2):382–9.
2. Rutter M, Saunders B, Wilkinson K, et al. Severity of inflammation is a risk factor for colorectal neoplasia in ulcerative colitis. Gastroenterology 2004;126(2):451–9.
3. Stidham R, Higgins P. Colorectal cancer in inflammatory bowel disease. Clin Colon Rectal Surg 2018;31(03):168–78.
4. Hurt LE. The relationship of chronic ulcerative colitis to malignancy. Ann Surg 1954;139(6):838–45.
5. Persson P-G, Karlén P, Bernell O, et al. Crohn's disease and cancer: A population-based cohort study. Gastroenterology 1994;107(6):1675–9.
6. Weedon DD, Shorter RG, Ilstrup DM, et al. Crohn's disease and cancer. New England Journal of Medicine 1973;289(21):1099–103.
7. Fiorillo C, Schena CA, Quero G, et al. Challenges in Crohn's disease management after gastrointestinal cancer diagnosis. Cancers (Basel) 2021;13(3):574.
8. Alpert L, Yassan L, Poon R, et al. Targeted mutational analysis of inflammatory bowel disease–associated colorectal cancers. Hum Pathol 2019;89:44–50.

9. Hartman DJ, Binion DG, Regueiro MD, et al. Distinct histopathologic and molecular alterations in inflammatory bowel disease-associated intestinal adenocarcinoma: c-MYC amplification is common and associated with mucinous/signet ring cell differentiation. Inflamm Bowel Dis 2018;24(8):1780–90.

10. Kim ER. Colorectal cancer in inflammatory bowel disease: The risk, pathogenesis, prevention and diagnosis. World J Gastroenterol 2014;20(29):9872.

11. Friedman S, Rubin PH, Bodian C, et al. Screening and surveillance colonoscopy in chronic Crohn's colitis: results of a surveillance program spanning 25 years. Clin Gastroenterol Hepatol 2008;6(9):993–8.

12. Ekbom A, Adami H-O, Helmick C, et al. Increased risk of large-bowel cancer in Crohn's disease with colonic involvement. Lancet 1990;336(8711):357–9.

13. Friedman S, Rubin PH, Bodian C, et al. Screening and surveillance colonoscopy in chronic Crohn's colitis. Gastroenterology 2001;120(4):820–6.

14. Canavan C, Abrams KR, Mayberry J. Meta-analysis: colorectal and small bowel cancer risk in patients with Crohn's disease. Aliment Pharmacol Ther 2006;23(8): 1097–104.

15. Olén O, Erichsen R, Sachs MC, et al. Colorectal cancer in Crohn's disease: a Scandinavian population-based cohort study. Lancet Gastroenterol Hepatol 2020;5(5):475–84.

16. Eaden JA. The risk of colorectal cancer in ulcerative colitis: a meta-analysis. Gut 2001;48(4):526–35.

17. Itzkowitz SH, Present DH. Consensus Conference: Colorectal cancer screening and surveillance in inflammatory bowel disease. Inflamm Bowel Dis 2005;11(3): 314–21.

18. Lutgens MWMD, Vleggaar FP, Schipper MEI, et al. High frequency of early colorectal cancer in inflammatory bowel disease. Gut 2008;57(9):1246–51.

19. Yvellez OV, Rai V, Sossenheimer PH, et al. Cumulative histologic inflammation predicts colorectal neoplasia in ulcerative colitis: a validation study. Inflamm Bowel Dis 2021;27(2):203–6.

20. Choi C-HR, Bakir I Al, Ding N-S, et al. Original article: Cumulative burden of inflammation predicts colorectal neoplasia risk in ulcerative colitis: a large single-centre study. Gut 2019;68(3):414–22.

21. Rubin DT, Huo D, Kinnucan J, et al. Inflammation is an independent risk factor for colonic neoplasia in patients with ulcerative colitis: a case-control study. Clin Gastroenterol Hepatol 2013;11(12):1601–8.e4.

22. Nieminen U, Jussila A, Nordling S, et al. Inflammation and disease duration have a cumulative effect on the risk of dysplasia and carcinoma in IBD: A case-control observational study based on registry data. Int J Cancer 2014;134(1):189–96.

23. Gupta RB, Harpaz N, Itzkowitz S, et al. Histologic inflammation is a risk factor for progression to colorectal neoplasia in ulcerative colitis: A cohort study. Gastroenterology 2007;133(4):1099–105.

24. Braden B, Halliday J, Aryasingha S, et al. Risk for colorectal neoplasia in patients with colonic Crohn's disease and concomitant primary sclerosing cholangitis. Clin Gastroenterol Hepatol 2012;10(3):303–8.

25. Lindström L, Lapidus A, Öst Å, et al. Increased risk of colorectal cancer and dysplasia in patients with Crohn's colitis and primary sclerosing cholangitis. Dis Colon Rectum 2011;54(11):1392–7.

26. Lightner AL, Vogler S, McMichael J, et al. Dysplastic progression to adenocarcinoma is equivalent in ulcerative colitis and Crohn's disease. J Crohns Colitis 2021;15(1):24–34.

27. Bernstein CN, Walld R, Marrie RA. Social determinants of outcomes in inflammatory bowel disease. Am J Gastroenterol 2020;115(12):2036–46.
28. D'Haens G, Kelly O, Battat R, et al. Development and validation of a test to monitor endoscopic activity in patients with crohn's disease based on serum levels of proteins. Gastroenterology 2020;158(3):515–26.e10.
29. Lichtenstein GR, Loftus EV, Isaacs KL, et al. ACG clinical guideline: management of crohn's disease in adults. Am J Gastroenterol 2018;113(4):481–517.
30. Rubin DT, Ananthakrishnan AN, Siegel CA, et al. ACG clinical guideline: ulcerative colitis in adults. Am J Gastroenterol 2019;114(3):384–413.
31. Colman RJ, Rubin DT. Histological inflammation increases the risk of colorectal neoplasia in ulcerative colitis: a systematic review. Intest Res 2016;14(3):202.
32. Shaffer SR, Erondu AI, Traboulsi C, et al. Achieving histologic normalization in ulcerative colitis Is associated with a reduced risk of subsequent dysplasia. Inflamm Bowel Dis 2021. https://doi.org/10.1093/ibd/izab130.
33. Krugliak Cleveland N, Colman RJ, Rodriquez D, et al. Surveillance of IBD using high definition colonoscopes does not miss adenocarcinoma in patients with low-grade dysplasia. Inflamm Bowel Dis 2016;22(3):631–7.
34. Rubin DT, Rothe JA, Hetzel JT, et al. Are dysplasia and colorectal cancer endoscopically visible in patients with ulcerative colitis? Gastrointest Endosc 2007; 65(7):998–1004.
35. Gondal B, Haider H, Komaki Y, et al. Efficacy of various endoscopic modalities in detecting dysplasia in ulcerative colitis: A systematic review and network meta-analysis. World J Gastrointest Endosc 2020;12(5):159–71.
36. Participants in the Paris Workshop. The Paris endoscopic classification of superficial neoplastic lesions: esophagus, stomach, and colon: November 30 to December 1, 2002. Gastrointest Endosc 2003;58(6):S3–43.
37. Endoscopic classification review group. Update on the paris classification of superficial neoplastic lesions in the digestive tract. Endoscopy 2005;37(6):570–8.
38. Murthy SK, Feuerstein JD, Nguyen GC, et al. AGA clinical practice update on endoscopic surveillance and management of colorectal dysplasia in inflammatory bowel diseases: expert review. Gastroenterology 2021;161(3):1043–51.e4.
39. Ten Hove JR, Shah SC, Shaffer SR, et al. Consecutive negative findings on colonoscopy during surveillance predict a low risk of advanced neoplasia in patients with inflammatory bowel disease with long-standing colitis: results of a 15-year multicentre, multinational cohort study. Gut 2019;68(4):615–22.
40. Krugliak Cleveland N, Ollech JE, Colman RJ, et al. Efficacy and follow-up of segmental or subtotal colectomy in patients with colitis-associated neoplasia. Clin Gastroenterol Hepatol 2019;17(1):205–6.
41. Wanders LK, Dekker E, Pullens B, et al. cancer risk after resection of polypoid dysplasia in patients with longstanding ulcerative colitis: a meta-analysis. Clin Gastroenterol Hepatol 2014;12(5):756–64.
42. Bogach J, Pond G, Eskicioglu C, et al. extent of surgical resection in inflammatory bowel disease associated colorectal cancer: a population-based study. J Gastrointest Surg 2021;25(10):2610–8.
43. Khan N, Cole E, Shah Y, et al. Segmental resection is a safe oncological alternative to total proctocolectomy in elderly patients with ulcerative colitis and malignancy. Colorectal Dis 2017;19(12):1108–16.
44. Shelton E, Laharie D, Scott FI, et al. Cancer recurrence following immunosuppressive therapies in patients with immune-mediated diseases: a systematic review and meta-analysis. Gastroenterology 2016;151(1):97–109.e4.

45. Laukoetter MG, Mennigen R, Hannig CM, et al. Intestinal cancer risk in Crohn's disease: a meta-analysis. J Gastrointest Surg 2011;15(4):576–83.

46. Uchino M, Ikeuchi H, Hata K, et al. Intestinal cancer in patients with Crohn's disease: A systematic review and meta-analysis. J Gastroenterol Hepatol 2021; 36(2):329–36.

47. Fields AC, Hu FY, Lu P, et al. Small bowel adenocarcinoma: is there a difference in survival for Crohn's versus sporadic cases? J Crohns Colitis 2020;14(3):303–8.

48. Cahill C, Gordon PH, Petrucci A, et al. Small bowel adenocarcinoma and Crohn's disease: Any further ahead than 50 years ago? World J Gastroenterol 2014; 20(33):11486.

49. Rubin DT, McVerry B, Hanauer SB. Small bowel cancer in Crohn's disease: The university of Chicago experience. Gastroenterology 2000;118(4):A121.

50. Widmar M, Greenstein AJ, Sachar DB, et al. Small bowel adenocarcinoma in Crohn's disease. J Gastrointest Surg 2011;15(5):797–802.

Fertility and Pregnancy in Crohn's Disease

Rishika Chugh, MD[a,b], Jill K.J. Gaidos, MD[a,c],*

KEYWORDS

• Crohn's disease • Pregnancy • Lactation

INTRODUCTION

The prevalence of inflammatory bowel disease (IBD) is continuing to increase world-wide.[1–3] A recent study examining more than 60 million people in the United States calculated a 123% increase in the prevalence of IBD among adults and a 133% increase among children from 2007 to 2016.[1] Crohn's disease (CD) seems to have a younger mean age of diagnosis when compared with ulcerative colitis, and in the adult population, the prevalence was noted to be higher in women compared with men.[1,2] Given the younger age of onset and increased prevalence in women, there is an overlap in the diagnosis of CD and childbearing years. Individuals with CD may have inaccurate perceptions regarding the rate of infertility, heritability, and the safety of taking therapies for Crohn's disease during pregnancy, all of which greatly affect their decisions surrounding family planning.[4] A recent survey study found that only a third of IBD providers are comfortable caring for pregnant patients and addressing family planning.[5] Given this area of need for both patients and providers, in this article, we have included the latest evidence on the impact of CD on fertility, heritability, pregnancy outcomes, and the safety of medications for Crohn's disease during pregnancy and lactation.

FERTILITY

The inability to conceive after 12 months of regular, unprotected sexual intercourse is the definition of infertility.[6] However, a referral to a fertility specialist is recommended after an inability to conceive for 6 months for those with IBD.[7] Psychological burdens associated with IBD can result in a decrease in libido, poor body image, and subsequently, a lower likelihood of engaging in sexual activity.[8] However, studies have

a Section of Digestive Diseases, Department of Medicine, Yale School of Medicine, Yale University, New Haven, CT, USA; b Gastroenterology, Department of Medicine, University of California San Francisco, 1701 Divisadero, San Francisco, CA 94115, USA; c Section of Digestive Diseases, Yale Inflammatory Bowel Disease Program, 40 Temple Street, Suite 1C, New Haven, CT 06510, USA
* Corresponding author. Section of Digestive Diseases, Yale Inflammatory Bowel Disease Program, 40 Temple Street, Suite 1C, New Haven, CT 06510.
E-mail address: jill.gaidos@yale.edu

Gastroenterol Clin N Am 51 (2022) 381–399
https://doi.org/10.1016/j.gtc.2021.12.012
0889-8553/22/© 2022 Elsevier Inc. All rights reserved.

not shown any decrease in fertility associated with CD in the absence of active inflammation or prior surgery.

Fertility in Men

A prior systematic review including three studies on fertility in men and CD reported an overall decrease of fertility in men with CD compared with controls.[6] However, only one of those studies differentiated between voluntary childlessness and involuntary infertility and discovered that fecundability was the same between the groups, suggesting that voluntary childlessness was the driving force behind this perceived discrepancy in fertility.[9]

Several medications for Crohn's disease, particularly methotrexate and sulfasalazine, can result in sexual dysfunction in men.[10] Although other 5-aminosalicyclic acid (5-ASA) regimens do not affect fertility,[11] sulfasalazine is associated with reversible oligospermia and should be discontinued 3 months before attempting conception.[12,13] The impact of methotrexate on fertility is controversial. A systematic review including 48 men with rheumatoid arthritis exposed to methotrexate found that only 2 developed oligospermia, which was noted to be reversible with discontinuation of the drug.[14,15] Although the association between oligospermia and methotrexate is unclear, there is evidence that methotrexate can reduce DNA integrity in sperm.[16] It is therefore recommended that methotrexate be discontinued at least 3 months before conception. Most biologics and thiopurines have not been shown to have any impact on fertility.[14,17] Data on the fertility risk of ustekinumab and tofacitinib are lacking at this time.

There are other common medications that can affect fertility, including psychotropic drugs and opioids. The prevalence of anxiety and depression is elevated in the IBD population; up to one-third may suffer from anxiety and one quarter from depression.[18] Medications used to treat these conditions, most commonly selective serotonin reuptake inhibitors, cause ejaculatory dysfunction, increased ejaculation latency, and alteration in circulating hormones.[19,20] The prescription of opiates in the CD population has also been noted to have increased over time.[21,22] Opioid analgesics significantly increase the risk of erectile dysfunction, and consideration should be given to weaning a patient off, especially when infertility is a concern.[23]

Complications from CD can also negatively impact fertility. Perianal diseases including abscess and fistula formation are common complications of CD and may require surgical intervention such as fistulotomy, seton placement, advancement flaps, and temporary stoma creation. The presence of these complications may negatively affect sexual activity, but these surgical treatments do not seem to affect fertility.[24] Nutritional deficiencies, another common complication, may also play a role in low fertility rates seen in men with CD, particularly with zinc deficiency.[25]

Fertility in Women

Studies have shown a decrease in ovarian reserve in women with CD more than 30 years of age; however, studies have not shown an associated decrease in fertility.[26] A large database study from the United Kingdom looked at fertility rates among women with IBD compared with women without IBD and found that women with CD had marginally lower fertility rates; however, the fertility rates were noted to further decrease in the setting of a flare and after surgery.[27] Among studies accounting for voluntary childlessness, infertility rates were reported to be similar: 2.5%–14% in controls compared with 3%–12% in women with CD.[9] The noted increased rate of voluntary childlessness is due to a lack of education about the safety of medication use during pregnancy, further stressing the need for providers to counsel women of child-bearing age.

Medications for the treatment of CD have not been shown to negatively affect fertility. Although tofacitinib is not yet approved for the treatment of CD, data on its impact on fertility and pregnancy are lacking at this time.[28,29] Most surgical management for CD does not impact fertility. However, total colectomy with ileal pouch anal anastomosis (IPAA) is associated with a 3-fold higher rate of infertility among women and a longer time to conception.[30] This is likely secondary to the pelvic dissection resulting in fallopian tube scarring. Studies suggest that using a laparoscopic approach may lead to lower infertility rates.[31,32] Importantly, assisted reproductive technologies (ARTs) can be successful for the treatment of infertility for women with CD.[7,33,34] However, pregnancy rates with ART are lower in women with CD who have undergone surgery compared with women with CD who have not undergone surgery.[7,35,36]

RISK OF IBD HERITABILITY

Addressing questions on the heritability of IBD is essential to correct misconceptions which can discourage men and women with CD from having children of their own. Genetics play a strong role in IBD, more so in CD compared with UC. The concordance rates for monozygotic twins range from 33.3% to 58.3% for CD and 13.4% to 27.9% for UC.[35] A Danish study demonstrated that up to 12% of patients with IBD have other relatives with IBD.[36] The risk of having a child who ultimately develops IBD is higher in those who have multiple relatives with IBD and is especially increased if both parents have IBD. It is important to note that studies on this subject suggest a possible environmental component to developing IBD as well, and an increased incidence of IBD in the offspring may be attributed to the gene–environment interaction as opposed to genetics alone.[35,37] Genetic testing, which is gaining popularity, cannot be reliably used at this time as there are more than 230 gene loci implicated in the development of IBD.[38]

PRECONCEPTION OPTIMIZATION
Disease Activity

Controlling disease activity is the key to increasing the chances of conception and maintaining a healthy pregnancy. Among patients with CD who conceive while their disease is active, one-third will go into remission, one-third will remain stably active, and the disease activity will worsen in the remaining one-third.[39,40] Active CD has been associated with an increased incidence of preterm birth, low birth weight, and small for gestational age infants.[41–43] Moderate to severe disease activity is also correlated with spontaneous abortion and the need for caesarean section delivery but not with an increased risk of preeclampsia.[44] However, in the setting of quiescent CD, pregnancy outcomes are the same as in the general population.[45,46] Further, active CD can lead to worsening malnutrition resulting in poor maternal weight gain, which is associated with intrauterine growth restriction and poor fetal outcomes.[42,46] Given the lower rate of conception and increased risk of adverse outcomes with active CD, women should achieve steroid-free disease remission at least 3–6 months before attempting conception to decrease these risks.[7,47]

Health care Maintenance

The recommendations for preventative care as delineated by the American College of Obstetrics and Gynecology also apply to all patients with IBD, such as recommendations for tobacco, illicit drug, and alcohol cessation during preconception and throughout pregnancy.[48] In addition, women with CD need nutritional assessment and close monitoring of their weight with the goal of achieving a body mass index (BMI) within the normal range. Both low and high BMI are associated with pregnancy and fetal complications.[48] In addition, assessment for nutritional deficiencies with repletion is important throughout pregnancy. Folate supplementation consisting of at least 400 μg of folic acid daily is unanimously recommended among those trying to conceive and throughout pregnancy. Vitamin D deficiency is commonly seen in patients with CD and can result in disease progression and low fertility rates.[49,50] Patients with malabsorption due to prior bowel resection may require additional vitamin or mineral supplementation.[48] Further, any pending cancer surveillance and recommended vaccinations should also be completed before conception (**Box 1**).[51,52]

Contraception

Continued use of contraception may be necessary while undergoing health optimization. Non-estrogen-containing contraception should be encouraged due to the increased risk of thromboembolic events in those with IBD that is further heightened with exogenous estrogen use. In addition, estrogen-containing contraception has been shown to increase the likelihood of a CD flare and need for surgical intervention.[53,54] It may therefore be reasonable to consider progestin-only containing oral contraception or intrauterine devices as first-line treatment. Women should be

---

Box 1
Preconception counseling checklist

Control Disease Activity
- Goal is 3–6 months of steroid-free remission before conception
- Counsel on continued use of medical therapies with the exception of methotrexate
- Establish care with high-risk obstetrician proactively

Nutrition
- Encourage working toward a healthy BMI before pregnancy
- Check vitamin D level in all patients and supplement accordingly
- In those with evidence of prior small bowel resection or disease involvement, check Vitamin B12, folate, and iron levels and supplement accordingly
- Supplement with folic acid 400 micrograms per day minimum. However, if there is evidence of small bowel involvement or resection or the patient is taking sulfasalazine, increase to 2 mg per day.

Health Maintenance
- If there is colonic involvement, ensure patient is up to date with colonoscopy for dysplasia screening before pregnancy
- Patient should have a pap smear completed before conception
- Patient should have an annual total body skin examination with dermatologist if taking thiopurine or biologic therapy
- Patients should be up to date with all vaccines. This includes both pneumococcal vaccines, Tdap, annual influenza vaccine, and consideration for the vaccine against SARS CoV-2. Serologic immunity against hepatitis B and hepatitis A should be verified, and if negative, a booster or full vaccination series should be administered.

Contraception
- If the patient is not in remission or not optimized for pregnancy, discuss contraception
- Non-estrogen-containing forms of contraception are preferred

Tdap: tetanus toxoid, reduced diphtheria toxoid, and acellular pertussis; SARS CoV-2: severe acute respiratory syndrome coronavirus 2.

made aware that the efficacy of oral contraceptive pills is theoretically reduced in those with rapid bowel transit, active small bowel inflammation, and prior small bowel resection.[7,55]

MANAGEMENT DURING PREGNANCY
A Team Approach

Management of a pregnant woman with CD should include a team of providers and specialists. Depending on geography and the local resources, having multiple specialists involved may not be possible. Ideally, a gastroenterologist, specifically one who specializes in IBD, should continue to follow the patient throughout pregnancy, with clinic visits at least once during the first or second trimester and as needed during the remainder of the pregnancy.[7] A maternal–fetal medicine doctor or a high-risk obstetrician is also key to proactively monitor for any pregnancy-related complications for women with CD. Open communication among all providers is needed to ensure that all members of the team are delivering a common message; this has been shown to improve maternal and fetal outcomes.[56,57]

Medication Use and Safety

Patients identify the safety of IBD medications as a priority topic of concern during the preconception and pregnancy phase.[58] Fortunately, most medical therapies used for CD management do not result in adverse pregnancy outcomes and should be continued throughout pregnancy to control disease activity. Methotrexate is

Table 1
IBD Medications and their impact on Fertility, Pregnancy, and Breastfeeding

Medications	Fertility Impact	Pregnancy Safety	Breastfeeding Considerations
5-ASA	Risk of oligospermia with sulfasalazine. All other 5-ASA agents have no impact	Low risk. Sulfasalazine okay with increase of folic acid	Avoid sulfasalazine due to hemolysis risk, especially if child has G6PD
Corticosteroids	Long-term use may result in decreased testosterone in men. No known impact in women[126]	Low risk Gestational diabetes and adrenal insufficiency with long-term use	IV steroids may temporarily suppress lactation
Antibiotics			
Ciprofloxacin	Animal studies show impact on spermatogenesis and decrease in LH and FSH	Low risk. Short-term use recommended	Low levels in breast milk
Metronidazole	Animal studies show impact on spermatogenesis and decrease in LH and FSH	Low risk Short-term use recommended	Can cause infant diarrhea. Avoid breastfeeding 12–24 h after dose

(continued on next page)

Table 1 (continued)			
Medications	**Fertility Impact**	**Pregnancy Safety**	**Breastfeeding Considerations**
Immunomodulators			
Methotrexate	Oligospermia in men and risk of teratogenicity. Stop 3 mo before conception	High risk. Stop 3 mo before conception	Subcutaneous weekly doses used in IBD are safe. Avoid breastfeeding 24 h following injection
Thiopurines			
6-Mercaptopurine	No known impact on fertility	Low risk Safe to continue, not recommended to start during pregnancy	Breast milk concentrations are undetectable
Azathioprine	No known impact on fertility	Low risk Safe to continue, not recommended to start during pregnancy	Breast milk concentrations are undetectable
Biologic Therapies			
Anti-TNF			
Adalimumab	No known impact on fertility	Low risk	Low levels present or undetectable in breast milk
Infliximab	No known impact on fertility	Low risk	Low levels present or undetectable in breast milk
Certolizumab pegol	No known impact on fertility	Low risk	Low levels present or undetectable in breast milk
Anti-integrin			
Natalizumab	No known impact on fertility	Low risk	Low levels present or undetectable in breast milk
Vedolizumab	No known impact on fertility	Low risk	Low levels present or undetectable in breast milk
Anti-IL 12/23			
Ustekinumab	No known impact on fertility	Low risk	Low levels present or undetectable in breast milk

Abbreviations: LH: lutenizing hormone. IV: intravenous. FSH: follicle stimulating hormone. NTPR: National Transplant Pregnancy Registry.

teratogenic and has to be stopped at least 3 months before conception. Discussion of other common CD medications is included in this section and summarized in **Table 1.**

5-ASA medications
Sulfasalazine is the only 5-ASA agent recommended for the treatment of mild to moderate colonic CD.[59] Sulfasalazine interferes with folate metabolism but can be safely

continued without increasing the risk of neural tube defects or other congenital abnormalities when given in combination with a higher dose of folic acid. All patients on sulfasalazine should be taking folic acid 1 mg daily, which needs to be increased to 2 mg daily preconception and during pregnancy.[60]

Corticosteroids
Corticosteroids may be indicated for short-term management of flares but should be avoided as long-term therapy for CD. Corticosteroid use during pregnancy is associated with an increased risk of gestational diabetes.[61] Per case reports, long-term use can further result in adrenal insufficiency in both the mother and child.[62,63] Data on budesonide are lacking, but due to its high first pass metabolism and minimal systemic absorption, no associated adverse risk during pregnancy or breastfeeding is expected. Case series on the use of budesonide including the MMX (extended release, multimatrix) formulation have demonstrated no negative outcomes in mothers or their children.[64,65]

Antibiotics
Short courses of antibiotics may be needed for specific conditions such as pouchitis, perianal disease, or infectious complications. Common antibiotics used in IBD include metronidazole and ciprofloxacin. Fluoroquinolones have a theoretic risk of causing cartilage damage and arthropathies in the fetus when taken during pregnancy based on animal studies; however, subsequent meta-analyses do not support these findings.[62,66] Short courses of nitroimidazoles seem to be safe for the mother and infant.[67]

Thiopurines: 6-MP and Azathioprine
Women who are taking thiopurines before conception to maintain remission can safely continue their use throughout pregnancy. However, thiopurines are not initiated during pregnancy because of possible adverse side effects associated with use of these therapies, including bone marrow suppression, hepatitis, and pancreatitis. Continued thiopurine use during pregnancy does not result in higher rates of spontaneous abortions, congenital malformations, low birth weight, or preterm birth.[68,69] Recent data from a large prospective multicenter study on patients from the Pregnancy in Inflammatory Bowel Disease and Neonatal Outcomes (PIANO) registry found that thiopurine use during pregnancy did not result in increased infant infections compared with the nonexposed group.[70] Neurodevelopmental outcomes in children for up to 4 years of follow-up were not impacted by the use of these drugs.[70]

Biologic Therapies
Biologic agents, including anti-tumor necrosis factor (anti-TNF) medications, anti-integrin agents, and anti-interleukin (IL) 12/23 medications, are monoclonal antibodies that are actively transported across the placenta and can be detected in the infant's blood for up to 9 months postpartum. Because of the difference in the structure of the medication, certolizumab pegol is only passively transported across the placenta, leading to much lower drug levels in cord blood and infant serum.[70–72] Data from the PIANO registry have demonstrated that the use of biologic therapies during pregnancy does not worsen pregnancy outcomes or increase the risk of labor complications such as spontaneous abortion, preterm birth, stillbirth, low birth weight, abruptio placenta, eclampsia, preeclampsia, need for cesarean section, or fetal distress. Further, these drugs do not alter neonatal outcomes including the risk for intensive care unit admission, infections, or developmental milestones.[69,70] Although we understand that vedolizumab, an anti-integrin therapy, and ustekinumab, an anti-IL 12/23 therapy, have overall better patient safety profiles, evidence suggests that the use of these drugs

during pregnancy results in maternal and fetal outcomes comparable to those seen with anti-TNF agents.[73,74]

Natalizumab and vedolizumab are integrin receptor antagonists used for induction and maintenance in CD. Natalizumab is not commonly prescribed for the treatment of CD because of concerns regarding reactivation of the John Cunningham virus and resultant progressive multifocal leukoencephalopathy.[75] In the PIANO registry, 41 subjects were exposed to vedolizumab and 15 to natalizumab without any increase in pregnancy or fetal complications.[70] Other studies have shown similar safety for vedolizumab use during pregnancy.[73,76] Earlier studies on the use of natalizumab during pregnancy in women with multiple sclerosis have demonstrated that natalizumab exposure did not increase the risk of spontaneous abortions or congenital malformations.[77,78]

Therapeutic drug monitoring is commonly used to guide treatment changes and ensure dose optimization on patients being treated with biologic agents. Physiologic changes during pregnancy seem to minimally alter drug concentrations, but the data we have to date suggest that dose adjustments or more frequent drug monitoring in the gravid patient are not of clinical benefit.[79,80]

Combination Thiopurine and Biologic Agent. Studies have shown an increased risk of infection within the first year of life for infants who were exposed in utero to combination thiopurine and anti-TNF medications.[81] However, a recent multicenter study did not find an increased prevalence of severe infections among children with intrauterine exposure to combination therapy compared with those exposed to anti-TNF monotherapy (12% vs 11%, $P > .05$).[82] Because of the potential increased risk of infection, consideration should be given for discontinuing the thiopurine and continuing the anti-TNF medication as monotherapy throughout pregnancy; however, this decision should be made on an individualized basis according to each woman's medication history and her disease severity. Data on the safety of continuing a thiopurine in combination with other biologic agents are lacking.

Small Molecule Agents

Although these medications are not yet approved by the Food and Drug Administration for the treatment of CD, use in CD is already occurring on an off-label basis. Tofacitinib is an oral, Janus kinase inhibitor that is approved for the treatment of UC. In animal studies, tofacitinib has been shown to have teratogenic effects. However, case reports of tofacitinib-exposed pregnant patients have reported no fetal or neonatal deaths or an increase in congenital malformations.[83]

Ozanimod is an oral, sphingosine-1-phosphate receptor agonist that was recently approved for the treatment of UC, with studies in CD still underway. In animal studies, ozanimod has shown to cause an increase in fetal malformations and other adverse effects on fetal development.[84] However, small observational human studies have demonstrated that early pregnancy exposure did not result in adverse effects with no noted increase in the rate of spontaneous abortion and no fetal abnormalities were noted.[85] Because of the limited data available on the safety of use in humans, the current recommendations are to discontinue ozanimod use for 3 months before conception.

Surgical Management of Crohn's Disease

Approximately 50% of patients with CD will require surgery.[86] The indications for surgery in pregnant patients with IBD are the same as those for nonpregnant patients; these include obstruction, perforation, abscess, severe hemorrhage, or acute severe refractory disease.[87] Notably, surgery during pregnancy is associated with significant morbidity and mortality for the mother and child, in utero and after birth.[88] This was most recently noted in a case series including 15 pregnant patients with CD undergoing surgery for penetrating or stricturing complications of their disease.[89] If surgical intervention is absolutely indicated during pregnancy, then the second trimester is preferred due to the possible increased risk of miscarriage when operating during the first trimester and increased risk of preterm birth with surgery during the third trimester.[90] At the same time, urgent surgery should not be delayed as this may further increase the risk of complications. With bowel resection, a temporary stoma may be preferred over a primary anastomosis to avoid any postoperative complications related to surgical manipulation within the pelvis.[88]

Monitoring Disease Activity and Management of a Flare

The lowest risk of having a CD flare during pregnancy is when CD is in remission for at least 3 months before conception.[91] However, flares can complicate up to a third of pregnancies in women with IBD.[92] Active CD during pregnancy has been shown to increase the risk of adverse pregnancy and neonatal outcomes. One Danish study evaluated 71 pregnant patients with IBD and demonstrated that the risk of preterm birth was two times higher in women with moderate to severe disease activity compared with those with low disease activity during pregnancy.[93] This has been further substantiated in other studies.[45,94]

Because of the high risk for complications with active CD during pregnancy, continued monitoring for disease activity in pregnant patients is recommended. Noninvasive methods are preferred; however, erythrocyte sedimentation rate and C-reactive protein may not be reliable in pregnant patients.[95] Fecal calprotectin does increase in correlation with disease activity, although no clear thresholds have been validated in the pregnant individual.[96,97] Gastrointestinal ultrasonography (GIUS) is an emerging noninvasive and safe method to monitor for active intestinal inflammation and may become a particularly useful tool for disease monitoring during pregnancy. One study of GIUS in pregnant patients described adequate ileal views in 93% of patients less than 20 weeks of gestation and adequate colon views in 91% of patients throughout gestation. Here, bowel wall thickness correlated with calprotectin (at a threshold of >100 µg/g) with a sensitivity of 74% and a specificity of 83%.[98–100]

Evaluation and treatment of a flare in pregnant patients with CD should be approached similar to any IBD flare, starting with measuring objective markers of inflammation and obtaining stool studies to assess for an infection. If endoscopy is needed for a diagnosis and the findings will dictate a change in therapy, a nonsedated flexible sigmoidoscopy can be safely performed throughout pregnancy.[101] If indicated, a full colonoscopy can be performed.[102] The current American Society for Gastrointestinal Endoscopy guidelines suggest that endoscopy be deferred to the second trimester when possible and that the patient be placed in the left lateral tilt position to avoid maternal hypotension and decreased placental perfusion via compression of the aorta or inferior vena cava.[103] Ultrasound is safe throughout pregnancy and MRI can be used starting in the second trimester if additional imaging is needed. Treatment can consist of a short course of steroids, if needed, or dose escalation of the patient's current Crohn's therapy that had previously led to disease remission.

Nutrition

Inadequate gestational weight gain is common for patients with CD. A Norwegian study revealed that out of a cohort of 117 women with CD, 34.3% had an inadequate gestational weight gain, which was approximately 2-fold higher than in pregnant women without IBD. Inadequate gestational weight gain is a risk factor for preterm birth and for having a small for gestational age fetus.[7,104,105]

Nutritional deficiencies of concern during pregnancy include iron, vitamin D, vitamin B12, and folate. Levels of these nutritional markers need to be checked during the first trimester and subsequently thereafter depending on the individual to ensure proper supplementation.[7,106–108] In patients with CD having small bowel involvement or a prior bowel resection, folate intake should be a minimum of 2 mg per day due to decreased absorption. In a recent study, 33% of patients with CD were noted to have vitamin B12 deficiency compared with 16% of patients with UC with risk factors being ileal inflammation or having a prior ileal resection, particularly when resection was greater than 20 cm[107,109] Iron deficiency is noted in patients with CD as well, and supplementation is warranted for those with iron deficiency anemia.[109]

DELIVERY
Mode of Delivery

In most cases, the mode of delivery should be determined by the obstetrician based on the patient and fetal factors on an individualized basis. Cesarean delivery is recommended, however, for women with active perianal disease or with a history of IPAA).[110,111] Vaginal delivery in the setting of active perianal disease increases the risk of fourth degree laceration that can lead to anal sphincter dysfunction in the future.[112,113] In general, vaginal delivery can increase the risk of anal sphincter injury as well as pudendal nerve injury,[114] both of which can lead to pouch dysfunction.[115] Because of the potential for injury to the anal sphincter with a vaginal delivery, consideration for a cesarean section delivery for women with a prior IPAA is recommended.[7,111] Of note, the mode of delivery does not seem to affect the risk of IBD in the offspring.[116,117]

Anticoagulation

Pregnancy and IBD independently serve as risk factors for venous thromboembolism (VTE). When combined with immobilization during a hospitalization and the increased inflammatory state associated with pregnancy and delivery, the possibility of VTE increases further. The incidence of VTE is increased in patients with IBD during pregnancy and for up to 6–12 weeks postpartum compared with pregnant patients without IBD.[118,119] It is therefore recommended that patients be managed with anticoagulation for prophylaxis while hospitalized and potentially for several weeks thereafter depending on their individual risk factors. Treatment with unfractionated heparin, low-molecular-weight heparin, and warfarin is recommended for breastfeeding women.[7,120]

POSTPARTUM CARE

Multiple studies have shown an approximate 30% risk of a flare within the first 6 months postpartum.[121,122] In a cohort of 105 patients with CD, 68% of whom were on a biologic therapy, 30% of the patients experienced a flare without a clear risk factor identified in most women.[121] Another study including 206 women with IBD noted that therapy de-escalation during or after pregnancy and active disease during the third trimester were predictors of a postpartum flare.[122] Biologic therapies can be resumed 24 hours after a vaginal delivery and 48 hours following a cesarean section if the timing interval is appropriate.[7,123]

Medications for Crohn's disease that were continued during pregnancy can be safely continued with breastfeeding (see **Table 1**). There are no longer any recommendations to time breastfeeding sessions around medication dosing or any need to "pump and dump." However, for infants who were exposed in utero to a biologic medication other than certolizumab pegol, administration of any live vaccines should be avoided in the first 6 months of life. In the United States, this only impacts the administration of the rotavirus vaccine which is given in two or three doses starting at the age of 2 months.[7,124]

Infant exposure to medical therapies used for CD either in utero or through breast milk, with the exception of methotrexate, has not been shown to result in any developmental delays. The PIANO study measured developmental milestones in children of mothers with IBD up to 4 years of age and found no differences when compared with validated population norms.[70] A more long-term study from the Danish National Birth Cohort observed childhood development up to 7 years of age in 391 patients born to mothers with IBD and found similar cognitive scores and motor development when compared with children born to mothers without IBD.[125]

SUMMARY

There is an increasing likelihood that gastroenterology providers will encounter a patient with CD who is planning for pregnancy or is already pregnant. Healthy outcomes for the mother and child are achieved first and foremost by ensuring control of disease activity on a steroid-free treatment regimen for 3–6 months before conception. Those with CD entering pregnancy with active disease are more likely to continue to have active disease throughout pregnancy, which can negatively affect pregnancy and fetal outcomes. Updating health maintenance and assessing nutritional status should also be completed in the preconception period. Multiple providers may need to be involved for close monitoring throughout pregnancy. The role of the gastroenterologist is to proactively monitor for an increased disease activity with treatment as appropriate. Other than methotrexate, our current therapies for Crohn's disease are safe to continue during pregnancy and breastfeeding. Providing patients with CD the most current evidence on fertility and the safety of medications for Crohn's disease during pregnancy is the first step to correcting any misinformation and may affect decisions regarding family planning.

CLINICS CARE POINTS

- Crohn's disease does not decrease fertility in women or men.
- Of the medications approved for use in Crohn's disease, methotrexate is the only medication that should be discontinued at least 3 months before conception.
- Women with Crohn's disease can have normal pregnancies and deliver healthy infants.
- During pregnancy, women with Crohn's disease should have a team of providers overseeing their care, all with a shared treatment plan.

DISCLOSURE

The authors have nothing to disclose.

REFERENCES

1. Ye Y, Manne S, Treem WR, et al. Prevalence of Inflammatory Bowel Disease in Pediatric and Adult Populations: Recent Estimates From Large National Databases in the United States, 2007-2016. Inflamm Bowel Dis 2020;26:619–25.

2. Sykora J, Pomahacova R, Kreslova M, et al. Current global trends in the incidence of pediatric-onset inflammatory bowel disease. World J Gastroenterol 2018;24:2741–63.

3. Murakami Y, Nishiwaki Y, Oba MS, et al. Estimated prevalence of ulcerative colitis and Crohn's disease in Japan in 2014: an analysis of a nationwide survey. J Gastroenterol 2019;54:1070–7.

4. Mountifield R, Bampton P, Prosser R, et al. Fear and fertility in inflammatory bowel disease: a mismatch of perception and reality affects family planning decisions. Inflamm Bowel Dis 2009;15:720–5.

5. Malter L, Jain A, Cohen BL, et al. Identifying IBD Providers' Knowledge Gaps Using a Prospective Web-based Survey. Inflamm Bowel Dis 2020;26:1445–50.

6. Vander Borght M, Wyns C. Fertility and infertility: Definition and epidemiology. Clin Biochem 2018;62:2–10.

7. Mahadevan U, Robinson C, Bernasko N, et al. Inflammatory Bowel Disease in Pregnancy Clinical Care Pathway: A Report From the American Gastroenterological Association IBD Parenthood Project Working Group. Inflamm Bowel Dis 2019;25:627–41.

8. Walentynowicz M, Van de Pavert I, Coenen S, et al. Worries and concerns of inflammatory bowel disease (IBD) patients in Belgium - a validation of the Dutch rating form. Scand J Gastroenterol 2020;55:1427–32.

9. Tavernier N, Fumery M, Peyrin-Biroulet L, et al. Systematic review: fertility in non-surgically treated inflammatory bowel disease. Aliment Pharmacol Ther 2013; 38:847–53.

10. Hammami MB, Mahadevan U. Men With Inflammatory Bowel Disease: Sexual Function, Fertility, Medication Safety, and Prostate Cancer. Am J Gastroenterol 2020;115:526–34.

11. O'Morain C, Smethurst P, Dore CJ, et al. Reversible male infertility due to sulphasalazine: studies in man and rat. Gut 1984;25:1078–84.

12. Collen MJ. Azulfidine-induced oligospermia. Am J Gastroenterol 1980;74: 441–2.

13. Birnie GG, McLeod TI, Watkinson G. Incidence of sulphasalazine-induced male infertility. Gut 1981;22:452–5.

14. Mouyis M, Flint JD, Giles IP. Safety of anti-rheumatic drugs in men trying to conceive: A systematic review and analysis of published evidence. Semin Arthritis Rheum 2019;48:911–20.

15. Sussman A, Leonard JM. Psoriasis, methotrexate, and oligospermia. Arch Dermatol 1980;116:215–7.

16. Ley D, Jones J, Parrish J, et al. Methotrexate Reduces DNA Integrity in Sperm From Men With Inflammatory Bowel Disease. Gastroenterology 2018;154: 2064–2067 e3.

17. Bermas BL. Paternal safety of anti-rheumatic medications. Best Pract Res Clin Obstet Gynaecol 2020;64:77–84.

18. Barberio B, Zamani M, Black CJ, et al. Prevalence of symptoms of anxiety and depression in patients with inflammatory bowel disease: a systematic review and meta-analysis. Lancet Gastroenterol Hepatol 2021;6:359–70.

19. Beeder LA, Samplaski MK. Effect of antidepressant medications on semen parameters and male fertility. Int J Urol 2020;27:39–46.

20. Montejo AL, Llorca G, Izquierdo JA, et al. Incidence of sexual dysfunction associated with antidepressant agents: a prospective multicenter study of 1022

outpatients. Spanish Working Group for the Study of Psychotropic-Related Sexual Dysfunction. J Clin Psychiatry 2001;62(Suppl 3):10–21.

21. Burr NE, Smith C, West R, et al. Increasing Prescription of Opiates and Mortality in Patients With Inflammatory Bowel Diseases in England. Clin Gastroenterol Hepatol 2018;16:534–541 e6.

22. Crocker JA, Yu H, Conaway M, et al. Narcotic use and misuse in Crohn's disease. Inflamm Bowel Dis 2014;20:2234–8.

23. Zhao S, Deng T, Luo L, et al. Association Between Opioid Use and Risk of Erectile Dysfunction: A Systematic Review and Meta-Analysis. J Sex Med 2017;14: 1209–19.

24. Riss S, Schwameis K, Mittlbock M, et al. Sexual function and quality of life after surgical treatment for anal fistulas in Crohn's disease. Tech Coloproctol 2013;17: 89–94.

25. El-Tawil AM. Zinc deficiency in men with Crohn's disease may contribute to poor sperm function and male infertility. Andrologia 2003;35:337–41.

26. Freour T, Miossec C, Bach-Ngohou K, et al. Ovarian reserve in young women of reproductive age with Crohn's disease. Inflamm Bowel Dis 2012;18:1515–22.

27. Ban L, Tata LJ, Humes DJ, et al. Decreased fertility rates in 9639 women diagnosed with inflammatory bowel disease: a United Kingdom population-based cohort study. Aliment Pharmacol Ther 2015;42:855–66.

28. Levy RA, de Jesus GR, de Jesus NR, et al. Critical review of the current recommendations for the treatment of systemic inflammatory rheumatic diseases during pregnancy and lactation. Autoimmun Rev 2016;15:955–63.

29. McConnell RA, Mahadevan U. Use of Immunomodulators and Biologics Before, During, and After Pregnancy. Inflamm Bowel Dis 2016;22:213–23.

30. Lee S, Crowe M, Seow CH, et al. The impact of surgical therapies for inflammatory bowel disease on female fertility. Cochrane Database Syst Rev 2019;7: CD012711.

31. Bartels SA, D'Hoore A, Cuesta MA, et al. Significantly increased pregnancy rates after laparoscopic restorative proctocolectomy: a cross-sectional study. Ann Surg 2012;256:1045–8.

32. Beyer-Berjot L, Maggiori L, Birnbaum D, et al. A total laparoscopic approach reduces the infertility rate after ileal pouch-anal anastomosis: a 2-center study. Ann Surg 2013;258:275–82.

33. Lavie I, Lavie M, Doyev R, et al. Pregnancy outcomes in women with inflammatory bowel disease who successfully conceived via assisted reproduction technique. Arch Gynecol Obstet 2020;302:611–8.

34. Nørgård BM, Larsen PV, Fedder J, et al. Live birth and adverse birth outcomes in women with ulcerative colitis and Crohn's disease receiving assisted reproduction: a 20-year nationwide cohort study. Gut 2016;65:767–76.

35. Annese V. Genetics and epigenetics of IBD. Pharm Res 2020;159:104892.

36. Moller FT, Andersen V, Wohlfahrt J, et al. Familial risk of inflammatory bowel disease: a population-based cohort study 1977-2011. Am J Gastroenterol 2015; 110:564–71.

37. Laharie D, Debeugny S, Peeters M, et al. Inflammatory bowel disease in spouses and their offspring. Gastroenterology 2001;120:816–9.

38. Turpin W, Goethel A, Bedrani L, et al. Determinants of IBD Heritability: Genes, Bugs, and More. Inflamm Bowel Dis 2018;24:1133–48.

39. Hashash JG, Kane S. Pregnancy and Inflammatory Bowel Disease. Gastroenterol Hepatol (N Y) 2015;11:96–102.

40. Miller JP. Inflammatory bowel disease in pregnancy: a review. J R Soc Med 1986;79:221–5.
41. Cornish J, Tan E, Teare J, et al. A meta-analysis on the influence of inflammatory bowel disease on pregnancy. Gut 2007;56:830–7.
42. Leung KK, Tandon P, Govardhanam V, et al. The Risk of Adverse Neonatal Outcomes With Maternal Inflammatory Bowel Disease: A Systematic Review and Meta-analysis. Inflamm Bowel Dis 2021;27:550–62.
43. O'Toole A, Nwanne O, Tomlinson T. Inflammatory Bowel Disease Increases Risk of Adverse Pregnancy Outcomes: A Meta-Analysis. Dig Dis Sci 2015;60: 2750–61.
44. Kim MA, Kim YH, Chun J, et al. The Influence of Disease Activity on Pregnancy Outcomes in Women With Inflammatory Bowel Disease: A Systematic Review and Meta-Analysis. J Crohns Colitis 2021;15:719–32.
45. Lee HH, Bae JM, Lee BI, et al. Pregnancy outcomes in women with inflammatory bowel disease: a 10-year nationwide population-based cohort study. Aliment Pharmacol Ther 2020;51:861–9.
46. Nguyen GC, Munsell M, Harris ML. Nationwide prevalence and prognostic significance of clinically diagnosable protein-calorie malnutrition in hospitalized inflammatory bowel disease patients. Inflamm Bowel Dis 2008;14:1105–11.
47. Pedersen N, Bortoli A, Duricova D, et al. The course of inflammatory bowel disease during pregnancy and postpartum: a prospective European ECCO-EpiCom Study of 209 pregnant women. Aliment Pharmacol Ther 2013;38: 501–12.
48. ACOG Committee Opinion No. 762. Prepregnancy Counseling. Obstet Gynecol 2019;133:e78–89.
49. Mentella MC, Scaldaferri F, Pizzoferrato M, et al. The Association of Disease Activity, BMI and Phase Angle with Vitamin D Deficiency in Patients with IBD. Nutrients 2019;11.
50. Fung JL, Hartman TJ, Schleicher RL, et al. Association of vitamin D intake and serum levels with fertility: results from the Lifestyle and Fertility Study. Fertil Steril 2017;108:302–11.
51. Farraye FA, Melmed GY, Lichtenstein GR, et al. ACG Clinical Guideline: Preventive Care in Inflammatory Bowel Disease. Am J Gastroenterol 2017;112:241–58.
52. Gaidos J, Moss AM, Serrano M. Health Maintenance Summary. In: Foundation CsaC, ed. Volume 2021, 2020.
53. Khalili H, Higuchi LM, Ananthakrishnan AN, et al. Oral contraceptives, reproductive factors and risk of inflammatory bowel disease. Gut 2013;62:1153–9.
54. Long MD, Hutfless S. Shifting Away From Estrogen-Containing Oral Contraceptives in Crohn's Disease. Gastroenterology 2016;150:1518–20.
55. Centers for Disease C, Prevention. U S. Medical Eligibility Criteria for Contraceptive Use, 2010. MMWR Recomm Rep 2010;59:1–86.
56. de Lima A, Zelinkova Z, Mulders AG, et al. Preconception Care Reduces Relapse of Inflammatory Bowel Disease During Pregnancy. Clin Gastroenterol Hepatol 2016;14:1285–1292 e1.
57. Selinger C, Carey N, Cassere S, et al. Standards for the provision of antenatal care for patients with inflammatory bowel disease: guidance endorsed by the British Society of Gastroenterology and the British Maternal and Fetal Medicine Society. Frontline Gastroenterol 2021;12:182–7.
58. Lichtenstein GR, Loftus EV, Isaacs KL, et al. ACG Clinical Guideline: Management of Crohn's disease in Adults. Am J Gastroenterol 2018;113(4):481–517.

59. Aboubakr A, Riggs AR, Jimenez D, et al. Identifying Patient Priorities for Preconception and Pregnancy Counseling in IBD. Dig Dis Sci 2021;66:1829–35.

60. Nørgärd B, Czeizel AE, Rockenbauer M, et al. Population-based case control study of the safety of sulfasalazine use during pregnancy. Aliment Pharmacol Ther 2001;15:483–6.

61. Leung YP, Kaplan GG, Coward S, et al. Intrapartum corticosteroid use significantly increases the risk of gestational diabetes in women with inflammatory bowel disease. J Crohns Colitis 2015;9:223–30.

62. Schulze H, Esters P, Dignass A. Review article: the management of Crohn's disease and ulcerative colitis during pregnancy and lactation. Aliment Pharmacol Ther 2014;40:991–1008.

63. Szymanska E, Kisielewski R, Kierkus J. Reproduction and Pregnancy in Inflammatory Bowel Disease - Management and Treatment Based on Current Guidelines. J Gynecol Obstet Hum Reprod 2021;50:101777.

64. Vestergaard T, Jorgensen SMD, Christensen LA, et al. Pregnancy outcome in four women with inflammatory bowel disease treated with budesonide MMX. Scand J Gastroenterol 2018;53:1459–62.

65. Beaulieu DB, Ananthakrishnan AN, Issa M, et al. Budesonide induction and maintenance therapy for Crohn's disease during pregnancy. Inflamm Bowel Dis 2009;15:25–8.

66. Acar S, Keskin-Arslan E, Erol-Coskun H, et al. Pregnancy outcomes following quinolone and fluoroquinolone exposure during pregnancy: A systematic review and meta-analysis. Reprod Toxicol 2019;85:65–74.

67. Burtin P, Taddio A, Ariburnu O, et al. Safety of metronidazole in pregnancy: a meta-analysis. Am J Obstet Gynecol 1995;172:525–9.

68. Kanis SL, de Lima-Karagiannis A, de Boer NKH, et al. Use of Thiopurines During Conception and Pregnancy Is Not Associated With Adverse Pregnancy Outcomes or Health of Infants at One Year in a Prospective Study. Clin Gastroenterol Hepatol 2017;15:1232–1241 e1.

69. Nielsen OH, Gubatan JM, Juhl CB, et al. Biologics for Inflammatory Bowel Disease and Their Safety in Pregnancy: A Systematic Review and Meta-analysis. Clin Gastroenterol Hepatol 2020;20(1):74–87.e3.

70. Mahadevan U, Long MD, Kane SV, et al. Pregnancy and Neonatal Outcomes After Fetal Exposure to Biologics and Thiopurines Among Women With Inflammatory Bowel Disease. Gastroenterology 2021;160:1131–9.

71. Porter C, Armstrong-Fisher S, Kopotsha T, et al. Certolizumab pegol does not bind the neonatal Fc receptor (FcRn): Consequences for FcRn-mediated in vitro transcytosis and ex vivo human placental transfer. J Reprod Immunol 2016;116:7–12.

72. Mahadevan U, Wolf DC, Dubinsky M, et al. Placental transfer of anti-tumor necrosis factor agents in pregnant patients with inflammatory bowel disease. Clin Gastroenterol Hepatol 2013;11:286–92.

73. Wils P, Seksik P, Stefanescu C, et al. Safety of ustekinumab or vedolizumab in pregnant inflammatory bowel disease patients: a multicentre cohort study. Aliment Pharmacol Ther 2021;53:460–70.

74. Moens A, van der Woude CJ, Julsgaard M, et al. Pregnancy outcomes in inflammatory bowel disease patients treated with vedolizumab, anti-TNF or conventional therapy: results of the European CONCEIVE study. Aliment Pharmacol Ther 2020;51:129–38.

75. Singh S, Proctor D, Scott FI, et al. AGA Technical Review on the Medical Management of Moderate to Severe Luminal and Perianal Fistulizing Crohn's Disease. Gastroenterology 2021;160:2512–2556 e9.

76. Mahadevan U, Vermeire S, Lasch K, et al. Vedolizumab exposure in pregnancy: outcomes from clinical studies in inflammatory bowel disease. Aliment Pharmacol Ther 2017;45:941–50.

77. Peng A, Qiu X, Zhang L, et al. Natalizumab exposure during pregnancy in multiple sclerosis: a systematic review. J Neurol Sci 2019;396:202–5.

78. Hellwig K, Haghikia A, Gold R. Pregnancy and natalizumab: results of an observational study in 35 accidental pregnancies during natalizumab treatment. Mult Scler 2011;17:958–63.

79. Picardo S, Seow CH. The impact of pregnancy on biologic therapies for the treatment of inflammatory bowel disease. Best Pract Res Clin Gastroenterol 2020;44-45:101670.

80. Flanagan E, Gibson PR, Wright EK, et al. Infliximab, adalimumab and vedolizumab concentrations across pregnancy and vedolizumab concentrations in infants following intrauterine exposure. Aliment Pharmacol Ther 2020;52:1551–62.

81. Julsgaard M, Christensen LA, Gibson PR, et al. Concentrations of Adalimumab and Infliximab in Mothers and Newborns, and Effects on Infection. Gastroenterology 2016;151:110–9.

82. Chaparro M, Verreth A, Lobaton T, et al. Long-Term Safety of In Utero Exposure to Anti-TNFalpha Drugs for the Treatment of Inflammatory Bowel Disease: Results from the Multicenter European TEDDY Study. Am J Gastroenterol 2018; 113:396–403.

83. Mahadevan U, Dubinsky MC, Su C, et al. Outcomes of Pregnancies With Maternal/Paternal Exposure in the Tofacitinib Safety Databases for Ulcerative Colitis. Inflamm Bowel Dis 2018;24:2494–500.

84. ZEPOSIA. Prescribinginformation. Volume 2021: Bristol-Myers Squibb Company, 2021. Available at: https://www.zeposiahcp.com/ulcerative-colitis/.

85. Sandborn WJ, Feagan BG, Hanauer S, et al. Long-Term Efficacy And Safety Of Ozanimod In Moderate-To-Severe Ulcerative Colitis: Results From The Open-Label Extension Of The Randomized, Phase 2 Touchstone Study. J Crohns Colitis 2021;15(7):1120–9.

86. Peyrin-Biroulet L, Loftus EV Jr, Colombel JF, et al. The natural history of adult Crohn's disease in population-based cohorts. Am J Gastroenterol 2010;105: 289–97.

87. van der Woude CJ, Ardizzone S, Bengtson MB, et al. The second European evidenced-based consensus on reproduction and pregnancy in inflammatory bowel disease. J Crohns Colitis 2015;9:107–24.

88. Chaparro M, Gisbert JP. Surgery for Crohn's disease during pregnancy: a difficult decision. United Eur Gastroenterol J 2020;8:633–4.

89. Germain A, Chateau T, Beyer-Berjot L, et al. Surgery for Crohn's disease during pregnancy: A nationwide survey. United Eur Gastroenterol J 2020;8:736–40.

90. Tolcher MC, Clark SL. Diagnostic Imaging and Outcomes for Nonobstetric Surgery During Pregnancy. Clin Obstet Gynecol 2020;63:364–9.

91. Bortoli A, Pedersen N, Duricova D, et al. Pregnancy outcome in inflammatory bowel disease: prospective European case-control ECCO-EpiCom study, 2003-2006. Aliment Pharmacol Ther 2011;34:724–34.

92. Caprilli R, Gassull MA, Escher JC, et al. European evidence based consensus on the diagnosis and management of Crohn's disease: special situations. Gut 2006;55(Suppl 1):i36–58.
93. Nørgärd B, Hundborg HH, Jacobsen BA, et al. Disease activity in pregnant women with Crohn's disease and birth outcomes: a regional Danish cohort study. Am J Gastroenterol 2007;102:1947–54.
94. Meyer A, Drouin J, Weill A, et al. Pregnancy in women with inflammatory bowel disease: a French nationwide study 2010-2018. Aliment Pharmacol Ther 2020; 52:1480–90.
95. Tandon P, Leung K, Yusuf A, et al. Noninvasive Methods For Assessing Inflammatory Bowel Disease Activity in Pregnancy: A Systematic Review. J Clin Gastroenterol 2019;53:574–81.
96. Kammerlander H, Nielsen J, Kjeldsen J, et al. Fecal Calprotectin During Pregnancy in Women With Moderate-Severe Inflammatory Bowel Disease. Inflamm Bowel Dis 2018;24:839–48.
97. Julsgaard M, Hvas CL, Gearry RB, et al. Fecal Calprotectin Is Not Affected by Pregnancy: Clinical Implications for the Management of Pregnant Patients with Inflammatory Bowel Disease. Inflamm Bowel Dis 2017;23:1240–6.
98. Flanagan E, Wright EK, Begun J, et al. Monitoring Inflammatory Bowel Disease in Pregnancy Using Gastrointestinal Ultrasonography. J Crohns Colitis 2020;14: 1405–12.
99. Kakkadasam Ramaswamy P, Vizhi NK, Yelsangikar A, et al. Utility of bowel ultrasound in assessing disease activity in Crohn's disease. Indian J Gastroenterol 2020;39:495–502.
100. Bryant RV, Friedman AB, Wright EK, et al. Gastrointestinal ultrasound in inflammatory bowel disease: an underused resource with potential paradigm-changing application. Gut 2018;67:973–85.
101. Ko MS, Rudrapatna VA, Avila P, et al. Safety of Flexible Sigmoidoscopy in Pregnant Patients with Known or Suspected Inflammatory Bowel Disease. Dig Dis Sci 2020;65:2979–85.
102. Cappell MS, Fox SR, Gorrepati N. Safety and efficacy of colonoscopy during pregnancy: an analysis of pregnancy outcome in 20 patients. J Reprod Med 2010;55:115–23.
103. Committee ASoP, Shergill AK, Ben-Menachem T, et al. Guidelines for endoscopy in pregnant and lactating women. Gastrointest Endosc 2012;76:18–24.
104. Bengtson MB, Martin CF, Aamodt G, et al. Inadequate Gestational Weight Gain Predicts Adverse Pregnancy Outcomes in Mothers with Inflammatory Bowel Disease: Results from a Prospective US Pregnancy Cohort. Dig Dis Sci 2017;62: 2063–9.
105. Bengtson MB, Aamodt G, Mahadevan U, et al. Inadequate Gestational Weight Gain, the Hidden Link Between Maternal IBD and Adverse Pregnancy Outcomes: Results from the Norwegian Mother and Child Cohort Study. Inflamm Bowel Dis 2017;23:1225–33.
106. Lee S, Metcalfe A, Raman M, et al. Pregnant Women with Inflammatory Bowel Disease Are at Increased Risk of Vitamin D Insufficiency: A Cross-Sectional Study. J Crohns Colitis 2018;12:702–9.
107. Ward MG, Kariyawasam VC, Mogan SB, et al. Prevalence and Risk Factors for Functional Vitamin B12 Deficiency in Patients with Crohn's Disease. Inflamm Bowel Dis 2015;21:2839–47.

108. Battat R, Kopylov U, Szilagyi A, et al. Vitamin B12 deficiency in inflammatory bowel disease: prevalence, risk factors, evaluation, and management. Inflamm Bowel Dis 2014;20:1120–8.

109. Rossi RE, Whyand T, Murray CD, et al. The role of dietary supplements in inflammatory bowel disease: a systematic review. Eur J Gastroenterol Hepatol 2016; 28:1357–64.

110. Lamb CA, Kennedy NA, Raine T, et al. British Society of Gastroenterology consensus guidelines on the management of inflammatory bowel disease in adults. Gut 2019;68:s1–106.

111. Nguyen GC, Seow CH, Maxwell C, et al. The Toronto Consensus Statements for the Management of Inflammatory Bowel Disease in Pregnancy. Gastroenterology 2016;150:734–757 e1.

112. Foulon A, Dupas JL, Sabbagh C, et al. Defining the Most Appropriate Delivery Mode in Women with Inflammatory Bowel Disease: A Systematic Review. Inflamm Bowel Dis 2017;23:712–20.

113. Hatch Q, Champagne BJ, Maykel JA, et al. Crohn's disease and pregnancy: the impact of perianal disease on delivery methods and complications. Dis Colon Rectum 2014;57:174–8.

114. Sultan AH, Kamm MA, Hudson CN, et al. Anal-sphincter disruption during vaginal delivery. N Engl J Med 1993;329:1905–11.

115. Remzi FH, Gorgun E, Bast J, et al. Vaginal delivery after ileal pouch-anal anastomosis: a word of caution. Dis Colon Rectum 2005;48:1691–9.

116. Bruce A, Black M, Bhattacharya S. Mode of delivery and risk of inflammatory bowel disease in the offspring: systematic review and meta-analysis of observational studies. Inflamm Bowel Dis 2014;20:1217–26.

117. Antao C, Teixeira C, Gomes MJ. OC28 - Effect of mode of delivery on early oral colonization and childhood dental caries: a systematic review. Nurs Child Young People 2016;28:74–5.

118. Kim YH, Pfaller B, Marson A, et al. The risk of venous thromboembolism in women with inflammatory bowel disease during pregnancy and the postpartum period: A systematic review and meta-analysis. Medicine (Baltimore) 2019;98: e17309.

119. Hansen AT, Erichsen R, Horvath-Puho E, et al. Inflammatory bowel disease and venous thromboembolism during pregnancy and the postpartum period. J Thromb Haemost 2017;15:702–8.

120. Bates SM, Middeldorp S, Rodger M, et al. Guidance for the treatment and prevention of obstetric-associated venous thromboembolism. J Thromb Thrombolysis 2016;41:92–128.

121. Bennett A, Mamunes A, Kim M, et al. The Importance of Monitoring the Postpartum Period in Moderate to Severe Crohn's Disease. Inflammatory Bowel Diseases 2021;104. https://doi.org/10.1093/ibd/izab104.

122. Yu A, Friedman S, Ananthakrishnan AN. Incidence and Predictors of Flares in the Postpartum Year Among Women With Inflammatory Bowel Disease. Inflamm Bowel Dis 2020;26:1926–32.

123. Mahadevan U, McConnell RA, Chambers CD. Drug Safety and Risk of Adverse Outcomes for Pregnant Patients With Inflammatory Bowel Disease. Gastroenterology 2017;152:451–462 e2.

124. Wodi AP, Ault K, Hunter P, et al. Advisory Committee on Immunization Practices Recommended Immunization Schedule for Children and Adolescents Aged 18

Years or Younger - United States, 2021. MMWR Morb Mortal Wkly Rep 2021;70: 189–92.

125. Friedman S, Nielsen J, Jolving LR, et al. Long-term motor and cognitive function in the children of women with inflammatory bowel disease. J Crohns Colitis 2020;14(12):1709–16.

126. Drobnis EZ, Nangia AK. Immunosuppressants and Male Reproduction. Adv Exp Med Biol 2017;1034:179–210.

Pediatric Management of Crohn's Disease

Elana B. Mitchel, MD, MSCE[a],*, Joel R. Rosh, MD[b]

KEYWORDS

- Crohn's disease • Pediatric • Children • Adolescents

KEY POINTS

- Pediatric CD is often more severe and dynamic, requires higher levels of immunosuppression, and is associated with greater morbidity than adult CD.
- Unique considerations in pediatric CD include growth impairment, pubertal delay, bone disease, longevity of disease burden, and the psychological impact of chronic disease on children and adolescents.
- Treatment options are limited. Anti-TNF therapy is the only FDA-approved biologic therapy; however, there is growing evidence to support off-label use of additional biologic therapies and work to enhance the study of medications in the pediatric population.
- Without effective therapy complications can occur including growth delay, bone disease, anemia, venous thromboembolism, infection, and malignancy.
- Pediatric CD is an area of tremendous potential for ongoing translational and clinical research and quality improvement and it is important that all gastroenterologists have an understanding of this complex and growing population.

INTRODUCTION

Twenty-five percent of individuals with inflammatory bowel disease (IBD) are diagnosed before 18 years of age and are considered to have pediatric-onset IBD.[1,2] Recent studies have demonstrated a rising incidence in children in North America, with the pediatric prevalence estimated at 77 per 100,000 in 2016.[2–4] The highest percentage increase is in young children less than 5 years of age.[3] Crohn's disease (CD) is nearly two times more prevalent than ulcerative colitis (45.9 vs 21.6 per 100,000).[2]

Although there are similarities to the presentation, diagnostic approach, and treatment of pediatric and adult CD, there are unique challenges and significant differences. Pediatric-onset CD is often more extensive with a more aggressive disease course.[5–9] It has been shown that patients with childhood-onset CD were more likely to have severe disease and higher immunosuppressant requirement compared with

[a] Children's Hospital of Philadelphia, 3401 Civic Center Boulevard, Suite 7NW, Philadelphia, PA 19104, USA; [b] Goryeb Children's Hospital/Atlantic Children's Health, 100 Madison Avenue, Morristown, NJ 07962, USA
* Corresponding author.
E-mail address: mitchele@chop.edu

Gastroenterol Clin N Am 51 (2022) 401–424
https://doi.org/10.1016/j.gtc.2021.12.013
0889-8553/22/© 2022 Elsevier Inc. All rights reserved.

gastro.theclinics.com

adult-onset patients.[6] In addition, pediatric-onset disease is more dynamic, often with change in disease location and behavior over time.[6–9] This dynamic quality can make it difficult to predict prognosis and response to therapy. Because of the longevity of disease burden, associated morbidity is also higher in pediatric IBD. Disease-related complications, such as growth impairment and delay in puberty, are a central focus. In addition, recognition of the psychological impact of chronic disease on children and their families is important.[6,7]

Although the average age at diagnosis is between 10 and 12 years of age, a growing population within pediatric IBD is the very early onset (VEO) IBD cohort, children who are diagnosed by 6 years of age.[10–12] This is a unique and challenging population with a disease phenotype that typically favors colonic distribution, is refractory to traditional therapies, and involves primary immunodeficiencies. Patients with VEO-IBD often have more severe disease with less improvement in growth during follow-up, higher likelihood of surgery and medication failure, and greater frequency for readmission to the hospital compared with older children diagnosed with IBD.[10] Monogenic causes of VEO-IBD have been identified and immunologic work-up and whole-exome sequencing are needed to allow for more targeted therapy in this subset of pediatric patients with IBD.[10–12]

Therapy in pediatric CD is focused on minimizing inflammation with a goal of mucosal healing and preventing disease-related complications while optimizing nutrition, growth, and quality of life. Individualized treatment plans based on age, disease phenotype, medication side effects, and extent of growth delay are imperative. Although this is an exciting time for IBD therapeutics as the treatment armamentarium expands, there are limited approved therapy options in pediatric CD despite the unique challenges and complexities of pediatric CD.[5] The juxtaposition of the growing prevalence, the recognized complexity, and still limited treatment options serve to highlight the importance for why gastroenterologists should be highly knowledgeable of how to optimize the care of those with pediatric-onset CD.

PATIENT EVALUATION OVERVIEW
Presentation

As in adults, pediatric-onset CD can present with abdominal pain, diarrhea, rectal bleeding, constipation, weight loss, mouth sores, fever, and joint pain. Symptoms are heterogeneous and often insidious.[13]

One of the major distinctions in pediatric IBD is the impact on growth and pubertal development. Growth retardation and pubertal delay are common in pediatric CD at the time of diagnosis and can be the first signs of disease. The cause of growth failure is multifactorial and primarily a result of increased energy expenditure and the metabolic consequences of inflammation with decreased oral intake and malabsorption also contributing.[7,14–16] Pubertal delay can include absence of breast development or testicular enlargement and delayed menarche. Given the impact that pediatric IBD has on growth, it is paramount to diagnose and intervene before puberty is complete to ensure optimization of the patient's growth potential.

Symptoms

The most common symptoms reported in CD include diarrhea, abdominal pain, and poor growth. Red flag symptoms that should be identified and explored include rectal bleeding, nocturnal stooling, fecal urgency, tenesmus, vomiting, and weight loss. As in adults, extraintestinal symptoms include dermatologic manifestations, such as erythema nodosum and pyoderma gangrenosum; rheumatologic conditions, such as arthritis and ankylosing spondylitis; ophthalmologic conditions, such as uveitis; hepatobiliary manifestations, such as primary sclerosing cholangitis and auto-immune hepatitis; urologic issues including nephrolithiasis; and hematologic issues, such as iron-deficiency anemia and venous thromboembolism (VTE). Some of these manifestations occur in the setting of active disease but others can occur when disease is under control. Many of these extraintestinal manifestations can impact treatment decisions and long-term outcomes.

Physical Examination

Physical examination is an important part of the work-up and diagnosis of pediatric CD. Assessment for weight loss and decreased height velocity should occur. In addition, assessment of pubertal status using Tanner staging is important. Evaluation for extraintestinal manifestations, such as oral ulcers, arthritis, digital clubbing, hepatomegaly, and rashes, is important. Careful abdominal and perianal examinations must be performed.

Laboratory Work-up

The laboratory evaluation for a patient suspected to have CD is outlined in **Table 1**. Importantly, normal laboratory studies do not exclude the diagnosis of IBD. Infectious

Table 1
Laboratory work-up for suspected IBD

Laboratory Test	Findings Consistent with CD
Blood tests	
Complete blood count	Elevated white blood cell count Microcytic anemia Elevated platelet count
Electrolytes	Elevated serum urea nitrogen to creatinine ratio caused by dehydration/gastrointestinal losses Acidosis
Hepatic chemistries	Hypoalbuminemia Elevated aspartate aminotransferase, alanine aminotransferase, and γ-glutamyltransferase
C-reactive protein	Elevated
Sedimentation rate	Elevated
Stool tests	
Stool calprotectin	Elevated
Stool culture	Rule out bacterial enteritis, such as salmonella and campylobacter
Stool *Clostridium difficile* toxin	Rule out *C difficile* infection
Giardia and cryptosporidium antigen	Rule out parasitic infections
Immunologic work-up[a]	
Immunoglobulins (IgA, IgM, IgE, IgG with subclasses)	Evaluate for antibody deficiencies
Dihydrorhodamine test	Evaluate for chronic granulomatous disease
Vaccine titers (pneumococcal, diphtheria, tetanus)	Evaluate for T- and B-cell memory

[a] Perform if VEO-IBD is suspected. Additional testing should be performed in collaboration with a pediatric immunologist.

stool studies must be performed to rule out other causes of chronic or bloody diarrhea before endoscopic evaluation. A positive infection does not rule out IBD; however, the patient should be treated or observed, as appropriate, before further evaluation. Fecal calprotectin is a useful noninvasive measure of bowel inflammation and is used to monitor response to therapy and disease recurrence.[17–20] It must be used thoughtfully, however, because it is not specific for IBD; reflects colonic inflammation better than small bowel; and is elevated with infectious enteritis, presence of intestinal blood, inflammatory polyps, nonsteroidal anti-inflammatory drug use, and oncologic process.[19,21] Calprotectin should not take the place of endoscopic evaluation.

In the work-up of very young children in whom there is a high suspicion for VEO-IBD additional immunologic testing is recommended.

Endoscopic Work-up

Upper gastrointestinal endoscopy and colonoscopy are used to make the definitive diagnosis of CD. Both the European Society for Pediatric Gastroenterology, Hepatology and Nutrition and North American Society for Pediatric Gastroenterology, Hepatology, and Nutrition and the Crohn's and Colitis Foundation recommend total colonoscopy with ileal intubation, upper endoscopy, multiple biopsies, and small bowel exploration to make the diagnosis of CD.[22,23] Intubation of the ileum is important because 9% of children with CD have isolated ileal disease.[24] In pediatrics, biopsy is essential to make the diagnosis with chronic inflammation on histology that is characteristic for IBD.

Small Bowel Imaging Work-up

Small bowel imaging is important for complete evaluation of the bowel. In addition, small bowel imaging can help to assess transmural complications, such as fistula and abscess. Imaging in the pediatric population requires multiple considerations including the patient's ability to tolerate the study with attention to duration of the study, need for sedation, ingestion of contrast, and radiation exposure. The pros and cons to each imaging modality are listed in **Table 2**.

Magnetic resonance enterography of the abdomen and pelvis has become the imaging modality of choice in the evaluation of pediatric CD. Magnetic resonance enterography has shown high specificity and sensitivity in detecting inflammatory changes in the intestinal wall and other disease complications. In addition, magnetic resonance enterography has no associated ionizing radiation exposure.[25,26] However, because of the long study duration, issues with claustrophobia, and discomfort involved in tolerating enteral contrast, magnetic resonance enterography is difficult to tolerate in certain populations, particularly young children or patients with developmental delay. Alternatively, computed tomography enterography or ultrasound with contrast are good options. Ultrasound with contrast is increasing in use, particularly among younger patients; however, it remains user dependent and there are no standardized norms.[27–29]

PHARMACOLOGIC OR MEDICAL TREATMENT OPTIONS

Treatment decisions are made based on disease severity, disease location, disease phenotype, growth and development status, patient and family preference, and impact on quality of life. As in adults, the goal of therapy is not only to induce and maintain clinical remission but to also achieve mucosal healing, which has been shown to decrease the risk for hospitalization, surgery, and disease complications, and in pediatrics, correct growth failure.[30–32] Use of effective therapy upfront is fundamental in

Table 2
Pros and cons of small bowel imaging modalities

Imaging Modality	Pros	Cons
Small bowel series	Available at most centers Inexpensive	Ionizing radiation exposure Long duration of examination Poor sensitivity for transmural complications
Bowel ultrasound ± contrast enhanced	No ionizing radiation Inexpensive Well-tolerated by young children	Operator dependent No standardized norms Difficult to visualize entire gastrointestinal tract Bowel gas and soft tissue can obscure view Decreased reproducibility
Computed tomography	Available at most centers Excellent visualization of bowel wall Short duration of examination Ideal imaging for emergencies	Ionizing radiation Need for intravenous and oral contrast
Magnetic resonance enterography	No ionizing radiation Can obtain cross-sectional imaging in different planes Excellent visualization of bowel wall Can evaluate inflammatory vs fibrotic bowel changes	Expensive Need for intravenous and oral contrast Long duration of examination Difficult to tolerate in young children and children with developmental delay Pediatric expertise may not be widely available
Video capsule endoscopy	No ionizing radiation In-depth evaluation of small bowel mucosa	Placed under anesthesia if cannot swallow capsule No standardized scoring system in pediatrics Can cause obstruction and lead to surgical emergency if undiagnosed stricture present Technologic issues including "overinterpretation" of findings

pediatric CD given the often more complex and aggressive phenotype. Further complicating IBD therapy in pediatrics are the limited Food and Drug Administration (FDA)-approved therapies. FDA-approved therapies, doses, administration form, and side effects are listed in **Table 3**.

Nonbiologic Therapies

The goal of 5-aminosalicylic acid therapy (5-ASA) is to provide a topical anti-inflammatory therapy to the site of inflammation while minimizing systemic absorption.

Table 3
Pediatric IBD medications and standard doses

Medication name	Dose	Route	Side Effects
5-aminosalicylate (mesalamine)	50–100 mg/kg/d, up to 4 g daily	Oral	Nausea, vomiting, abdominal pain, bloody diarrhea, interstitial nephritis, pancreatitis
Antibiotics	Based on specific antibiotic	Oral or intravenous	Based on specific antibiotic
Immunomodulators			
Azathioprine	2–3 mg/kg/d	Oral	Myelosuppression, pancreatitis, lymphoma
6-Mercaptopurine	1–1.5 mg/kg/d	Oral	
Methotrexate	10–15 mg/m^2/d, maximum 25 mg/d	Oral or subcutaneous	Nausea, hepatotoxicity, pulmonary fibrosis
Prednisone	1–2 mg/kg/d, maximum 40 mg/d	Oral or intravenous	Infection, secondary adrenal insufficiency, growth suppression, bone demineralization, mood lability, sleep disturbance, acne
Budesonide	3–9 mg/d	Oral	Possible similar effects as prednisone, need to swallow capsule
Infliximab (standard dosing)	Induction: 5 mg/kg at 0, 2, 6 wk Maintenance: 5 mg/kg every 8 wk Maintenance interval can be shortened and/or dose increased based on clinical response and/or therapeutic drug monitoring	Intravenous	Infection, psoriasis, allergic reaction, lymphoma, immunogenicity
Adalimumab (standard dosing)	Induction: <40 kg: 80 mg on Day 0, 40 mg on Day 14, 20 mg on Day 28; ≥40 kg: 160 mg on Day 0, 80 mg on Day 14, 40 mg on Day 28 Maintenance: <40 kg: 20 mg; ≥40 kg: 40 mg every 14 d Maintenance interval can be shortened and/or dose increased based on clinical response and/or therapeutic drug monitoring	Subcutaneous	

Vedolizumab[a]	Induction: <40 kg: 5 mg/kg; ≥40 kg: 300 mg at 0, 2, 6 wk Maintenance: <40 kg: 5 mg/kg; ≥40 kg: 300 mg every 8 wk Maintenance interval can be shorted based on clinical response	Intravenous	Infection, allergic reaction
Ustekinumab[a]	Induction: 40–55 kg: 260 mg, 56–85 kg: 390 mg, ≥86 kg: 520 mg Maintenance: <40 kg: 45 mg; ≥40 kg: 90 mg every 8 wk Maintenance interval can be shortened based on clinical response	Induction dose: intravenous Maintenance dose: subcutaneous	Infection, allergic reaction

[a] Not yet FDA approved for pediatric CD, off-label use in children.

The role of 5-ASA therapy in pediatric CD is extremely limited to select patients with mild, uncomplicated, and predominantly colonic disease.[33] Overall the literature has shown that 5-ASA is not a suitable maintenance therapy for pediatric patients with CD and is associated with more exacerbations and longer steroid courses.[34,35] 5-ASA therapy is further limited in its use because there are no liquid preparations, a barrier for pediatric patients who cannot swallow pills. Certain capsule formulations can be opened and mixed into food, such as Pentasa and Colazal; however, the efficacy of this practice has not been studied.

Antibiotics are used in multiple ways in CD therapy, including treatment of perianal disease and penetrating disease, such as fistulae and intra-abdominal abscess.[33,36] In pediatric CD there is also some evidence for their use in treating active disease, primarily colonic.[37,38] Antibiotics are thought to combat the intestinal dysbiosis that impacts the pathogenesis of IBD and through immunomodulation.[13,37–40] The risks and benefits must be weighed because some studies have suggested that antibiotic exposure may contribute to the development of IBD and each antibiotic has its own side effects.[41,42]

Immunomodulators, thiopurine analogues (azathioprine and 6-mercaptopurine) and methotrexate, are used for maintenance therapy in CD.[33] This medication class was one of the first to show maintenance of clinical remission and decreased rates of hospitalization, steroid use, and surgery in patients with CD.[43] However, because of their side effect profile, lack of impact on growth restoration, and growing confidence in biologic therapies, immunomodulator monotherapy use has decreased overtime, especially in North America.[31,33,43,44] This has been most apparent in pediatric CD because thiopurines were found to have an increased risk of non-Hodgkin lymphoma and hepatosplenic T-cell lymphoma, particularly in adolescent boys.[45] Although immunomodulators do not play as much of a primary role in the treatment of pediatric CD, they are still often used in combination with anti–tumor necrosis factor (TNF) therapy to improve circulating drug levels.[46] Although methotrexate has not been as extensively studied, it has not been shown to be associated with hepatosplenic T-cell lymphoma and is therefore more commonly used in practice in pediatric CD.[47–49]

Corticosteroids are considered an effective treatment of induction of remission in children with moderate to severe CD. However, because of their significant side effect profile, including growth failure, increased risk of infection, secondary adrenal insufficiency, bone demineralization, and sleep disturbance, steroids are not a long-term therapy option. When patients require ongoing steroid therapy and are deemed steroid dependent, a change in therapy or surgical evaluation should be considered.[13,50] Nonsystemic steroid therapy, such as budesonide, which is released in the ileum or colon based on the formulation, is a way to provide targeted steroid therapy without systemic side effects. In a 12-week randomized controlled trial (RCT), comparing budesonide with prednisone in children with mild to moderate CD, there was no difference in rate of clinical remission (47% budesonide vs 50% prednisone); however, side effects were more common in the prednisone group (31.6% budesonide vs 71.4% prednisone; $P < .05$).[51] Budesonide is also not considered an effective maintenance therapy in pediatric CD.[33]

Anti–Tumor Necrosis Factor-α Agents

Infliximab and adalimumab, two of the anti-TNF agents, are the only biologic therapies that are FDA-approved for the treatment of pediatric CD. The efficacy and safety of anti-TNF therapy have been extensively studied in adult CD using placebo-controlled studies. In pediatrics, randomized placebo-controlled studies are lacking; however, open-label induction and dose-ranging nonplacebo-controlled studies have shown efficacy of infliximab and adalimumab in pediatric CD. The Randomized, Multicenter, Open Label Study to Evaluate the Safety and Efficacy of Anti-TNF Chimeric Monoclonal Antibody in Pediatric Subjects with Moderate-to-Severe Crohn's Disease (REACH) trial was the first study in pediatric CD to show clinical response and remission with infliximab at induction and maintenance. Clinical remission was achieved in 59% of patients at Week 10 postinduction and 55.8% with maintenance therapy every 8 weeks at 1 year.[52] Similar findings in efficacy and safety have been illustrated with adalimumab.[53,54] The Multicenter, Double-Blind Study to Evaluate the Safety, Efficacy and Pharmacokinetics of the Human Anti-TNF Monoclonal Antibody Adalimumab in Pediatric Subjects with Moderate to Severe Crohn's Disease (IMAgINE-1) trial was a double-blinded RCT comparing efficacy of a higher- and lower-dose adalimumab in infliximab-exposed and infliximab-naive patients. Clinical remission occurred in 33.5% of patients at 1 year. Infliximab-naive patients had higher rates of remission at 1 year compared with patients who had been previously treated with infliximab (45.1 vs 19.0%, respectively).[53] In the recent Pediatric Crohn's Disease Adalimumab Level-based Optimization Treatment (PAILOT) trial, a pediatric RCT to evaluate therapeutic drug monitoring with adalimumab in infliximab-naive patients with CD, clinical remission rates ranged from 48% to 82%.[54] These higher remission rates in infliximab-naive patients in IMAgINE-1 and PAILOT support the idea that optimization of the first biologic agent is important.[53–56]

Mucosal healing has become a central focus in studies of anti-TNF therapy given the positive impact that mucosal healing has on CD-related outcomes in adults. In pediatrics, only a few observational studies have demonstrated mucosal healing with anti-TNF therapy.[37,57,58] In addition, early use of anti-TNF therapy has been linked to higher likelihood of mucosal healing and improved CD-related outcomes.[31,37,41,59,60] The RISK inception cohort, which followed pediatric patients prospectively over 3 years, demonstrated the importance of early anti-TNF therapy, particularly in decreasing penetrating complications.[41] These findings have helped to change therapeutic approach with early use of anti-TNF therapy, often as first line.

Of importance in pediatric CD, anti-TNF therapy has also been shown to restore growth. The REACH trial showed that anti-TNF therapy allowed for catch-up growth.[52] Walters and colleagues[31] showed that patients with CD treated with early anti-TNF therapy had a significantly greater rate of linear growth normalization, compared with those on immunomodulator only (85.3% vs 60.3%; $P = .0017$).

Side effects and safety of anti-TNF therapy is important to discuss with pediatric patients. Overall, the rate of serious infections in pediatric patients is low and most infections do not require hospitalization or use of intravenous antibiotics. Pediatric patients being treated in combination with steroid or immunomodulator have higher risk of infection. In addition, rates of infection are higher in adults compared with children.[61–63] It is important to counsel patients that although anti-TNF therapy can lead to infection, untreated disease can lead to disease complications that increase risk of infection as well. There have also been reports of increased risk for lymphoproliferative disorders, such as hepatosplenic T-cell lymphoma, with anti-TNF therapy. Although most of the literature in pediatrics is limited by small sample size and retrospective design, the Multicenter, Prospective, Long-term, Observational Registry of Pediatric Patients with Inflammatory Bowel Disease (DEVELOP) registry, a prospective registry to monitor pediatric patients exposed and unexposed to anti-TNF therapy, showed that thiopurines rather than anti-TNF therapy increased the risk for malignancy.[45] Overall, more safety data and close monitoring of pediatric patients are needed.

Vedolizumab

Vedolizumab is currently used off-label in pediatric patients with CD because it is not FDA approved for this indication. Although the efficacy and safety of vedolizumab in adult patients with CD has been rigorously studied, the evidence in pediatrics is limited to real-world and retrospective studies with heterogenous populations and small sample size. Despite this, results have been positive and similar to those in adults. Clinical remission rates at 14 weeks have ranged between 37% and 76% and at 22 weeks between 34% and 71%.[64–67] Remission rates have been higher in patients with ulcerative colitis compared with CD and in anti-TNF-naive patients, with up to 100% of anti-TNF-naive patients achieving steroid-free remission in one study.[65,67] In a pediatric cohort study, mucosal healing was shown in 51% of patients, especially in the anti-TNF-naive group (66% vs 40%; P = .03, respectively).[65] In the ongoing prospective, multicenter study, Predicting Response to Vedolizumab in Pediatric Inflammatory Bowel Diseases (VEDOKIDS), an interim analysis showed clinical remission rates at Week 14 and 30 of 35% and 30%, respectively, for patients with CD. In addition, the mean height z-score improved slightly from baseline, although this was not significant.[68]

Overall, the safety profile of this gut-specific biologic is favorable. However, this is mainly extrapolated from adult studies and the data in pediatrics are limited. The Pediatric IBD Porto Group of European Society for Pediatric Gastroenterology, Hepatology and Nutrition published on 64 children with median follow-up time of 24 months and reported no adverse events.[66] In the interim analysis of VEDOKIDS, there were five adverse events that were graded as possibly related to vedolizumab in the 43 children enrolled. These included back pain, parotitis, myalgia, upper respiratory infection, and leukocytoclastic vasculitis.[68] More data are needed to fully understand the long-term risk.

Given vedolizumab's favorable side effect profile, it is an appealing choice of therapy; however, it can take time to work and so often a bridge therapy, such as antibiotics or corticosteroid, is needed.

Ustekinumab

Ustekinumab is used off-label in pediatric CD, mainly extrapolating from adult studies in which it has been shown to be efficacious and safe, leading to clinical remission and endoscopic healing.[69–72] There have been a few retrospective and small pediatric studies to date that have shown similar results to adult studies. In a study of 20 biologic-exposed pediatric patients (16 with CD), 52% showed clinical response by Week 6 and 45% by median follow-up time at Week 26.[73] Similar rates of clinical response were found in a multicenter retrospective study of 44 children with 47.8% clinical response and 38.6% clinical remission at 1 year.[74] Dayan and colleagues[75] showed similar rates of clinical remission but also showed increased efficacy in biologic-naive compared with biologic-exposed patients (90% vs 50%; P = .03).

There is an ongoing double-blind induction dose-ranging clinical trial, the Pharmacokinetic Study of Ustekinumab in Pediatric Subjects with Moderately to Severely Active Crohn's Disease (UniStar), to understand the pharmacokinetics, safety, and efficacy of ustekinumab in pediatric CD. At Week 16, 22% of patients receiving a lower dose and 29% of patients receiving a higher dose achieved clinical remission. The pharmacokinetics and safety profile were similar to those from adult studies with the exception of children less than 40 kg who had lower serum ustekinumab concentration levels, suggesting they may require a different dosing regimen.[76]

Overall data from adult studies have demonstrated a favorable safety profile.[69,71,72] In the UniStar trial, interim data reported serious adverse events in 16% of patients with disease exacerbation being the most frequent.[76] At this time, because of lack of approval, ustekinumab is used for refractory CD in patients who have failed anti-TNF or other biologic therapy or in those who cannot tolerate anti-TNF therapy.

NONPHARMACOLOGIC OR SURGICAL/INTERVENTIONAL TREATMENT OPTIONS
Nutritional Therapy

Dietary therapy for induction and maintenance of remission in CD is often appealing to families because it does not involve pharmacologic agents that are associated with potential side effects and may require injection or intravenous placement. However, dietary therapies are restrictive and greatly impact the patient's lifestyle. Therefore, before beginning dietary therapy, commitment from the patient and family is essential.

The goal of dietary therapy is to decrease inflammation through alteration in the gut microbiome, restoring the intestinal bacterial composition, mucous layers, and epithelial tight junctions.[33,77] Exclusive enteral nutrition (EEN), in which 80% to 100% of caloric needs are provided by formula, has been shown to induce remission and decrease steroid exposure in children and adolescents with CD.[78–81] In one small RCT, EEN was superior at Week 10 in inducing clinical and endoscopic remission compared with corticosteroids.[82] There has been no difference shown between the efficacy of polymeric and elemental formulas, and whereas EEN was thought to be more effective in patients with small bowel disease historically, EEN has been shown to induce remission in patients with luminal disease regardless of the site of inflammation.[66,83,84] There are no data to support the use of EEN for extraintestinal manifestations, oral CD, perianal, or penetrating disease.[33]

Partial enteral nutrition, in which patients ingest 50% of their calories from formula with an otherwise free diet, has not been shown to lead to remission.[85] However, the Crohn's Disease Exclusion Diet (CDED), a structured anti-inflammatory diet coupled with partial enteral nutrition, has been shown to have similar response and remission rates as EEN with more tolerable and better sustained remission rates than EEN.[86] A recent study showed that EEN and CDED with partial enteral nutrition induced rapid clinical response (85% and 82%, respectively) by Week 3 and that most patients were in remission by Week 6, with no difference between the diets.[87]

There are other dietary approaches, including the specific carbohydrate diet and low FODMAP diet, which are mainly recommended in combination with other IBD therapies.[77] There is no strong evidence to support these diets; however, research is ongoing. Overall, in pediatrics in which growth is emphasized, a restrictive diet can often lead to unintended issues and so the decision to pursue such therapies should be done with the specific patient in mind and in discussion with a dietician.

Surgical Treatment

Surgical intervention in pediatric CD occurs for disease-related complications and disease refractory to medical therapy. In a recent large observational study in pediatric CD, the 10-year surgery rate was 37.7%.[88] Patients may require intestinal resection, most commonly ileocectomy caused by stricturing or penetrating disease. Postoperative recurrence is common after intestinal resection, with clinical and endoscopic recurrence rates of 20% to 25% and 65% to 90% in adult CD, respectively.[33] In one pediatric study, clinical disease recurrence was present in 18.9%, 49.2%, and 71% of patients at 1, 5, and 10 years. Endoscopic recurrence occurred in 9%, 52%, and 71% at 1, 5, and 10 years, respectively.[89] Risk factors for recurrence in pediatric CD include younger age at resection, site of disease, and operative complications at the initial surgery.[90] Postoperative clinical monitoring, endoscopic surveillance, and medical therapy are recommended.[33] The postoperative therapy of choice has yet to be determined and research in pediatric CD is lacking; however, adult studies have shown that anti-TNF therapy can prevent clinical and endoscopic recurrence and is superior to 5-ASA and thiopurines.[91,92]

In patients with severe, refractory colonic CD or perianal disease, diverting ileostomy may be used as a temporizing measure. One small retrospective pediatric study showed improvement in height and weight velocity, increase in hemoglobin, and decrease in blood transfusion requirement, chronic steroid use, and hospitalization rate with diverting ileostomy.[93] This approach requires discussion with the family and close monitoring to determine when and if reanastamosis is appropriate. Finally, perianal surgery, including abscess drainage and seton placement, to allow for healing and avoid premature closure of fistulae, are common. These surgical approaches are most often complementary to medical therapy.

Risk factors for surgical complications include colonic disease, emergency surgery, poor nutritional status, anemia, concomitant steroid exposure, and microscopically positive resection margins.[89,94] Studies have not linked use of biologic therapy to increased surgical complications.[95] Surgical planning in a controlled setting to allow the family to meet and discuss the approach with a pediatric-focused surgeon is preferred.

COMBINATION THERAPIES

Combination therapy with use of anti-TNF therapy and an immunomodulator should be considered in children and adolescents who have experienced loss of response to anti-TNF therapy, subtherapeutic biologic drug concentrations, or those thought to benefit from the synergistic effect of both agents. Although the mechanism by which combination therapy works is not well understood, early adult studies, such as the SONIC trial, showed that higher rates of clinical and endoscopic remission could be achieved with combination therapy.[46] However, post hoc analysis of the SONIC trial and the results from two pediatric RCTs, IMAgINE-1 and PAILOT, have shown that there is no significant difference in rates of clinical remission between those treated with combination therapy compared with anti-TNF monotherapy when therapeutic drug levels are monitored and goal concentrations are achieved.[53,54,96–98] This finding emphasizes the role of therapeutic drug monitoring as a strategy to improve the effectiveness and durability of anti-TNF therapy. Overall, the risks and benefits of combination therapy should be weighed against the risks involved in immunomodulator use, including increased risk of malignancy, infection, and drug toxicity.

Use of combination therapy with immunomodulator and other biologic agents, such as ustekinumab and vedolizumab, has been studied in adults. Overall immunogenicity is lower with these biologic agents and these studies have not found a benefit to use of combination therapy.[99–101] Therefore, combination therapy is not recommended with use of ustekinumab and vedolizumab at this time. There are no pediatric studies to evaluate the utility of combination therapy with these newer biologic agents and therefore practice is extrapolated from adult data. An immunomodulator may be added to these agents in patients with refractory and aggressive disease for synergistic effect when other options are limited.

TREATMENT RESISTANCE/COMPLICATIONS

Untreated or undertreated CD can lead to disease-related complications. It is important to look for and recognize these issues in pediatric patients with CD.

Growth, Nutrition, and Bone Health

Growth failure is a unique aspect of pediatric CD and greatly impacts treatment decisions and quality of life.[50] It involves delay in skeletal maturation and puberty.[50,102] Accurate assessment of height and weight at diagnosis including a standardized z-score for age and sex and radiologic bone age is necessary. In addition, pubertal assessment should be obtained and a bone density scan (dual X-ray absorptiometry) considered.[102]

Up to 80% of CD children have some degree of weight loss at the time of diagnosis. The cause of undernutrition and growth failure is multifactorial and involves the metabolic consequences of inflammation, inadequate intake, and malabsorption.[103] Nutritional support by a trained dietician with close monitoring of calorie and nutrient intake, weight trajectory, and bone health is important. Clear guidelines of specific foods and nutritionally complete formulas to boost calories and protein intake can help restore nutritional status in patients with CD.[50,103]

Specific micronutrient and vitamin deficiencies are encountered in pediatric CD. Although there are no guidelines for screening for these deficiencies, assessment should be considered on an individual basis based on disease location and/or history of surgical resection.[50] Vitamin B_{12} deficiency can occur after terminal ileal resection and folate deficiency with small intestinal disease. Zinc deficiency should be considered with significant diarrhea or high-output fistula.[104] Vitamin D deficiency is more often seen in patients with IBD compared with healthy control subjects, although this is not specific to a disease phenotype or location. Vitamin D has been found to be beneficial for bone health but may also have effects on morbidity, disease severity, and hospitalization frequency.[105,106] Other nutrient deficiencies include vitamin A, vitamin E, magnesium, selenium, and beta-carotene.[50,103,104]

Overall, optimization of growth in children with CD is achieved through early diagnosis, assessment of dietary intake, and treatment of inflammatory disease. There is a narrow window for intervention; this occurs before the cessation of puberty and the pubertal growth spurt. Treatment with infliximab and surgical resection have been shown to significantly improve growth. Infliximab has also been shown to improve bone mineral density.[31,52,107]

Anemia

Anemia is one of the most common complications of IBD and is often caused by multiple etiologies including iron deficiency, anemia of chronic disease, vitamin deficiencies, hemolysis, or CD medications.[108] The incidence of anemia in children with IBD is 78% with 58% attributed to iron deficiency anemia.[109] The incidence of anemia is higher in children than adults with CD.[108–110] Risk factors for anemia in pediatric patients with CD include low albumin, elevated inflammatory markers, low body mass index, acute onset of severe disease, extensive colitis, and female sex. Providers should be aware of the presenting symptoms of anemia including dizziness, fatigue, decreased exercise tolerance, nausea, and poor concentration. More severe and uncompensated anemia can lead to tachycardia, syncope, systolic murmur, and even cardiovascular failure.[108]

The recent North American Society for Pediatric Gastroenterology, Hepatology, and Nutrition position paper on anemia recommends regularly screening for anemia and iron deficiency every 3 months in patients with active disease and every 6 to 12 months for inactive disease. Testing should include complete blood count, iron, total iron binding capacity, and ferritin. Vitamin B_{12} and folate should be assessed every year. Treatment of anemia should be based on the severity of anemia, cost and availability of medications, and medication side effects and tolerance. In patients with mild anemia and/or quiescent disease, oral iron is trialed first. Parenteral iron is indicated when oral iron is not effective or tolerated well and for severe iron deficiency. IBD therapy also should be optimized.[108]

Venous Thromboembolism

IBD is an independent risk factor for VTE.[111–113] Although studies in adults have established this risk, studies in pediatrics have been limited and there is much less known about overall risk of VTE in pediatric patients with IBD. The incidence in pediatric patients with IBD is estimated between 0.09% and 1.9%, lower than in adults.[114–117] In a cohort study, children hospitalized with IBD flare were estimated to have a six-fold increased risk for VTE compared with hospitalized children without CD.[115] In another large cohort study, the relative risk for VTE was 2.37 (95% confidence interval [CI], 2.16–2.61) in patients with CD.[116] Pediatric patients with IBD with VTE incur longer hospital stay, increased likelihood of intensive care unit admission, and greater risk for recurrent admission and death.[118]

Risk factors for VTE include increased disease activity, malnutrition, dehydration, hypoalbuminemia, immobility, surgery, presence of central venous catheter, total parenteral nutrition, and steroid exposure.[119,120] Despite well-recognized guidelines for thromboprophylaxis in adult patients with IBD, there are no established guidelines for thromboprophylaxis in pediatric IBD.[121] Thus more work is needed in this area.

Malignancy

Malignancy in pediatric CD is extremely rare. However, it is recognized that duration of disease is linked to increased risk of cancer, putting patients with pediatric-onset IBD at greater risk for development of malignancy over their lifetime. In one population-based cohort study, malignancy rates were increased in patients with pediatric-onset CD compared with the general population with a standardized incidence ratio (SIR) of 2.6 (95% CI, 1.8–3.7).[122] In another cohort study assessing long-term outcomes in patients with pediatric-onset CD, the crude cancer incidence was 1.1% with an SIR 3.3 (95% CI, 1.2–7.0). Cancers included basal cell carcinoma, genital cancer, leukemia, cholangiocarcinoma, and adenocarcinoma of the colon.[123] It is important for providers to discuss this increased risk with patients at diagnosis and during their transition to adult providers.

Non-Hodgkin lymphoma and hepatosplenic T-cell lymphoma have been associated with use of thiopurines and possibly anti-TNF therapy. Cases have been rare but most reported cases have been in males less than 35 years of age.[45,61,124] Therefore, currently it is recommended that patients and their families are counseled about the risks of using thiopurines as monotherapy or combination therapy.

Psychosocial

CD can have a significant impact on the mental health and quality of life of pediatric patients. There are unique features of IBD that can have a significant psychological impact including short stature, pubertal delay, perianal disease, embarrassment of symptoms, frequent use of the bathroom, and the unpredictability of symptoms. A meta-analysis concluded that depressive disorders were more common in young patients with IBD compared with other chronic illnesses (odds ratio, 5.80; 95% CI, 1.6–21.0).[125] In addition, increased disease severity has been linked to increased risk of depression, decreased quality of life, and increased parental stress.[126] A multidisciplinary approach is key to ensuring that these issues are identified and addressed.[50]

Mortality

There is minimal data available about mortality and CD in pediatric patients. This is mainly because it is an extremely rare event. Studies have suggested that mortality in pediatric patients with IBD is no different than the general population.[123] This was supported by a recent population-based study of patients with pediatric-onset CD in which five deaths were reported over a median follow-up time of 11 years, with a mortality rate of 0.93% and SIR 1.6 (95% CI, 0.5–3.8).[123] However, in another large cohort study, there was an increased mortality rate in pediatric CD compared with the general population (SIR 2.2; 95% CI, 1.4–3.4). Strikingly, the leading causes of mortality in this population were cancer-related (1 in 4008 person-years) and suicide (1 in 4509 person-years), underlying the importance of cancer surveillance and mental health care in pediatric CD.[122]

EVALUATION OF OUTCOME AND/OR LONG-TERM RECOMMENDATIONS

Outcomes are assessed based on clinical symptoms, normalization of growth, biochemical markers, and endoscopic assessment. Although there are no published guidelines on the interval at which clinicians should reassess disease state and response to therapy, there are general parameters that are followed in pediatric patients with CD. At the time of diagnosis and initiation of therapy and in times of active disease, close monitoring is needed to assess response and determine if a change must be made in management. As patients improve and achieve remission, monitoring generally becomes less intensive.

After diagnosis and/or at the time of initiation of a new therapy, laboratory studies should be checked at least 4 to 8 weeks after to assess response and ensure patient safety. Fecal calprotectin is used after initiation of therapy to trend response. Endoscopy should be performed 6 to 18 months after initiation of a new therapy, or sooner if the patient does not have clinical response to therapy. Patients should be followed closely by their health care team after diagnosis and/or after starting a new therapy. The follow-up interval can vary but it should be more frequent until growth is completed.

SUMMARY

Pediatric-onset CD is often more aggressive, extensive, severe, and dynamic with a higher immunosuppressant requirement and associated morbidity than adult CD. Growth impairment, pubertal delay, poor nutritional status, and the negative psychological impact of chronic disease in childhood are important for clinicians to understand and recognize in pediatric CD. Although the incidence and prevalence of pediatric-onset CD is increasing, especially the VEO-IBD population, there are limited FDA-approved therapeutic options available to pediatric patients with CD. Off-label use of biologics is often necessary. Understanding the therapies available to pediatric patients with CD, the data to support off-label use of certain biologic therapies, and the side effect profiles of these therapies is important. There is work being done to improve the study of therapeutics in this challenging patient population. As more is understood about the interplay between the immune system, genetics, microbiome, and additional environmental factors, a more advanced and personalized therapy approach will be achieved. This is an area with tremendous potential for ongoing improvement and it is imperative that all gastroenterologists understand this complex patient population.

CLINIC CARE POINTS

- 25% of individuals diagnosed with IBD are diagnosed before the age of 18 years old and are considered to have pediatric-onset IBD.

- Pediatric CD is often more severe and dynamic, requires higher levels of immunosuppression, and is associated with greater morbidity than adult CD.

- Unique considerations in pediatric CD include growth impairment, pubertal delay, bone disease, longevity of disease burden, and the psychological impact of chronic disease on children and adolescents.

- Treatment is limited given the select FDA-approved therapies.

- Anti-TNF therapy (infliximab and adalimumab) is the only FDA-approved biologic therapy and has been shown to lead to mucosal healing, restoration in weight and height, improvement in bone disease, and increase in quality of life.

- Alternative therapies, such as dietary therapy and surgery, are also effective treatment interventions in pediatric CD.

- Without effective therapy complications can occur including growth delay, bone disease, anemia, venous thromboembolism, infection, and malignancy.

- Pediatric CD is an area of tremendous potential for ongoing translational and clinical research and quality improvement and it is important that all gastroenterologists have an understanding of this complex and growing population.

DISCLOSURE

E.B. Mitchel: None J.R. Rosh: Grant/Research Support: AbbVie, Janssen; Advisory Boards/Consultant: BMS, Celgene, Lilly, Pfizer.

REFERENCES

1. Sartor RB. Mechanisms of disease: pathogenesis of Crohn's disease and ulcerative colitis. Nat Clin Pract Gastroenterol Hepatol 2006;3:390–407.
2. Ye Y, Manne S, Treem WR, et al. Prevalence of inflammatory bowel disease in pediatric and adult populations: recent estimates from large national databases in the United States, 2007-2016. Inflamm Bowel Dis 2020;26: 619–25.
3. Benchimol EI, Bernstein CN, Bitton A, et al. Trends in epidemiology of pediatric inflammatory bowel disease in Canada: distributed network analysis of multiple population-based provincial health administrative databases. Am J Gastroenterol 2017;112:1120–34.
4. Malmborg P, Grahnquist L, Lindholm J, et al. Increasing incidence of paediatric inflammatory bowel disease in northern Stockholm County, 2002-2007. J Pediatr Gastroenterol Nutr 2013;57:29–34.
5. Turner D, Griffiths AM, Wilson D, et al. Designing clinical trials in paediatric inflammatory bowel diseases: a PIBDnet commentary. Gut 2020;69:32–41.
6. Pigneur B, Seksik P, Viola S, et al. Natural history of Crohn's disease: comparison between childhood- and adult-onset disease. Inflamm Bowel Dis 2010;16: 953–61.
7. Rosen MJ, Dhawan A, Saeed SA. Inflammatory bowel disease in children and adolescents. JAMA Pediatr 2015;169:1053–60.

8. Van Limbergen J, Russell RK, Drummond HE, et al. Definition of phenotypic characteristics of childhood-onset inflammatory bowel disease. Gastroenterology 2008;135:1114–22.

9. Vernier-Massouille G, Balde M, Salleron J, et al. Natural history of pediatric Crohn's disease: a population-based cohort study. Gastroenterology 2008; 135:1106–13.

10. Kelsen JR, Conrad MA, Dawany N, et al. The unique disease course of children with very early onset-inflammatory bowel disease. Inflamm Bowel Dis 2020;26: 909–18.

11. Kelsen JR, Dawany N, Moran CJ, et al. Exome sequencing analysis reveals variants in primary immunodeficiency genes in patients with very early onset inflammatory bowel disease. Gastroenterology 2015;149:1415–24.

12. Kelsen JR, Sullivan KE, Rabizadeh S, et al. North American Society for Pediatric Gastroenterology, Hepatology, and Nutrition position paper on the evaluation and management for patients with very early-onset inflammatory bowel disease. J Pediatr Gastroenterol Nutr 2020;70:389–403.

13. Conrad MA, Rosh JR. Pediatric inflammatory bowel disease. Pediatr Clin North Am 2017;64:577–91.

14. Sanderson IR. Growth problems in children with IBD. Nat Rev Gastroenterol Hepatol 2014;11:601–10.

15. Ghersin I, Khateeb N, Katz LH, et al. Anthropometric measures in adolescents with inflammatory bowel disease: a population-based study. Inflamm Bowel Dis 2019;25:1061–5.

16. Ley D, Duhamel A, Behal H, et al. Growth pattern in paediatric Crohn disease is related to inflammatory status. J Pediatr Gastroenterol Nutr 2016;63:637–43.

17. Alibrahim B, Aljasser MI, Salh B. Fecal calprotectin use in inflammatory bowel disease and beyond: a mini-review. Can J Gastroenterol Hepatol 2015;29: 157–63.

18. Schoepfer AM, Beglinger C, Straumann A, et al. Fecal calprotectin correlates more closely with the Simple Endoscopic Score for Crohn's disease (SES-CD) than CRP, blood leukocytes, and the CDAI. Am J Gastroenterol 2010;105:162–9.

19. Vernia F, Di Ruscio M, Stefanelli G, et al. Is fecal calprotectin an accurate marker in the management of Crohn's disease? J Gastroenterol Hepatol 2020;35:390–400.

20. Foster AJ, Smyth M, Lakhani A, et al. Consecutive fecal calprotectin measurements for predicting relapse in pediatric Crohn's disease patients. World J Gastroenterol 2019;25:1266–77.

21. D'Arcangelo G, Imondi C, Terrin G, et al. Is fecal calprotectin a useful marker for small bowel Crohn disease? J Pediatr Gastroenterol Nutr 2021;73:242–6.

22. Ibd Working Group of the European Society for Paediatric Gastroenterology H. Nutrition. Inflammatory bowel disease in children and adolescents: recommendations for diagnosis: the Porto criteria. J Pediatr Gastroenterol Nutr 2005;41:1–7.

23. North American Society for Pediatric Gastroenterology, Hepatology, and Nutrition; Colitis Foundation of America, Bousvaros A, Antonioli DA, Colletti RB, et al. Differentiating ulcerative colitis from Crohn disease in children and young adults: report of a working group of the North American Society for Pediatric Gastroenterology, Hepatology, and Nutrition and the Crohn's and Colitis Foundation of America. J Pediatr Gastroenterol Nutr 2007;44:653–74.

24. Sawczenko A, Lynn R, Sandhu BK. Variations in initial assessment and management of inflammatory bowel disease across Great Britain and Ireland. Arch Dis Child 2003;88:990–4.

25. Anupindi SA, Grossman AB, Nimkin K, et al. Imaging in the evaluation of the young patient with inflammatory bowel disease: what the gastroenterologist needs to know. J Pediatr Gastroenterol Nutr 2014;59:429–39.

26. Schooler GR, Hull NC, Mavis A, et al. MR imaging evaluation of inflammatory bowel disease in children: where are we now in 2019. Magn Reson Imaging Clin N Am 2019;27:291–300.

27. Fraquelli M, Castiglione F, Calabrese E, et al. Impact of intestinal ultrasound on the management of patients with inflammatory bowel disease: how to apply scientific evidence to clinical practice. Dig Liver Dis 2020;52:9–18.

28. Dilillo D, Zuccotti GV, Galli E, et al. Noninvasive testing in the management of children with suspected inflammatory bowel disease. Scand J Gastroenterol 2019;54:586–91.

29. Pecere S, Holleran G, Ainora ME, et al. Usefulness of contrast-enhanced ultrasound (CEUS) in inflammatory bowel disease (IBD). Dig Liver Dis 2018;50: 761–7.

30. Bouguen G, Levesque BG, Feagan BG, et al. Treat to target: a proposed new paradigm for the management of Crohn's disease. Clin Gastroenterol Hepatol 2015;13:1042–10450 e2.

31. Walters TD, Kim MO, Denson LA, et al. Increased effectiveness of early therapy with anti-tumor necrosis factor-alpha vs an immunomodulator in children with Crohn's disease. Gastroenterology 2014;146:383–91.

32. Shah SC, Colombel JF, Sands BE, et al. Systematic review with meta-analysis: mucosal healing is associated with improved long-term outcomes in Crohn's disease. Aliment Pharmacol Ther 2016;43:317–33.

33. Ruemmele FM, Veres G, Kolho KL, et al. Consensus guidelines of ECCO/ES-PGHAN on the medical management of pediatric Crohn's disease. J Crohns Colitis 2014;8:1179–207.

34. Cezard JP, Munck A, Mouterde O, et al. Prevention of relapse by mesalazine (Pentasa) in pediatric Crohn's disease: a multicenter, double-blind, randomized, placebo-controlled trial. Gastroenterol Clin Biol 2009;33:31–40.

35. Mesker T, van Rheenen PF, Norbruis OF, et al. Pediatric Crohn's disease activity at diagnosis, its influence on pediatrician's prescribing behavior, and clinical outcome 5 years later. Inflamm Bowel Dis 2009;15:1670–7.

36. Su JW, Ma JJ, Zhang HJ. Use of antibiotics in patients with Crohn's disease: a systematic review and meta-analysis. J Dig Dis 2015;16:58–66.

37. Breton J, Kastl A, Conrad MA, et al. Positioning biologic therapies in the management of pediatric inflammatory bowel disease. Gastroenterol Hepatol (N Y) 2020;16:400–14.

38. Turner D, Levine A, Kolho KL, et al. Combination of oral antibiotics may be effective in severe pediatric ulcerative colitis: a preliminary report. J Crohns Colitis 2014;8:1464–70.

39. Levine A, Turner D. Combined azithromycin and metronidazole therapy is effective in inducing remission in pediatric Crohn's disease. J Crohns Colitis 2011;5: 222–6.

40. Breton J, Kastl A, Hoffmann N, et al. Efficacy of combination antibiotic therapy for refractory pediatric inflammatory bowel disease. Inflamm Bowel Dis 2019;25: 1586–93.

41. Kugathasan S, Denson LA, Walters TD, et al. Prediction of complicated disease course for children newly diagnosed with Crohn's disease: a multicentre inception cohort study. Lancet 2017;389:1710–8.

42. Lewis JD, Chen EZ, Baldassano RN, et al. Inflammation, antibiotics, and diet as environmental stressors of the gut microbiome in pediatric Crohn's disease. Cell Host Microbe 2015;18:489–500.

43. Markowitz J, Grancher K, Kohn N, et al. A multicenter trial of 6-mercaptopurine and prednisone in children with newly diagnosed Crohn's disease. Gastroenterology 2000;119:895–902.

44. Pfefferkorn M, Burke G, Griffiths A, et al. Growth abnormalities persist in newly diagnosed children with Crohn disease despite current treatment paradigms. J Pediatr Gastroenterol Nutr 2009;48:168–74.

45. Hyams JS, Dubinsky MC, Baldassano RN, et al. Infliximab is not associated with increased risk of malignancy or hemophagocytic lymphohistiocytosis in pediatric patients with inflammatory bowel disease. Gastroenterology 2017;152: 1901–1914 e3.

46. Colombel JF, Sandborn WJ, Reinisch W, et al. Infliximab, azathioprine, or combination therapy for Crohn's disease. N Engl J Med 2010;362:1383–95.

47. Sunseri W, Hyams JS, Lerer T, et al. Retrospective cohort study of methotrexate use in the treatment of pediatric Crohn's disease. Inflamm Bowel Dis 2014;20:1341–5.

48. Turner D, Grossman AB, Rosh J, et al. Methotrexate following unsuccessful thiopurine therapy in pediatric Crohn's disease. Am J Gastroenterol 2007;102:2804–12.

49. Willot S, Noble A, Deslandres C. Methotrexate in the treatment of inflammatory bowel disease: an 8-year retrospective study in a Canadian pediatric IBD center. Inflamm Bowel Dis 2011;17:2521–6.

50. Oliveira SB, Monteiro IM. Diagnosis and management of inflammatory bowel disease in children. BMJ 2017;357:j2083.

51. Levine A, Weizman Z, Broide E, et al. A comparison of budesonide and prednisone for the treatment of active pediatric Crohn disease. J Pediatr Gastroenterol Nutr 2003;36:248–52.

52. Hyams J, Crandall W, Kugathasan S, et al. Induction and maintenance infliximab therapy for the treatment of moderate-to-severe Crohn's disease in children. Gastroenterology 2007;132:863–73, quiz 1165-6.

53. Hyams JS, Griffiths A, Markowitz J, et al. Safety and efficacy of adalimumab for moderate to severe Crohn's disease in children. Gastroenterology 2012;143: 365–374 e2.

54. Assa A, Matar M, Turner D, et al. Proactive monitoring of adalimumab trough concentration associated with increased clinical remission in children with Crohn's disease compared with reactive monitoring. Gastroenterology 2019; 157:985–996 e2.

55. Hazlewood GS, Rezaie A, Borman M, et al. Comparative effectiveness of immunosuppressants and biologics for inducing and maintaining remission in Crohn's disease: a network meta-analysis. Gastroenterology 2015;148:344–354 e5.

56. Cholapranee A, Hazlewood GS, Kaplan GG, et al. Systematic review with meta-analysis: comparative efficacy of biologics for induction and maintenance of mucosal healing in Crohn's disease and ulcerative colitis controlled trials. Aliment Pharmacol Ther 2017;45.1291–302.

57. Nobile S, Gionchetti P, Rizzello F, et al. Mucosal healing in pediatric Crohn's disease after anti-TNF therapy: a long-term experience at a single center. Eur J Gastroenterol Hepatol 2014;26:458–65.

58. Santha SL, Shankar PR, Pan A, et al. Mucosal healing in clinical practice: a single-center pediatric IBD experience. Inflamm Bowel Dis 2017;23:1447–53.

59. Kang B, Choi SY, Kim HS, et al. Mucosal healing in paediatric patients with moderate-to-severe luminal Crohn's disease under combined immunosuppression: escalation versus early treatment. J Crohns Colitis 2016;10:1279–86.

60. Lee YM, Kang B, Lee Y, et al. Infliximab "top-down" strategy is superior to "step-up" in maintaining long-term remission in the treatment of pediatric Crohn disease. J Pediatr Gastroenterol Nutr 2015;60:737–43.

61. de Ridder L, Turner D, Wilson DC, et al. Malignancy and mortality in pediatric patients with inflammatory bowel disease: a multinational study from the Porto pediatric IBD group. Inflamm Bowel Dis 2014;20:291–300.

62. Dulai PS, Thompson KD, Blunt HB, et al. Risks of serious infection or lymphoma with anti-tumor necrosis factor therapy for pediatric inflammatory bowel disease: a systematic review. Clin Gastroenterol Hepatol 2014;12:1443–51.

63. Singh S, Facciorusso A, Dulai PS, et al. Comparative risk of serious infections with biologic and/or immunosuppressive therapy in patients with inflammatory bowel diseases: a systematic review and meta-analysis. Clin Gastroenterol Hepatol 2020;18:69–81 e3.

64. Conrad MA, Stein RE, Maxwell EC, et al. Vedolizumab therapy in severe pediatric inflammatory bowel disease. Inflamm Bowel Dis 2016;22:2425–31.

65. Jossen J, Kiernan BD, Pittman N, et al. Anti-tumor necrosis factor-alpha exposure impacts vedolizumab mucosal healing rates in pediatric inflammatory bowel disease. J Pediatr Gastroenterol Nutr 2020;70:304–9.

66. Ledder O, Assa A, Levine A, et al. Vedolizumab in paediatric inflammatory bowel disease: a retrospective multi-centre experience from the paediatric IBD Porto Group of ESPGHAN. J Crohns Colitis 2017;11:1230–7.

67. Singh N, Rabizadeh S, Jossen J, et al. Multi-center experience of vedolizumab effectiveness in pediatric inflammatory bowel disease. Inflamm Bowel Dis 2016; 22:2121–6.

68. Shavit-Brunschwig ZLO, Focht G, Urlep D, et al. P538 Vedolizumab is effective in real life paediatric inflammatory bowel disease: report from the prospective, multi-centre VEDOKIDS cohort study. J Crohn's Colitis 2019;13:S383.

69. Feagan BG, Sandborn WJ, Gasink C, et al. Ustekinumab as induction and maintenance therapy for Crohn's disease. N Engl J Med 2016;375:1946–60.

70. Rutgeerts P, Gasink C, Chan D, et al. Efficacy of ustekinumab for inducing endoscopic healing in patients with Crohn's disease. Gastroenterology 2018;155: 1045–58.

71. Sandborn WJ, Feagan BG, Fedorak RN, et al. A randomized trial of ustekinumab, a human interleukin-12/23 monoclonal antibody, in patients with moderate-to-severe Crohn's disease. Gastroenterology 2008;135:1130–41.

72. Sandborn WJ, Gasink C, Gao LL, et al. Ustekinumab induction and maintenance therapy in refractory Crohn's disease. N Engl J Med 2012;367:1519–28.

73. Fusillo SJ, Chang V, Stein RE, et al. Ustekinumab responders versus non-responders in refractory pediatric inflammatory bowel disease. Gastroenterology 2018;154:S82.

74. Chavannes M, Martinez-Vinson C, Hart L, et al. Management of paediatric patients with medically refractory Crohn's disease using ustekinumab: a multi-centred cohort study. J Crohns Colitis 2019;13:578–84.

75. Dayan JR, Dolinger M, Benkov K, et al. Real world experience with ustekinumab in children and young adults at a tertiary care pediatric inflammatory bowel disease center. J Pediatr Gastroenterol Nutr 2019;69:61–7.

76. Rosh JR, Turner D, Griffiths A, et al. Ustekinumab in pediatric patients with moderately to severely active Crohn's disease pharmacokinetics, safety, and

efficacy results from UniStar, a phase 1 study. J Crohns Colitis 2021;15(11): 1931–42.

77. Levine A, Rhodes JM, Lindsay JO, et al. Dietary guidance from the international organization for the study of inflammatory bowel diseases. Clin Gastroenterol Hepatol 2020;18:1381–92.

78. Grover Z, Lewindon P. Two-year outcomes after exclusive enteral nutrition induction are superior to corticosteroids in pediatric Crohn's disease treated early with thiopurines. Dig Dis Sci 2015;60:3069–74.

79. Gupta K, Noble A, Kachelries KE, et al. A novel enteral nutrition protocol for the treatment of pediatric Crohn's disease. Inflamm Bowel Dis 2013;19:1374–8.

80. Lee D, Albenberg L, Compher C, et al. Diet in the pathogenesis and treatment of inflammatory bowel diseases. Gastroenterology 2015;148:1087–106.

81. Levine A, Turner D, Pfeffer Gik T, et al. Comparison of outcomes parameters for induction of remission in new onset pediatric Crohn's disease: evaluation of the Porto IBD group "growth relapse and outcomes with therapy" (GROWTH CD) study. Inflamm Bowel Dis 2014;20:278–85.

82. Borrelli O, Cordischi L, Cirulli M, et al. Polymeric diet alone versus corticosteroids in the treatment of active pediatric Crohn's disease: a randomized controlled open-label trial. Clin Gastroenterol Hepatol 2006;4:744–53.

83. Ludvigsson JF, Krantz M, Bodin L, et al. Elemental versus polymeric enteral nutrition in paediatric Crohn's disease: a multicentre randomized controlled trial. Acta Paediatr 2004;93:327–35.

84. Buchanan E, Gaunt WW, Cardigan T, et al. The use of exclusive enteral nutrition for induction of remission in children with Crohn's disease demonstrates that disease phenotype does not influence clinical remission. Aliment Pharmacol Ther 2009;30:501–7.

85. Johnson T, Macdonald S, Hill SM, et al. Treatment of active Crohn's disease in children using partial enteral nutrition with liquid formula: a randomised controlled trial. Gut 2006;55:356–61.

86. Levine A, Wine E, Assa A, et al. Crohn's disease exclusion diet plus partial enteral nutrition induces sustained remission in a randomized controlled trial. Gastroenterology 2019;157:440–450 e8.

87. Sigall Boneh R, Van Limbergen J, Wine E, et al. Dietary therapies induce rapid response and remission in pediatric patients with active Crohn's disease. Clin Gastroenterol Hepatol 2021;19:752–9.

88. Kurowski JA, Milinovich A, Ji X, et al. Differences in biologic utilization and surgery rates in pediatric and adult Crohn's disease: results from a large electronic medical record-derived cohort. Inflamm Bowel Dis 2021;27:1035–44.

89. Diederen K, de Ridder L, van Rheenen P, et al. Complications and disease recurrence after primary ileocecal resection in pediatric Crohn's disease: a multicenter cohort analysis. Inflamm Bowel Dis 2017;23:272–82.

90. Abdelaal K, Jaffray B. Colonic disease site and perioperative complications predict need for later intestinal interventions following intestinal resection in pediatric Crohn's disease. J Pediatr Surg 2016;51:272–6.

91. Yang Z, Ye X, Wu Q, et al. A network meta-analysis on the efficacy of 5-aminosalicylates, immunomodulators and biologics for the prevention of postoperative recurrence in Crohn's disease. Int J Surg 2014;12:516–22.

92. Yoshida K, Fukunaga K, Ikeuchi H, et al. Scheduled infliximab monotherapy to prevent recurrence of Crohn's disease following ileocolic or ileal resection: a 3-year prospective randomized open trial. Inflamm Bowel Dis 2012;18:1617–23.

93. Maxwell EC, Dawany N, Baldassano RN, et al. Diverting ileostomy for the treatment of severe, refractory, pediatric inflammatory bowel disease. J Pediatr Gastroenterol Nutr 2017;65:299–305.

94. Michailidou M, Nfonsam VN. Preoperative anemia and outcomes in patients undergoing surgery for inflammatory bowel disease. Am J Surg 2018;215:78–81.

95. Mitsuya JB, Gonzalez R, Thomas R, et al. The effect of biologics on postoperative complications in children with inflammatory bowel disease and bowel resection. J Pediatr Gastroenterol Nutr 2019;68:334–8.

96. Colombel JF, Adedokun OJ, Gasink C, et al. Combination therapy with infliximab and azathioprine improves infliximab pharmacokinetic features and efficacy: a post hoc analysis. Clin Gastroenterol Hepatol 2019;17:1525–1532 e1.

97. Hyams JS, Dubinsky M, Rosh J, et al. The effects of concomitant immunomodulators on the pharmacokinetics, efficacy and safety of adalimumab in paediatric patients with Crohn's disease: a post hoc analysis. Aliment Pharmacol Ther 2019;49:155–64.

98. Matar M, Shamir R, Turner D, et al. Combination therapy of adalimumab with an immunomodulator is not more effective than adalimumab monotherapy in children with Crohn's disease: a post hoc analysis of the PAILOT randomized controlled trial. Inflamm Bowel Dis 2020;26:1627–35.

99. Hu A, Kotze PG, Burgevin A, et al. Combination therapy does not improve rate of clinical or endoscopic remission in patients with inflammatory bowel diseases treated with vedolizumab or ustekinumab. Clin Gastroenterol Hepatol 2021;19:1366–1376 e2.

100. Van den Berghe N, Verstockt B, Tops S, et al. Immunogenicity is not the driving force of treatment failure in vedolizumab-treated inflammatory bowel disease patients. J Gastroenterol Hepatol 2019;34:1175–81.

101. Adedokun OJ, Xu Z, Gasink C, et al. Pharmacokinetics and exposure response relationships of ustekinumab in patients with Crohn's disease. Gastroenterology 2018;154:1660–71.

102. Heuschkel R, Salvestrini C, Beattie RM, et al. Guidelines for the management of growth failure in childhood inflammatory bowel disease. Inflamm Bowel Dis 2008;14:839–49.

103. Kappelman MD, Bousvaros A. Nutritional concerns in pediatric inflammatory bowel disease patients. Mol Nutr Food Res 2008;52:867–74.

104. Hwang C, Ross V, Mahadevan U. Micronutrient deficiencies in inflammatory bowel disease: from A to zinc. Inflamm Bowel Dis 2012;18:1961–81.

105. Kabbani TA, Koutroubakis IE, Schoen RE, et al. Association of vitamin D level with clinical status in inflammatory bowel disease: a 5-year longitudinal study. Am J Gastroenterol 2016;111:712–9.

106. Pappa HM, Gordon CM, Saslowsky TM, et al. Vitamin D status in children and young adults with inflammatory bowel disease. Pediatrics 2006;118:1950–61.

107. Thayu M, Leonard MB, Hyams JS, et al. Improvement in biomarkers of bone formation during infliximab therapy in pediatric Crohn's disease: results of the REACH study. Clin Gastroenterol Hepatol 2008;6:1378–84.

108. Goyal A, Zheng Y, Albenberg LG, et al. Anemia in children with inflammatory bowel disease: a position paper by the IBD Committee of the North American Society of Pediatric Gastroenterology, Hepatology and Nutrition. J Pediatr Gastroenterol Nutr 2020;71:563–82.

109. Pels LP, Van de Vijver E, Waalkens HJ, et al. Slow hematological recovery in children with IBD-associated anemia in cases of "expectant management. J Pediatr Gastroenterol Nutr 2010;51:708–13.

110. Sjoberg D, Holmstrom T, Larsson M, et al. Anemia in a population-based IBD cohort (ICURE): still high prevalence after 1 year, especially among pediatric patients. Inflamm Bowel Dis 2014;20:2266–70.

111. Faye AS, Wen T, Ananthakrishnan AN, et al. Acute venous thromboembolism risk highest within 60 days after discharge from the hospital in patients with inflammatory bowel diseases. Clin Gastroenterol Hepatol 2020;18:1133–1141 e3.

112. Grainge MJ, West J, Card TR. Venous thromboembolism during active disease and remission in inflammatory bowel disease: a cohort study. Lancet 2010;375: 657–63.

113. Nguyen GC, Bernstein CN, Bitton A, et al. Consensus statements on the risk, prevention, and treatment of venous thromboembolism in inflammatory bowel disease: Canadian Association of Gastroenterology. Gastroenterology 2014; 146:835–848 e6.

114. Diamond CE, Hennessey C, Meldau J, et al. Catheter-related venous thrombosis in hospitalized pediatric patients with inflammatory bowel disease: incidence, characteristics, and role of anticoagulant thromboprophylaxis with enoxaparin. J Pediatr 2018;198:53–9.

115. Kappelman MD, Horvath-Puho E, Sandler RS, et al. Thromboembolic risk among Danish children and adults with inflammatory bowel diseases: a population-based nationwide study. Gut 2011;60:937–43.

116. Nylund CM, Goudie A, Garza JM, et al. Venous thrombotic events in hospitalized children and adolescents with inflammatory bowel disease. J Pediatr Gastroenterol Nutr 2013;56:485–91.

117. Zitomersky NL, Levine AE, Atkinson BJ, et al. Risk factors, morbidity, and treatment of thrombosis in children and young adults with active inflammatory bowel disease. J Pediatr Gastroenterol Nutr 2013;57:343–7.

118. Chien KA, Cooley V, Prishtina F, et al. Health and financial burdens associated with venous thrombosis in hospitalized children with inflammatory bowel disease. J Pediatr Gastroenterol Nutr 2021;72:748–51.

119. Mitchel EB, Rosenbaum S, Gaeta C, et al. Venous thromboembolism in pediatric inflammatory bowel disease: a case-control study. J Pediatr Gastroenterol Nutr 2021;72:742–7.

120. Turner D, Ruemmele FM, Orlanski-Meyer E, et al. Management of paediatric ulcerative colitis, part 2: acute severe colitis-an evidence-based consensus guideline from the European Crohn's and Colitis Organization and the European Society of Paediatric Gastroenterology, Hepatology and Nutrition. J Pediatr Gastroenterol Nutr 2018;67:292–310.

121. Chien KA, Hammad HT, Gerber L, et al. Pediatric gastroenterologists' approach to venous thromboembolism prophylaxis in pediatric inflammatory bowel disease. J Pediatr Gastroenterol Nutr 2018;66:286–8.

122. Malham M, Jakobsen C, Paerregaard A, et al. The incidence of cancer and mortality in paediatric onset inflammatory bowel disease in Denmark and Finland during a 23-year period: a population-based study. Aliment Pharmacol Ther 2019;50:33–9.

123. Fumery M, Pariente B, Sarter H, et al. Long-term outcome of pediatric-onset Crohn's disease: a population-based cohort study. Dig Liver Dis 2019;51: 496–502.

124. Kotlyar DS, Osterman MT, Diamond RH, et al. A systematic review of factors that contribute to hepatosplenic T-cell lymphoma in patients with inflammatory bowel disease. Clin Gastroenterol Hepatol 2011;9:36–41 e1.

125. Greenley RN, Hommel KA, Nebel J, et al. A meta-analytic review of the psychosocial adjustment of youth with inflammatory bowel disease. J Pediatr Psychol 2010;35:857–69.
126. Gourdonneau A, Bruneau L, Ruemmele FM, et al. Clinical remission and psychological management are major issues for the quality of life in pediatric Crohn disease. J Pediatr Gastroenterol Nutr 2021;72:74–9.

Crohn's Disease of the Elderly
Unique Biology and Therapeutic Efficacy and Safety

Simon J. Hong, MD*, Jonathan Galati, MD, Seymour Katz, MD

KEYWORDS

- Inflammatory bowel disease • Crohn's disease • Elderly • Phenotype • Frailty
- COVID-19 • Treatment

KEY POINTS

- Patients with elderly-onset Crohn's disease (CD) have a unique phenotype, natural history, and baseline immunophysiology compared with patients with adult-onset CD.
- Frailty in elderly patients with inflammatory bowel disease (IBD) is associated with increased rates of infection, hospital readmission, and mortality and may be a more accurate measure of risk than chronologic age alone.
- The risk profile of biologic therapy has evolved over time with higher-quality data, identification of risk modifiers such as frailty, and the development of more targeted biologic and small molecule therapies.

OVERVIEW

There is increasing recognition that inflammatory bowel disease (IBD) diagnosed at an elderly age (age >60 years), or elderly-onset IBD, is a distinct phenotype from IBD with disease onset during adulthood.[1] This review discusses the unique biology of the elderly patient with Crohn's disease (CD), the distinct phenotype of elderly patients with CD, the emergence of frailty as an important risk marker, updates on biologic effectiveness and safety, and special considerations regarding the ongoing coronavirus disease 2019 (COVID-19) pandemic in the elderly patient with IBD.

DISTINCT DISEASE PHENOTYPE AND NATURAL HISTORY

Elderly-onset CD has a distinct phenotype and disease presentation with some variation in different regions of the world. In Western populations, it is characterized by

Division of Gastroenterology and Hepatology, Inflammatory Bowel Disease Center at New York University Langone Health, 305 East 33rd St, New York, NY 10016, USA
* Corresponding author.
E-mail address: Simon.hong@nyulangone.org

Gastroenterol Clin N Am 51 (2022) 425–440
https://doi.org/10.1016/j.gtc.2021.12.014
0889-8553/22/© 2022 Elsevier Inc. All rights reserved.

a predominance of colonic disease, with 65% of elderly patients with CD having colonic involvement, and 25% and 10% with ileocolonic or ileal disease, respectively, in the French-based Registre Epidemiologique des Maladies de l'Appareil Digestif (EPIMAD) registry.[2] In contrast, in a large cohort study from Hong Kong, 39% of elderly-onset patients with CD had ileocolonic disease followed by 31% with ileal and 30% with colonic disease.[3] In all studied populations of elderly-onset CD, disease behavior tends to be predominantly inflammatory, with 64% to 78% of patients having a nonstricturing, nonpenetrating phenotype.[2,3] Elderly patients also tend to have lower rates of penetrating (12% vs 19%) and perianal (17% vs 23%) disease than their adult-onset counterparts.[4] Change in disease location is rare in elderly-onset CD, with a stable location over time reported in 92% of patients.[2,5] Disease behavior also remains stable, with only 9% of patients progressing from inflammatory to stricturing or penetrating disease.[2] Differences in clinical symptoms exist as well, as elderly patients with CD generally present with more rectal bleeding and less diarrhea and abdominal pain than younger patients.[2]

Despite having less extensive, penetrating, and stricturing disease, elderly-onset patients with CD do not necessarily have a more benign disease course. Rates of surgery are similar when comparing adult- versus elderly-onset patients with CD. In one systematic review and meta-analysis, the risk of surgery in elderly patients with CD was similar to that of adult-onset patients (odds ratio [OR], 0.70; 95% confidence interval [CI], 0.40 to 1.22), and similar findings have been reported in other multicenter studies and meta-analyses.[1,6–8]

UNIQUE BIOLOGY OF THE ELDERLY: GENETICS, IMMUNOPHYSIOLOGY, AND MICROBIOME

Patients with elderly-onset CD appear to have a unique biologic underpinning as well (**Fig. 1**). The pathophysiology of IBD involves an inappropriate immune reaction to environmental factors in the setting of underlying genetic susceptibility.[9] However, genetics appear to have a less important role in elderly-onset IBD than it does in adult- or pediatric-onset disease. A family history of IBD is reported in only 7% of elderly-onset CD compared with 14% of patients with adult-onset disease.[2] Pediatric-onset IBD (onset before the age of 18) has been linked with several susceptibility genes, including NOD2, POUF5F1, TNFSF15, and HLA DRB *501, but no such genetic mutations have been identified that correlate with elderly-onset IBD.[10]

In contrast to decreased genetic susceptibility, aging is associated with an increased risk of physiologic function decline over time, which is theorized to contribute to the development of IBD. These pathophysiologic alterations include cellular immunosenescence, progenitor cell dysfunction, and chronic inflammation.[11] A decrease in hematopoiesis may lead to immunosenescence, an impairment of the innate and adaptive immune systems. Subsequent impairment in T- and B-cell responses promotes an aberrant immune response to environmental antigens, which may trigger the onset of IBD.[12] Aging is also associated with an increase of proinflammatory cytokines, which can lead to a chronic state of low-grade inflammation.[11,13,14]

Increasing age is also associated with changes in the gut microbiome.[15] In the elderly, there is a decrease in the diversity and abundance of obligate anaerobes, such as *Bifidobacteria*, and an increase in facultative anaerobes, such as *Enterobacteriaceae*, *Streptococci*, and *Staphylococci*, changes which have been associated with IBD.[16,17] These changes are thought to be related to physiologic changes of

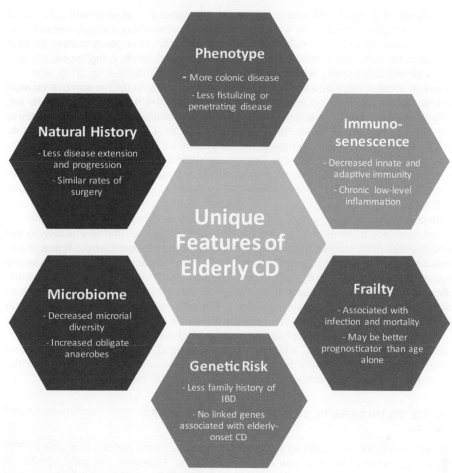

Fig. 1. Unique features of CD in the elderly.

aging, which include prolonged transit time, decreased intestinal motility, fecal retention, an increase in the use of laxatives or antibiotics, and a decrease in dietary fiber.[18]

FRAILTY: THE NEW RISK ASSESSMENT

Frailty is increasingly recognized as an important risk factor for adverse health outcomes in elderly patients. Frailty is defined as a decline in multiple physiologic systems and homeostatic reserve which results in a state of increased vulnerability.[19,20] This is often the consequence of an acute stressor, such as an infection, hospitalization, or surgery, which precipitates the onset of a state of accelerated functional decline.[21] The decline may manifest as a decrease in function, adaptive capacity, and resiliency in several interrelated physiologic systems, including the brain, endocrine system, immune system, skeletal muscle, and the gut microbiome.[21–23]

Although there is growing recognition of the importance of frailty, it remains an often neglected part of the routine assessment of elderly patients with IBD and is likely underdiagnosed in a considerable proportion of patients.[24] In one study of 135 patients with IBD aged ≥65 who underwent frailty screening assessments, 23% had reduced handgrip strength and 44% had increased vulnerability and impairment.[25] In another prospective study of 405 elderly patients with IBD undergoing routine geriatric assessments, 40% had moderate and 8% had severe deficits. A higher clinical and biomarker disease activity was correlated with worse deficits.[26]

Several studies have shown that the presence of frailty in IBD is associated with adverse outcomes. Frailty is associated with increased risk of infection in elderly patients who start antitumor necrosis factor (anti-TNF) therapy (adjusted risk ratio [aRR], 2.05; 95% CI, 1.07–3.93) or an immunomodulator (aOR, 1.81; 95% CI, 1.22–2.70), as well as an overall increase in mortality (OR, 2.90; 95% CI, 2.29–3.68).[27,28] Frailty is also an independent predictor of 30-day readmission (absolute risk reduction [aRR], 1.16; 95% CI, 1.14–1.17), readmission for severe IBD (adjusted hazard ratio [aHR], 1.22; 95% CI, 1.16–1.29), and 30-day readmission mortality (aRR, 1.12; 95% CI, 1.02–1.23).[29,30]

Despite the known impact of frailty on morbidity and mortality in IBD, data are limited regarding interventions to prevent or alter the disease course of frailty. In the general population, studies have shown that cognitive, nutritional, and physical interventions can be effective in improving frailty.[31,32] Preoperative frailty indices can be predictive of postoperative complications, but data have not clearly shown that interventions in those with preoperative frailty decrease the risk of these complications.[33,34] A systematic review examining the effectiveness of prehabilitation on postoperative outcomes found a decrease in overall morbidity (OR, 0.63; 95% CI, 0.46–0.87), but no difference in the 6-minute walking test (weighted mean difference, 9.06; 95% CI, −35.68–53.81), which is a commonly used measure of frailty.[35] Further studies are required to identify the optimal frailty assessment tools in patients with IBD and the most effective interventions to improve long-term outcomes.

UPDATES ON THERAPEUTIC SAFETY: THE PREBIOLOGIC ERA
Overview

The last 2 decades have seen an expansion in the therapeutic options available for IBD with the approval of several new classes of therapy. However, the safety profile of these agents in the elderly remains a major concern. This section provides an update on the effectiveness and safety of therapeutics in the elderly CD patient.

Aminosalicylates

Aminosalicylates are generally not recommended for the treatment of CD, but substantial proportions of elderly patients with CD (36%–77%) remain on them, likely because of their relatively benign safety profile.[36–39] In previous reports, 5-aminosalicylates (5-ASA) have been linked to interstitial nephritis, but more recent data bring this association into question. Studies suggest that renal injury in patients with IBD may actually be related to underlying inflammatory disease, not 5-ASA use.[40,41] The main risk of 5-ASA in elderly patients with CD is likely inadequate long-term control of inflammation owing to the overall lack of effect of this class of therapies in CD.[42]

Corticosteroids

Steroids are also frequently used in elderly patients with IBD despite their considerable side effects, which include heart failure, hypertension, osteoporosis, glaucoma, diabetes, psychosis, and infection.[43] Despite these risks, elderly patients with IBD are more likely to receive corticosteroids and less likely to receive immunomodulators or biologics than their younger counterparts.[37,44] In the aforementioned EPIMAD registry, the cumulative probability of receiving corticosteroids over a 10-year period was 47%, compared with a 27% probability of receiving immunomodulators or biologics.[2]

This reliance on steroids in the elderly IBD patient may be misdirected, as the adverse risks of corticosteroids are substantial. In the prospective TREAT (Crohn's Therapy, Resource, Evaluation, and Assessment Tool) registry of 6290 patients with IBD, over a mean follow-up of 5.2 years, there was an overall 3% case-mortality rate. The predictors of mortality under multivariable analysis were increasing age, and corticosteroid or narcotic use.[45] In a population-based study of 3552 elderly-onset patients with IBD in Quebec, Canada, corticosteroids use within the past 45 days was associated with a 2.8-fold increased risk of serious infections.[46] Other significant adverse events associated with corticosteroids in the elderly patients with IBD include increased risk of fractures, venous thromboembolism, depression, anxiety, and sleep disturbance.[46,47] Given all of these risks, systemic corticosteroids in the elderly should only be initiated for short-term use with an "exit strategy" for an alternative agent for long-term maintenance therapy.

Budesonide is a corticosteroid that is available as an ileal-release or multi-matrix-release formulation, effective for ileocecal CD and ulcerative colitis (UC), respectively.[48,49] Budesonide exhibits a high first-pass metabolism, with approximately 80% to 85% of drug metabolized by the hepatic cytochrome p450 system, which results in a low (10%–15%) systemic bioavailability.[49] Because of its limited systemic absorption, budesonide is associated with fewer side effects in both pediatric and adult patients with IBD.[50,51] Data regarding the safety benefit of budesonide specifically in the elderly patient with IBD are lacking, but nevertheless if corticosteroids are required, budesonide may be a preferred alternative for this population.

Immunomodulators

Immunomodulators are proven to be effective for the maintenance of remission in CD.[39] However, real-world usage of thiopurines in the elderly patient with IBD remains low, with only 3% of patients starting thiopurines (azathioprine or 6-mercaptopurine) within the first year of diagnosis and 16% over the course of their lifetimes in the EPI-MAD registry.[2,52]

These low rates of usage are due largely to concerns about the substantial side-effect profile of thiopurines. Thiopurine use is in elderly patients is associated with an increased risk of infection. In a French nationwide study, patients aged 65 or older who were exposed to thiopurine monotherapy had a 2- to 3-fold higher absolute risk of infection than younger patients.[53] Large prospective observational studies have also demonstrated that exposure to thiopurines is associated with an increased risk of several malignancies, which include nonmelanoma skin cancer (NMSC), acute myeloid leukemia (AML), myelodysplastic syndromes (MDS), and lymphoproliferative disorders (both Hodgkin and non-Hodgkin lymphoma).[54–57] Interestingly, a recent Veterans Administration (VA) study of 56,314 patients with a mean age of 58 years found that the risk of AML and MDS reverted to baseline in patients who discontinued thiopurines greater than 6 months prior, which suggests that the risk of malignancy may be mitigated by cessation of therapy.[58]

Current guidelines recommend methotrexate for maintenance of remission in patients with Crohn's as either monotherapy or combination therapy.[59,60] Despite this, the use of methotrexate is even lower than that of thiopurines in elderly patients with IBD, with only 1% to 2% of elderly patients with IBD treated with methotrexate over the course their lifetime.[2,44] Methotrexate does not appear to increase the risk of lymphoma, but use of this agent may be limited by common side effects of nausea, fatigue, rash, stomatitis, hepatotoxicity, and bone marrow suppression.[61] Supplementation with folic acid can mitigate these risks and is imperative when using this therapy.[62] Data on the use of methotrexate in the elderly patient with IBD are sparse, but experience from its use in older patients with psoriasis and rheumatoid arthritis has shown that gastrointestinal and hematologic toxicity is more likely in older patients.[63] Methotrexate is mainly excreted by the kidneys, which can be impacted by decreased glomerular filtration rate related to age, nonsteroidal anti-inflammatory drugs, or loop diuretic use.[64]

UPDATES ON THERAPEUTIC EFFICACY AND SAFETY: THE BIOLOGIC ERA

Since the advent of the biologic era, there are now several novel biologic and small molecule classes available for treatment of CD. However, elderly patients generally make up a small proportion of those enrolled in registration trials. Further studies are required to determine the effectiveness and safety of these agents specifically in the elderly CD patient. The following section discusses the existing data regarding efficacy and safety of biologics in elderly patients with CD (**Table 1**).

Anti-Tumor Necrosis Factor agents

In the elderly patient with IBD, anti-TNF therapy requires a prolonged time to full treatment effect, but long-term efficacy rates are similar to those of their younger counterparts.[65,66] Despite similar effectiveness, long-term rates of discontinuation are 3 times higher in older patients than in younger patients (25% vs 7%, respectively; $P<.05$), with infection being the most common reason for treatment discontinuation.[67] Given their broad immunosuppressive effect, concerns about the side effects of anti-TNF biologics remain at the forefront of both physicians' and patients' consideration. Studies have reported overall infection rates ranging from 11% to 22% in elderly patients with IBD on anti-TNFs, and rates of severe infections are as high as 15%.[65,67,68] Furthermore, infection rates are consistently 2- to 4-fold higher than those of younger patients.[4,67]

Emerging data have provided new insights into the risks of anti-TNFs in the elderly IBD population. In one recent study, Kochar and colleagues found that frailty was independently associated with infection in elderly patients on anti-TNF (OR, 2.32; 95% CI, 1.23–4.37) even after adjusting for age. This suggests that even more than chronologic age , the presence of frailty may be a major determinant of adverse outcomes in elderly patients with IBD.[69]

The risk of malignancy is also a concern for elderly patients with IBD on chronic immunosuppression, as earlier studies have reported a 3-fold increase in the risk of lymphoma associated with anti-TNF therapy. However, prior study populations were confounded by concomitant immunomodulator exposure, and more recent studies have not clearly demonstrated an increased risk of malignancy.[70–73] In the TREAT Registry, the risk of lymphoma with anti-TNF monotherapy was similar to those who were anti-TNF naïve over a mean follow-up of 5 years.[72] Recent studies have also shown that anti-TNF therapy does not increase the risk of new or recurrent cancer in patients with a previous history of cancer.[74]

Mortality has been reported to be increased in elderly patients on anti-TNF, but in one single-center study, mortality was not increased after adjusting for comorbidities, and a greater number of deaths in this study were attributable to cardiovascular complications.[65] Kochar and colleagues[28] showed that frailty is an independent predictor of mortality in patients with IBD, again suggesting that frailty may be the more reliable marker of risk in these patients than age.

Table 1
Updates on effectiveness and safety of therapeutics in elderly patients with Crohn's disease

	Effectiveness	Risk Profile
Aminosalicylates	• Not recommended for induction or maintenance of remission in CD	• Previously linked to acute interstitial nephritis, but more recent data suggest may be consequence of underlying IBD • Risk of undertreatment of elderly CD
Corticosteroids	• Effective for induction of remission, but need alternative long-term maintenance strategy, that is, "exit plan"	• Increased mortality and infections • Increased complications (osteoporosis, fractures, venous thromboembolism, diabetes, psychological disturbance) • Budesonide may be a safer alternative, given its decreased systemic absorption
Thiopurines[a]	• Effective for maintenance of remission	• Increased infections • Increased malignancy (NMSC, leukemia, MDS, Hodgkin and non-Hodgkin lymphoma) • Risk of AML/MDS may revert to baseline after cessation of therapy
Methotrexate	• Effective for maintenance of remission	• Risk of gastrointestinal and hepatoxicity can be mitigated by folic acid supplementation • No increase in lymphoma risk
Anti-TNF[b]	• May take 6–12 mo for maximal improvement • Equivalent long-term effectiveness as younger patients	• Earlier studies showed 3-fold increase in lymphoma, but more recent studies suggest TNF-α monotherapy (without immunomodulator) may *not* increase malignancy risk • Associated with increased infections and mortality, but frailty may be more prognostic than chronologic age alone
Vedolizumab	• Similar rates of remission, clinical and endoscopic response at 52 wk as younger patients • Slower onset of action than TNF-α at 3 mo, but similar effectiveness at 6 and 12 mo	• Theoretically safer due to gut-selective nature, but conflicting real-world data • Possible increase in nonsevere infections compared with younger patients • Lower rates of serious infections compared with TNF-α
Ustekinumab	• Similar responses rates in elderly in retrospective studies	• No difference in infusion reactions, infection, or postsurgical complications based on age

[a] 6-Mercaptopurine and azathioprine.
[b] Infliximab, adalimumab, and certolizumab.

Given the evolving understanding of the physiology of the elderly and the impact of frailty on adverse outcomes, future studies should focus on more accurately stratifying the true independent risk of anti-TNF therapy in elderly patients. It is possible that further elucidation of the interaction between chronologic age, frailty, immunosenescence, and underlying comorbidities will enable more accurate identification of elderly patients who are at increased risk of adverse events with anti-TNF therapy.

Vedolizumab

Vedolizumab is a monoclonal antibody that targets the integrin subunit α4β7, thereby preventing the migration of lymphocytes into the intestinal lumen.[75,76] Given its gut-selective nature, it is largely viewed as a favorable option for elderly patients, and evidence suggests that it is effective in this population. In post hoc analyses of the GEMINI 2 registry trial, vedolizumab was similarly effective across 3 different age groups (age ≤35 years, 35–55 years, ≥55 years), with 33% versus 27% versus 29% of patients with CD, respectively, achieving corticosteroid-free remission at 52 weeks.[77] A multicenter retrospective cohort study of 284 patients reported similar clinical and endoscopic response rates at week 52 between elderly (age 60 or older) and younger (age 40 or younger) patients.[78] When compared with anti-TNF, vedolizumab was associated with a lower remission rate at 3 months (38% vs 50%; $P = .07$), but was comparable at 6 (45% vs 54%; $P = .23$) and 12 months (54% vs 58%; $P = .63$), which suggests a slow onset of action but equivalent long-term effectiveness and durability of response.[66]

Despite the presumed safety benefit of vedolizumab in the elderly, real-world data are somewhat conflicting. In the GEMINI post hoc analyses, rates of malignancy and infection in older patients (age ≥55) were similar to their younger counterparts.[77] Cohen and colleagues[78] reported an increased risk of infections in the elderly compared with younger patients (12% vs 2%, $P = .002$), all of which were nonfatal infections (predominantly of the nasopharynx, urinary tract, skin, and vulva, or *Clostridioides difficile*). In contrast, Adar and colleagues[66] reported that rates of significant infections were modestly lower in vedolizumab compared with anti-TNF (17% vs 20%), as were rates of *C difficile* (18% vs 21%), but these differences were not statistically significant. Further studies are required to better characterize the potential safety benefit of vedolizumab over other biologic classes.

Ustekinumab

Ustekinumab is a monoclonal antibody that targets the p40 subunit of interleukin (IL)-12/23 and has demonstrated efficacy and safety in CD.[79] However, in the UNITI/IM-UNITI registry trial, outcomes were not stratified by age, and the study population was relatively young, with a mean age range of 37 to 42 years old in all treatment arms.

A recently published retrospective study of 117 elderly patients with CD treated with ustekinumab noted that age was not associated with decreased response rates. There were no differences in infusion reactions (2.6% vs 6.4%; $P = .77$), infection (5.2% vs 7.7%; $P = .70$), or postsurgical complications ($P = .99$) based on older age.[80] A study by the same group also reported that vedolizumab and ustekinumab had similar rates of steroid-free remission (35.3% vs 30%; $P = .08$), infusion/injection reactions (2.6% vs 2.6%; $P = .98$), and infection (5.2% vs 2.6%; $P = .39$).[81] These data suggest that ustekinumab is effective and has an overall favorable safety profile, but more studies are needed to determine the real-world effectiveness and safety of ustekinumab in elderly patients with IBD.

Emerging Biologic and Small Molecule Agents

An in-depth discussion of emerging novel biologic and small molecule therapies is beyond the scope of this review, but several new promising therapeutic agents are on the horizon for CD. Risankizumab, a selective IL-23 blocker that binds the p19 subunit (in contrast to the dual inhibition of IL-12/23 by ustekinumab), has been shown to be effective in phase III trials for CD and to be superior to ustekinumab in trials for plaque psoriasis.[82–84] Oral small molecules targeting the Janus kinase (JAK) pathway represent another promising class of therapeutic agents. Tofacitinib, a pan-JAK blocker approved for UC, did not show efficacy for CD, but the more selective JAK-1 inhibitor upadacitinib was effective for CD in phase II trials and is currently undergoing evaluation in phase III trials.[85] Ozanimod, an oral sphingosine-1 phosphate receptor modulator that increases sequestration of lymphocytes in peripheral lymphoid tissues, is approved for UC and is undergoing phase III trials for CD.[86] The future for IBD therapeutics is promising, but future studies must consider the unique disease characteristics and risk factors of the elderly CD population, which may impact treatment outcomes and the risk profiles of these new agents.

CORONAVIRUS DISEASE 2019 AND THE ELDERLY INFLAMMATORY BOWEL DISEASE PATIENT

Severe acute respiratory syndrome coronavirus 2 (SARS-CoV-2) is a novel virus that emerged in late 2019 and quickly spread to become the deadly global pandemic known as coronavirus disease 2019 (COVID-19). The mortality of COVID-19 is much higher in older patients, with 80% of deaths in the United States occurring in patients aged 65 or older. Data from China revealed a case fatality rate of 8% in patients aged 70 to 79 years and 15% in those older than age 80, compared with 2% in the general population.[87,88]

Given the underlying immune dysregulation of IBD and the increased mortality risk associated with advanced age, there is understandable concern about the impact of COVID-19 on elderly patients with IBD. The mechanism of cell entry for SARS-CoV-2 is via angiotensin-converting enzyme-2 (ACE-2) receptors, which are found throughout the body, including in the enterocytes of the ileum and colon.[88–90] Furthermore, ACE-2 receptor expression is upregulated in IBD, creating a biological basis by which patients with IBD might theoretically be particularly susceptible to COVID-19.[91]

Despite these underlying pathophysiologic links between IBD and COVID-19, evidence thus far does not suggest that IBD alone portends a worse COVID-19 prognosis.[92,93] In regards to the impact of age, increasing age in patients with IBD was not associated with higher rates of COVID-19 in a nationwide VA cohort study of 37,857 patients.[94] In patients with IBD who develop COVID-19, increasing age and number of comorbidities are independently associated with severe outcome of intensive care unit admission, ventilator use, and death based on data from the international SECURE-IBD registry.[95] However, when assessing the impact of age in the same registry, IBD disease activity was independently correlated with severe outcomes in younger patients but not in older ones, which suggests that increasing age may modify the effect of IBD disease activity in patients with COVID-19.[96]

Immunosuppressive therapies in patients with IBD with COVID-19 are another source of concern, given their effect on inhibiting the intracellular signaling cascades needed to fight infection.[91] Thus far, corticosteroids are the only IBD-related immunosuppressants consistently associated with worsened outcomes. Reassuringly, immunomodulators and anti-TNFs do not appear to increase the risk of COVID-19.[92,95] A retrospective Italian study of elderly patients with IBD with COVID-19 showed similar mortality rates among those on immunomodulators and those not on any immunosuppression.[97] A recent meta-analysis of 249,095 patients showed that patients with IBD on anti-TNFs actually had a lower average pooled incidence of COVID-19 (0.68 per 1000 patients) than those not on therapy (1.93 per 1000), which suggest the possibility that anti-TNF use may be protective against COVID-19.[98] Furthermore, data from the SECURE-IBD registry and US-based studies report that anti-TNF use was not associated with worse outcomes, even after adjusting for age in multivariable regression modeling.[95,98,99] The COVID-19 pandemic has highlighted the importance of early assessment, collaborative research, and practice optimization caring for immunologically vulnerable populations, such as elderly patients with IBD.[100]

SUMMARY

The phenotypic and physiologic differences between elderly- and adult-onset CD have an important impact on therapeutic management and outcomes. An improving understanding of altered biology, frailty, and natural history continues to inform care of the elderly CD patient and assessment of therapeutic risks. Newer biologics have increasingly improved safety profiles, but further studies are needed to clarify these risks in the elderly CD population. Last, as new global health challenges such as COVID-19 emerge, it is important to be aware of their unique impact on the elderly IBD population.

CLINICS CARE POINTS

- Elderly-onset Crohn's disease must be considered in elderly patients with unexplained or new-onset symptoms of diarrhea, rectal bleeding, or abdominal pain, as Crohn's disease is no longer just a "disease of the young".

- Elderly patients with Crohn's disease may have less aggressive disease phenotypes, but their risk of surgery is similar to younger patients, and adequate control of inflammation remains a priority for this population.

- Determining whether a patient is frail or not may predict more accurately the risk of medical or surgical intervention than a patient's age alone.

- A "start low and go slow" approach is emphasized, but if a patient is not responding to initial treatment, practitioners should not hesitate to escalate therapy.

- Physiologic differences, polypharmacy, and drug-drug interactions must be considered in the elderly, but newer biologics are relatively effective, safe, and well tolerated.

- Inflammatory bowel disease and its related non-corticosteroid therapies do not impact on COVID-19 risk and severity, but elderly age remains an independent risk factor for worse outcomes.

REFERENCES

1. Jeuring SFG, van den Heuvel TRA, Zeegers MP, et al. Epidemiology and long-term outcome of inflammatory bowel disease diagnosed at elderly age-an increasing distinct entity? Inflamm Bowel Dis 2016;22(6):1425–34.
2. Charpentier C, Salleron J, Savoye G, et al. Natural history of elderly-onset inflammatory bowel disease: a population-based cohort study. Gut 2014;63(3): 423–32.

3. Mak JWY, Lok Tung Ho C, Wong K, et al. Epidemiology and natural history of elderly-onset inflammatory bowel disease: results from a territory-wide Hong Kong IBD Registry. J Crohns Colitis 2021;15(3):401–8.
4. Mañosa M, Calafat M, de Francisco R, et al. Phenotype and natural history of elderly onset inflammatory bowel disease: a multicentre, case-control study. Aliment Pharmacol Ther 2018;47(5):605–14.
5. Gower-Rousseau C, Vasseur F, Fumery M, et al. Epidemiology of inflammatory bowel diseases: new insights from a French population-based registry (EPI-MAD). Dig Liver Dis 2013;45(2):89–94.
6. Ananthakrishnan AN, Shi HY, Tang W, et al. Systematic review and meta-analysis: phenotype and clinical outcomes of older-onset inflammatory bowel disease. J Crohns Colitis 2016;10(10):1224–36.
7. Kochar B, Long MD, Galanko J, et al. Inflammatory bowel disease is similar in patients with older onset and younger onset. Inflamm Bowel Dis 2017;23(7): 1187–94.
8. Rozich JJ, Dulai PS, Fumery M, et al. Progression of elderly onset inflammatory bowel diseases: a systematic review and meta-analysis of population-based cohort studies. Clin Gastroenterol Hepatol 2020;18(11):2437–47.
9. Kaser A, Zeissig S, Blumberg RS. Inflammatory bowel disease. Annu Rev Immunol 2010;28:573–621.
10. Connelly TM, Berg AS, Harris L, et al. Genetic determinants associated with early age of diagnosis of IBD. Dis Colon Rectum 2015;58(3):321–7.
11. Pignolo RJ, Nath KA. Introduction to thematic reviews on aging and geriatric medicine. Mayo Clin Proc 2020;95(6):1102–4.
12. Kugelberg E. T cell memory: the effect of ageing on CD8(+) T cells. Nat Rev Immunol 2013;14(1):3.
13. Franceschi C, Garagnani P, Vitale G, et al. Inflammaging and "Garb-aging". Trends Endocrinol Metab 2017;28(3):199–212.
14. Cambier J. Immunosenescence: a problem of lymphopoiesis, homeostasis, microenvironment, and signaling. Immunol Rev 2005;205:5–6.
15. Cucchiara S, Iebba V, Conte MP, et al. The microbiota in inflammatory bowel disease in different age groups. Dig Dis 2009;27(3):252–8.
16. Biagi E, Candela M, Fairweather-Tait S, et al. Aging of the human metaorganism: the microbial counterpart. Age (Dordr) 2012;34(1):247–67.
17. Taleban S, Colombel J-F, Mohler MJ, et al. Inflammatory bowel disease and the elderly: a review. J Crohns Colitis 2015;9(6):507–15.
18. Tiihonen K, Ouwehand AC, Rautonen N. Human intestinal microbiota and healthy ageing. Ageing Res Rev 2010;9(2):107–16.
19. Khezrian M, Myint PK, McNeil C, et al. A review of frailty syndrome and its physical, cognitive and emotional domains in the elderly. Geriatrics (Basel) 2017;2(4).
20. Kojima G, Liljas AEM, Iliffe S. Frailty syndrome: implications and challenges for health care policy. Risk ManagHealthc Policy 2019;12:23–30.
21. Clegg A, Young J, Iliffe S, et al. Frailty in elderly people. Lancet 2013;381(9868): 752–62.
22. Lightner AL, Regueiro M, Click B. Special considerations for colorectal surgery in the elderly IBD patient. Curr Treat Options Gastroenterol 2019;17(4):449–56.
23. van Tongeren SP, Slaets JPJ, Harmsen HJM, et al. Fecal microbiota composition and frailty. Appl Environ Microbiol 2005;71(10):6438–42.
24. Asscher VER, Lee-Kong FVY, Kort ED, et al. Systematic review: components of a comprehensive geriatric assessment in inflammatory bowel disease-a

potentially promising but often neglected risk stratification. J Crohns Colitis 2019;13(11):1418–32.

25. Asscher V, Meijer L, Waars S, et al. P732 disability in older IBD patients. J Crohn's Colitis 2018;12(Suppl_1):S481–2.

26. Asscher VER, Waars SN, van der Meulen-de Jong AE, et al. Deficits in geriatric assessment associate with disease activity and -burden in older patients with inflammatory bowel disease. Clin Gastroenterol Hepatol 2021 Jun;19. S1542-3565(21)00643-1.

27. Kochar B, Cai W, Cagan A, et al. Pretreatment frailty is independently associated with increased risk of infections after immunosuppression in patients with inflammatory bowel diseases. Gastroenterology 2020;158(8):2104–11.

28. Kochar B, Cai W, Cagan A, et al. Frailty is independently associated with mortality in 11 001 patients with inflammatory bowel diseases. Aliment Pharmacol Ther 2020;52(2):311–8.

29. Faye AS, Wen T, Soroush A, et al. Increasing prevalence of frailty and its association with readmission and mortality among hospitalized patients with IBD. Dig Dis Sci 2021. https://doi.org/10.1007/s10620-020-06746-w.

30. Qian AS, Nguyen NH, Elia J, et al. Frailty is independently associated with mortality and readmission in hospitalized patients with inflammatory bowel diseases. Clin Gastroenterol Hepatol 2021 Oct;19(10):2054–63.

31. Tarazona-Santabalbina FJ, Gómez-Cabrera MC, Pérez-Ros P, et al. A multicomponent exercise intervention that reverses frailty and improves cognition, emotion, and social networking in the community-dwelling frail elderly: a randomized clinical trial. J Am Med Dir Assoc 2016;17(5):426–33.

32. Ng TP, Feng L, Nyunt MSZ, et al. Nutritional, physical, cognitive, and combination interventions and frailty reversal among older adults: a randomized controlled trial. Am J Med 2015;128(11):1225–36.

33. McIsaac DI, Jen T, Mookerji N, et al. Interventions to improve the outcomes of frail people having surgery: a systematic review. PLoS One 2017;12(12): e0190071.

34. Birkelbach O, Mörgeli R, Spies C, et al. Routine frailty assessment predicts postoperative complications in elderly patients across surgical disciplines - a retrospective observational study. BMC Anesthesiol 2019;19(1):204.

35. Hughes MJ, Hackney RJ, Lamb PJ, et al. Prehabilitation before major abdominal surgery: a systematic review and meta-analysis. World J Surg 2019;43(7): 1661–8.

36. Kurti Z, Vegh Z, Golovics PA, et al. Nationwide prevalence and drug treatment practices of inflammatory bowel diseases in Hungary: a population-based study based on the National Health Insurance Fund database. Dig Liver Dis 2016; 48(11):1302–7.

37. Everhov ÅH, Halfvarson J, Myrelid P, et al. Incidence and treatment of patients diagnosed with inflammatory bowel diseases at 60 years or older in Sweden. Gastroenterology 2018;154(3):518–28.

38. Holko P, Kawalec P, Stawowczyk E. Prevalence and drug treatment practices of inflammatory bowel diseases in Poland in the years 2012-2014: an analysis of nationwide databases. Eur J Gastroenterol Hepatol 2018;30(4):456–64.

39. Lichtenstein GR, Loftus EV, Isaacs KL, et al. ACG clinical guideline: management of Crohn's disease in adults. Am J Gastroenterol 2018;113(4):481–517.

40. Van Staa TP, Travis S, Leufkens HGM, et al. 5-Aminosalicylic acids and the risk of renal disease: a large British epidemiologic study. Gastroenterology 2004; 126(7):1733–9.

41. Vajravelu RK, Copelovitch L, Osterman MT, et al. Inflammatory bowel diseases are associated with an increased risk for chronic kidney disease, which decreases with age. Clin Gastroenterol Hepatol 2020;18(10):2262–8.
42. Akobeng AK, Gardener E. Oral 5-aminosalicylic acid for maintenance of medically-induced remission in Crohn's disease. Cochrane Database Syst Rev 2005;(1):CD003715.
43. Fleischer DE, Grimm IS, Friedman LS. Inflammatory bowel disease in older patients. Med Clin North Am 1994;78(6):1303–19.
44. Juneja M, Baidoo L, Schwartz MB, et al. Geriatric inflammatory bowel disease: phenotypic presentation, treatment patterns, nutritional status, outcomes, and comorbidity. Dig Dis Sci 2012;57(9):2408–15.
45. Lichtenstein GR, Feagan BG, Cohen RD, et al. Serious infection and mortality in patients with Crohn's disease: more than 5 years of follow-up in the TREAT™ registry. Am J Gastroenterol 2012;107(9):1409–22.
46. Brassard P, Bitton A, Suissa A, et al. Oral corticosteroids and the risk of serious infections in patients with elderly-onset inflammatory bowel diseases. Am J Gastroenterol 2014;109(11):1795–802.
47. LeBlanc J-F, Wiseman D, Lakatos PL, et al. Elderly patients with inflammatory bowel disease: updated review of the therapeutic landscape. World J Gastroenterol 2019;25(30):4158–71.
48. Travis SPL, Danese S, Kupcinskas L, et al. Once-daily budesonide MMX in active, mild-to-moderate ulcerative colitis: results from the randomised CORE II study. Gut 2014;63(3):433–41.
49. Rutgeerts P, Löfberg R, Malchow H, et al. A comparison of budesonide with prednisolone for active Crohn's disease. N Engl J Med 1994;331(13):842–5.
50. Levine A, Weizman Z, Broide E, et al. A comparison of budesonide and prednisone for the treatment of active pediatric Crohn disease. J Pediatr Gastroenterol Nutr 2003;36(2):248–52.
51. D'Haens G, Verstraete A, Cheyns K, et al. Bone turnover during short-term therapy with methylprednisolone or budesonide in Crohn's disease. Aliment Pharmacol Ther 1998;12(5):419–24.
52. Duricova D, Pariente B, Sarter H, et al. Impact of age at diagnosis on natural history of patients with elderly-onset ulcerative colitis: a French population-based study. Dig Liver Dis 2018;50(9):903–9.
53. Kirchgesner J, Lemaitre M, Carrat F, et al. Risk of serious and opportunistic infections associated with treatment of inflammatory bowel diseases. Gastroenterology 2018;155(2):337–46.
54. Lopez A, Mounier M, Bouvier A-M, et al. Increased risk of acute myeloid leukemias and myelodysplastic syndromes in patients who received thiopurine treatment for inflammatory bowel disease. Clin Gastroenterol Hepatol 2014;12(8):1324–9.
55. Peyrin-Biroulet L, Khosrotehrani K, Carrat F, et al. Increased risk for nonmelanoma skin cancers in patients who receive thiopurines for inflammatory bowel disease. Gastroenterology 2011;141(5):1621–8.
56. Beaugerie L, Brousse N, Bouvier AM, et al. Lymphoproliferative disorders in patients receiving thiopurines for inflammatory bowel disease: a prospective observational cohort study. Lancet 2009;374(9701):1617–25.
57. Lemaitre M, Kirchgesner J, Rudnichi A, et al. Association between use of thiopurines or tumor necrosis factor antagonists alone or in combination and risk of lymphoma in patients with inflammatory bowel disease. JAMA 2017;318(17):1679–86.

58. Khan N, Patel D, Trivedi C, et al. Incidence of acute myeloid leukemia and myelodysplastic syndrome in patients with inflammatory bowel disease and the impact of thiopurines on their risk. Am J Gastroenterol 2021;116(4):741–7.
59. Feuerstein JD, Ho EY, Shmidt E, et al. AGA Clinical Practice Guidelines on the medical management of moderate to severe luminal and perianal fistulizing Crohn's disease. Gastroenterology 2021;160(7):2496–508.
60. Patel V, Macdonald JK, McDonald JW, et al. Methotrexate for maintenance of remission in Crohn's disease. Cochrane Database Syst Rev 2009;(4):CD006884.
61. Subramaniam K, D'Rozario J, Pavli P. Lymphoma and other lymphoproliferative disorders in inflammatory bowel disease: a review. J Gastroenterol Hepatol 2013;28(1):24–30.
62. Shea B, Swinden MV, Ghogomu ET, et al. Folic acid and folinic acid for reducing side effects in patients receiving methotrexate for rheumatoid arthritis. J Rheumatol 2014;41(6):1049–60.
63. Morgacheva O, Furst DE. Use of MTX in the elderly and in patients with compromised renal function. Clin Exp Rheumatol 2010;28(5 Suppl 61):S85–94.
64. Bourré J. Methotrexate drug interactions in the treatment of rheumatoid arthritis: a systematic review. J Rheumatol 2010;37(7):1416–21.
65. Lobatón T, Ferrante M, Rutgeerts P, et al. Efficacy and safety of anti-TNF therapy in elderly patients with inflammatory bowel disease. Aliment Pharmacol Ther 2015;42(4):441–51.
66. Adar T, Faleck D, Sasidharan S, et al. Comparative safety and effectiveness of tumor necrosis factor α antagonists and vedolizumab in elderly IBD patients: a multicentre study. Aliment Pharmacol Ther 2019;49(7):873–9.
67. Desai A, Zator ZA, de Silva P, et al. Older age is associated with higher rate of discontinuation of anti-TNF therapy in patients with inflammatory bowel disease. Inflamm Bowel Dis 2013;19(2):309–15.
68. Cottone M, Kohn A, Daperno M, et al. Advanced age is an independent risk factor for severe infections and mortality in patients given anti-tumor necrosis factor therapy for inflammatory bowel disease. Clin Gastroenterol Hepatol 2011;9(1):30–5.
69. Faye AS, Colombel J-F. Age is just a number-frailty associates with outcomes of patients with inflammatory bowel disease. Gastroenterology 2020;158(8):2041–3.
70. Nyboe Andersen N, Pasternak B, Basit S, et al. Association between tumor necrosis factor-α antagonists and risk of cancer in patients with inflammatory bowel disease. JAMA 2014;311(23):2406–13.
71. Williams CJM, Peyrin-Biroulet L, Ford AC. Systematic review with meta-analysis: malignancies with anti-tumour necrosis factor-α therapy in inflammatory bowel disease. Aliment Pharmacol Ther 2014;39(5):447–58.
72. Lichtenstein GR, Feagan BG, Cohen RD, et al. Drug therapies and the risk of malignancy in Crohn's disease: results from the TREAT™ Registry. Am J Gastroenterol 2014;109(2):212–23.
73. Siegel CA, Marden SM, Persing SM, et al. Risk of lymphoma associated with combination anti-tumor necrosis factor and immunomodulator therapy for the treatment of Crohn's disease: a meta-analysis. Clin Gastroenterol Hepatol 2009;7(8):874–81.
74. Axelrad J, Bernheim O, Colombel J-F, et al. Risk of new or recurrent cancer in patients with inflammatory bowel disease and previous cancer exposed to immunosuppressive and anti-tumor necrosis factor agents. Clin Gastroenterol Hepatol 2016;14(1):58–64.

75. Sandborn WJ, Feagan BG, Rutgeerts P, et al. Vedolizumab as induction and maintenance therapy for Crohn's disease. N Engl J Med 2013;369(8):711–21.
76. Feagan BG, Rutgeerts P, Sands BE, et al. Vedolizumab as induction and maintenance therapy for ulcerative colitis. N Engl J Med 2013;369(8):699–710.
77. Yajnik V, Khan N, Dubinsky M, et al. Efficacy and safety of vedolizumab in ulcerative colitis and crohn's disease patients stratified by age. Adv Ther 2017;34(2): 542–59.
78. Cohen NA, Plevris N, Kopylov U, et al. Vedolizumab is effective and safe in elderly inflammatory bowel disease patients: a binational, multicenter, retrospective cohort study. United Eur Gastroenterol J 2020;8(9):1076–85.
79. Feagan BG, Sandborn WJ, Gasink C, et al. Ustekinumab as induction and maintenance therapy for Crohn's disease. N Engl J Med 2016;375(20):1946–60.
80. Garg R, Aggarwal M, Butler R, et al. Real-World effectiveness and safety of ustekinumab in elderly Crohn's disease patients. Dig Dis Sci 2021. https://doi.org/ 10.1007/s10620-021-07117-9.
81. Garg R, Aggarwal M, Mohammed A, et al. Sa580 real-world effectiveness and safety of ustekinumab and vedolizumab in elderly patients with Crohn's disease. Gastroenterology 2021;160(6):S560.
82. Papp KA, Blauvelt A, Bukhalo M, et al. Risankizumab versus ustekinumab for moderate-to-severe plaque psoriasis. N Engl J Med 2017;376(16):1551–60.
83. Gordon KB, Strober B, Lebwohl M, et al. Efficacy and safety of risankizumab in moderate-to-severe plaque psoriasis (UltIMMa-1 and UltIMMa-2): results from two double-blind, randomised, placebo-controlled and ustekinumab-controlled phase 3 trials. Lancet 2018;392(10148):650–61.
84. Bai F, Li GG, Liu Q, et al. Short-term efficacy and safety of IL-17, IL-12/23, and IL-23 inhibitors brodalumab, secukinumab, ixekizumab, ustekinumab, guselkumab, tildrakizumab, and risankizumab for the treatment of moderate to severe plaque psoriasis: a systematic review and network meta-analysis of randomized controlled trials. J Immunol Res 2019;2546161.
85. Sandborn WJ, Feagan BG, Loftus EV, et al. Efficacy and safety of upadacitinib in a randomized trial of patients with crohn's disease. Gastroenterology 2020; 158(8):2123–38.
86. Feagan BG, Sandborn WJ, Danese S, et al. Ozanimod induction therapy for patients with moderate to severe Crohn's disease: a single-arm, phase 2, prospective observer-blinded endpoint study. Lancet Gastroenterol Hepatol 2020;5(9): 819–28.
87. Wu Z, McGoogan JM. Characteristics of and important lessons from the coronavirus disease 2019 (COVID-19) outbreak in China: summary of a report of 72 314 cases from the Chinese Center for Disease Control and Prevention. JAMA 2020;323(13):1239–42.
88. Shahid Z, Kalayanamitra R, McClafferty B, et al. COVID-19 and older adults: what we know. J Am Geriatr Soc 2020;68(5):926–9.
89. Vaduganathan M, Vardeny O, Michel T, et al. Renin-angiotensin-aldosterone system inhibitors in patients with Covid-19. N Engl J Med 2020;382(17):1653–9.
90. Zheng S, Fan J, Yu F, et al. Viral load dynamics and disease severity in patients infected with SARS-CoV-2 in Zhejiang Province, China, January-March 2020: retrospective cohort study. BMJ 2020;369:m1443.
91. Neurath MF. COVID-19 and immunomodulation in IBD. Gut 2020;69(7):1335–42.
92. Singh S, Khan A, Chowdhry M, et al. Risk of severe coronavirus disease 2019 in patients with inflammatory bowel disease in the United States: a multicenter research network study. Gastroenterology 2020;159(4):1575–8.e4.

93. Hong S, Malter L, Bosworth BP, et al. S0717 Inflammatory bowel disease is not associated with severe outcomes of COVID -19: a cohort study from the United States epicenter. Am J Gastroenterol 2020;115(1):S360.

94. Khan N, Patel D, Xie D, et al. Impact of anti-tumor necrosis factor and thiopurine medications on the development of COVID-19 in patients with inflammatory bowel disease: a nationwide Veterans Administration Cohort Study. Gastroenterology 2020;159(4):1545–6.

95. Brenner EJ, Ungaro RC, Gearry RB, et al. Corticosteroids, but not TNF antagonists, are associated with adverse COVID-19 outcomes in patients with inflammatory bowel diseases: results from an international registry. Gastroenterology 2020;159(2):481–91.

96. Ricciuto A, Lamb C, Kuenzig E, et al. Fr493 Disease activity is associated with Covid-19 outcomes in IBD patients with effect modification by age. Gastroenterology 2021;160(6):S330–1.

97. Calafat M, González-Muñoza C, Fortuny M, et al. Impact of immunosuppressants on SARS-CoV-2 infection in elderly patients with inflammatory bowel disease. Aging Clin Exp Res 2021;33(8):2355–9.

98. Lee MH, Ng CH, Chin YH, et al. Incidence of SARS-CoV-2 infection in inflammatory bowel disease. J Gastroenterol Hepatol 2020;35(11):2021–2.

99. Axelrad JE, Malter L, Hong S, et al. From the American epicenter: coronavirus disease 2019 in patients with inflammatory bowel disease in the New York City metropolitan area. Inflamm Bowel Dis 2020;27(5):662–6.

100. Allen T, Murray KA, Zambrana-Torrelio C, et al. Global hotspots and correlates of emerging zoonotic diseases. Nat Commun 2017;8(1):1124.

Health Care Maintenance in Patients with Crohn's Disease

Jana G. Hashash, MD, MSc*, Francis A. Farraye, MD, MSc

KEYWORDS

- Preventative care • Vaccinations • Health care maintenance • Screening
- Inflammatory bowel disease

KEY POINTS

- Health care maintenance of patients with inflammatory bowel disease is a vital part in their management.
- Inactive vaccines can be administered to all patients regardless of immune status.
- Live vaccines should be avoided in patients with inflammatory bowel disease who are on immunosuppression, and exceptions should be individualized.
- Vaccination is not associated with increase in disease activity.
- Physician and patient education about health care maintenance is extremely important in optimizing successful completion of these important tasks.

INTRODUCTION

Preventive care is as important as actual treatment of certain diseases. All individuals should receive preventive care. For those people, with an underlying medical condition, especially if it increases their risk for certain vaccine preventable diseases or malignancies, health care maintenance becomes even more critical. Examples of preventive care for patients with inflammatory bowel disease (IBD) include vaccination against vaccine preventable diseases and screening for malignancies, mood disorders, and osteoporosis, among other conditions.

It is not uncommon for patients with IBD to receive immunosuppressive therapy in the form of biological agents, small molecules, corticosteroids, and immunomodulators. Such treatments immunosuppress patients, increasing their susceptibility to certain vaccine preventable diseases and malignancies and for developing a more

Funding: none available.
Division of Gastroenterology and Hepatology, Inflammatory Bowel Disease Center, Mayo Clinic, 4500 San Pablo Rd S, Jacksonville, FL 32224, USA
* Corresponding author.
E-mail address: AlHashash.Jana@mayo.edu

Gastroenterol Clin N Am 51 (2022) 441–455
https://doi.org/10.1016/j.gtc.2021.12.015
0889-8553/22/© 2021 Elsevier Inc. All rights reserved.

severe and complicated course.[1] In addition, several of these treatments may blunt the immune response to vaccines subsequently decreasing their efficacy. As such, it is very important for gastroenterologists caring for patients with IBD to be aware of the preventive care recommendations of these patients and to offer vaccinations early in the course of a patient's disease. Gastroenterologists should not only know what vaccines to give, but know the best time to vaccinate, and the contraindications of administering certain vaccines is imperative in order to optimize patient safety.[2] Equally as important, health care maintenance also involves screening and surveillance for certain cancers, mood disorders, osteoporosis, and smoking.

Rates of preventive care have been shown to be lower among patients with IBD compared with the general population, due to many barriers.[1,3,4] One of the major reasons contributing to this low rate is the lack of knowledge of gastroenterologists as well as primary care physicians about health care maintenance in patients with IBD. A survey in 2017 showed that only 2.5% of primary care physicians correctly recommended vaccinations.[5] It was shown that primary care physicians were more likely to make recommendations about vaccinations to patients who are not receiving immunosuppressive medications.[5] Another study showed that 20% to 30% of gastroenterologists incorrectly recommended live vaccines to immunosuppressed patients.[6] In order to overcome the knowledge barrier, guideline statements as well as checklists that can be easily used in clinical practice have been published and made available to treating physicians.[7–10] In addition, gastroenterology guidelines advise that the treating gastroenterologist take ownership of making vaccination recommendations to their patients with IBD.[7] Although patients may not be receiving the vaccines at their gastroenterologist's office due to space issues, storage, cost, and lack of staff to administer the vaccines in the gastroenterology practices, patients can be referred to a local pharmacy with clear direction from their gastroenterologist to ensure appropriate vaccination.[11] In addition to lack of knowledge, it has been shown that physicians are less comfortable recommending vaccinations to immunosuppressed patients, and this may contribute further to the lower vaccination rates.[7]

In this review the authors discuss the health care maintenance recommendations for patients with IBD. These recommendations include vaccinations, screening for select malignancies, screening for osteoporosis, addressing tobacco use, as well as screening for mental health disorders. Special vaccinations required for international travel will not be addressed in this article, and the reader is advised to refer to the Centers for Disease Control and Prevention (CDC) Web site and the American College of Gastroenterology (ACG) preventive care clinical guidelines for direction in that regard.[7,12,13]

Vaccine Preventable Diseases

Vaccines have proved to play a vital role for the prevention of several infectious illnesses.[14] Vaccinations are important for all individuals at all ages and particularly those who are immunosuppressed. From birth and until advanced ages, there are scheduled vaccines that an individual is recommended to receive as detailed by the Advisory Committee on Immunization Practices (ACIP).[15] There are also recommendations and checklists available to increase vaccination awareness and uptake among patients with IBD.[7–9,14] Currently, it is recommended that all patients with IBD be brought up to date with their vaccinations soon after the time of diagnosis to avoid delays in treatment in case immunosuppressive medications are needed, as these medications may affect response to vaccination.[16] There have been no convincing data showing an association between vaccinations causing subsequent flare ups of known

IBD.[17–19] IBD experts advise a cocoon vaccination strategy whereby family members of patients with IBD are also vaccinated.[7]

Vaccines are classified as either nonlive or live. Administration of live vaccines are typically contraindicated in patients who are immunosuppressed, although newer data suggest individualization of such cases.[20] Per the CDC, highly/severely immunosuppressed status that precludes live vaccination includes (1) oral prednisone ($\geq$ 20 mg per day for at least 14 days), (2) thiopurines ($\geq$1.5 mg/kg of 6 mercaptopurine or $\geq$ 3 mg/kg of azathioprine), (3) methotrexate ($\geq$ 0.4 mg/kg weekly), (4) patient receiving biologics or small molecules, or (5) patient receiving transplant-related immunosuppressive medications (cyclosporine, tacrolimus, mycophenolate).[12,21] Nonlive vaccines are safe and can be administered to all patients, even if immunosuppressed.[15,22–24] Currently recommended vaccines include the inactivated influenza vaccine, pneumococcal vaccines (pneumococcal conjugate vaccine [PCV-13], pneumococcal polysaccharide vaccine [PPSV23]), tetanus diphtheria and pertussis (Tdap), meningococcus vaccine, hepatitis A and hepatitis B vaccines, human papilloma virus (HPV), the inactivated recombinant herpes zoster vaccine (Shingrix), and more recently, the coronavirus disease 2019 (COVID-19) vaccine.[7]

Table 1 summarizes the recommended vaccines for adult patients with IBD.[25]

Inactive Vaccines

Influenza vaccine

Patients with IBD are at a slightly increased risk of developing influenza (incidence rate ratio 1.54; 95% confidence interval 1.49–1.63) and demonstrate higher rates of hospitalization from the infection, compared with non-IBD controls (5.4% vs 1.85%; $P < .001$).[14] The risk of developing influenza is associated with steroid use.[26] The use of immunosuppressive medications was associated with a more severe and complicated course from this infection, including higher rates of hospitalization and superimposed pneumonia.[27]

The influenza vaccine has not been shown to increase risk of IBD flare.[18,28] For patients receiving biological therapy, timing of influenza vaccination should not be affected by the timing of biological administration, especially antitumor necrosis factor (anti-TNF) medications. Although the immune response elicited from the influenza vaccine among immunosuppressed patients with IBD may be blunted, particularly in patients receiving combination therapy with an anti-TNF and thiopurine, patients still develop some degree of protection.[28–33] Even the use of anti-TNF monotherapy blunted a patient's immune response to the influenza vaccine, and furthermore, persistence of serum protection was lower.[30,33–35] A study showed that of the patients with IBD who were receiving infliximab and who received the influenza vaccine, 80% mounted a serologic response.[33] When comparing vedolizumab with healthy controls, vaccine responses were comparable between both groups.[36] For patients with rheumatoid arthritis, holding methotrexate for 2 weeks after administration of the influenza vaccine showed improvement in immune response.[37]

Current recommendations are for all patients with IBD, regardless of immunosuppression status, to receive the inactivated nonlive influenza vaccine on an annual basis.[7] Patients aged 65 years and older should receive the high-dose influenza vaccine. In a recent expert review, it was recommended that in patients with IBD who are receiving anti-TNF agents, high-dose inactivated influenza vaccine should be used, as it leads to higher antibody levels when compared with the standard dose influenza vaccine.[36,38]

Table 1
Immunizations for adults with inflammatory bowel disease[a]

Infectious Pathogen	Vaccine		Dosing Schedule	Special Considerations
Influenza	Inactive influenza vaccines	Inactivated standard dose (SD) quadrivalent influenza vaccine (multiple formulations)	Annually	—
		Inactivated high-dose (HD) influenza vaccine (Fluzone)	Annually	Preferred for patients ≥ 65 y or 18–64 y who are on anti-TNF monotherapy
	Live attenuated influenza vaccine	Live attenuated intranasal influenza vaccine (FluMist)	Contraindicated in immunosuppressed patients	
Streptococcus pneumonia	Inactivated pneumococcal vaccines	Pneumococcal conjugate 13 valent (PCV13 Prevnar) Polysaccharide 23 valent (PPSV23 Pneumovax)	All ages ≥18 y; PCV13 followed by PPSV23 8 wk later if immunosuppressed or 1 y later if immunocompetent; repeat PPSV23 5 y after initial dose with third dose at age 65 y	
Herpes zoster virus	Inactivated/recombinant	Recombinant zoster vaccine (Shingrix)	Two doses (2–6 mo apart) for all ≥19 y who are or will be at increased risk due to immunodeficiency or immunosuppression caused by disease or therapy[b]	
Human papillomavirus (HPV)	Inactivated HPV vaccine	9 valent HPV (Gardasil, Cervarix)	Two-dose series (0, 6–12 mo) if initiated at ages 9 through 14 y; three doses: 0, 1–2, and 6 mo schedule for ages between 15 and 26 y and if immunocompromised; individualize for patients 27–45 y[b]	

Severe acute respiratory syndrome coronavirus 2 (SARS-CoV-2)	Messenger RNA vaccines	Pfizer BioNTech	Two doses 21 d apart, third dose 6 mo after second dose for select populations[d]	Patients ≥ 12 y
		Moderna	Two doses 28 d apart	Patients ≥ 16 y
	Viral vector vaccine	Johnson and Johnson	Single dose	Patients ≥ 18 y
Corynebacterium diphtheria, Clostridium tetani, Bordetella pertussis	Inactivated tetanus, diphtheria, pertussis (Tdap or Td) vaccine	Tdap or Td (Daptacel, Infanrix)	A single dose of Tdap between 11–64 y then Td or Tdap every 10 y	1 Tdap during the third trimester of each pregnancy
Hepatitis A virus	Inactivated vaccine	Hepatitis A (Havrix, Vaqta)	Two dose series 6–12 mo apart	
		Hepatitis A/Hepatitis B (Twinrix)	Three dose series at 0, 1, 6 mo or 4 doses accelerated dosing schedule 0, 7, 21–30 d, and 12 mo	Accelerated dosing for patients who start the vaccination series but are unable to complete the 3-dose schedule due to high-risk travel
Hepatitis B virus[c]	Inactivated vaccine	Hepatitis B virus (Engerix-B, Recombivax)	Three dose series on 0, 1, 6 mo	Check antibody to the surface antigen (antiHBs) 4–8 wk after completing series
		Hepatitis A/Hepatitis B (Twinrix)	Three dose series at 0, 1, 6 mo or 4 doses accelerated dosing schedule 0, 7, 21–30 d, and 12 mo	Accelerated dosing for patients who start the vaccination series but are unable to complete the 3-dose schedule due to high-risk travel
		Heplisav	2-dose series (HepB-CpG) at 0 and 1 mo	Check antibody to the surface antigen (antiHBs) 4–8 wk after completing series

(continued on next page)

Table 1
(continued)

Infectious Pathogen	Vaccine		Dosing Schedule	Special Considerations
Measles, mumps, and rubella	Live attenuated vaccine	MMR (M-M-R II)	2 doses at least 4 wk apart if not previously vaccinated or 1 dose if previously received 1 dose MMR	Contraindicated in patients on immunosuppressive therapy
Varicella	Live attenuated vaccine	Varicella vaccine (Varivax)	2 doses 4–8 wk apart if not previously vaccinated or if did not develop varicella or herpes zoster infection previously	Contraindicated in patients on immunosuppressive therapy
Neisseria meningitidis	Inactivated vaccine	Meningococcal A, C, W, Y (MenACWY) (multiple formulations)	1 or 2 doses depending on indication	Recommended only for adults with certain risk factors
		Meningococcal B (MenB) (multiple formulations)	A 2- or 3-dose series depending on vaccine and indication	Please see ACIP recommendations for more details

[a] The aforementioned recommendations do not apply to pregnant women with IBD.

[b] See text.

[c] For patients with a previous history of hepatitis B immunization, a single dose of hepatitis B vaccine is given followed by a hepatitis B surface antibody titer check 3 to 4 weeks later. If the quantitative hepatitis B surface antibody titer is < 10, then the complete hepatitis B vaccination immunization series is given.

[d] US Food and Drug Administration amended the emergency use authorization to allow for use of a single third dose for individuals 18 through 64 years of age who are at high risk of severe COVID-19 (to include immunocompromised patients with IBD), individuals 65 years and older, and individuals whose frequent institutional or occupational exposure to SARS-CoV-2 puts them at high risk of serious complications of COVID-19.

As for the live attenuated influenza vaccine, this is contraindicated in immunosuppressed patients with IBD. It is only recommended by the ACIP for healthy nonpregnant individuals between the ages of 2 and 49 years.

Pneumococcal vaccine

Similar to the influenza infection, patients with IBD are at an increased risk for acquiring pneumococcal pneumonia, compared with individuals without IBD.[39] The risk of complicated invasive pneumococcal disease is higher when comparing patients with IBD with those without IBD.[14] Immunosuppressive medications including anti-TNF agents and steroids were not shown to increase risk of complicated pneumonia (invasive pneumococcal disease).[40]

The current ACG recommendations state that all immunosuppressed patients or those in whom immunosuppressive therapy is planned should receive the pneumococcal vaccine.[7] The 2021 European Crohn's and Colitis Organization guidelines make a statement that the pneumococcal vaccination should be recommended for all patients with IBD, regardless of immunosuppression status.[14] For patients who are already immunocompromised, the pneumococcal polysaccharide PPSV23 vaccine (Pneumovax 23) should be given 8 weeks after the conjugate vaccine PCV13 (Prevnar 13). If the PPSV23 vaccine is given before the PCV13 vaccine, patients should be then given the PCV13 vaccine 1 year later. In immunocompetent individuals, PPSV23 is given 1 year after PCV-13. PPSV23 should be repeated after 5 years and then again at the age of 65 years.

As with the influenza vaccine, patients who are receiving immunosuppressive medications, especially those receiving combination therapy with anti-TNF agents and an immunosuppressive drug, have a blunted response to the pneumococcal vaccine and a diminished immune persistence.[41] In addition, timing of the biological agent administration should not interfere with pneumococcal vaccine administration.

Human papilloma virus vaccine

Although data are limited, rates of HPV infections have been shown to be higher among patients with IBD compared with patients with no IBD.[14] Immunosuppression with immunomodulators and/or combination therapy increases the risk of high-risk HPV infections and leads to persistence of HPV infection, which in itself increases the risk of cervical dysplasia and cervical cancer.[42–44] Studies have demonstrated that vaccination against HPV decreases HPV-related cancers by at least 90% in the general population.[14]

There are 3 available HPV vaccines; a quadrivalent vaccine, a bivalent vaccine, and a nonavalent vaccine. The latter, the recombinant HPV-9 valent vaccine (Gardasil 9) is the preferred vaccine. The Food and Drug Association (FDA) approved Gardasil 9 for women and men between the ages of 9 and 45 years.[45] The ACIP of the CDC recommends vaccination up to the age of 26 years, as by that age most women have been exposed to HPV. This committee advises that for individuals between the ages of 27 and 45 years, personalization and shared clinical decision-making between the patient and provider as to the risk for acquiring HPV should dictate the decision about vaccination.[46,47] Based on the FDA recommendations, all women and men with IBD who are between the ages of 9 and 26 years should receive the HPV vaccine with recommendations for individuals aged 27 to 45 years be made based on the patient's unique personal situation and risk of acquiring HPV infection.

Herpes zoster vaccine

The risk for herpes zoster is increased in patients with IBD, more so in those with Crohn's disease as compared with ulcerative colitis.[39,48] This risk is even higher in patients who are receiving immunosuppressive therapy.[49] Among patients with Crohn's disease, corticosteroids have been shown to increase this risk, whereas in patients with ulcerative colitis, this risk was found to also be increased with the use of anti-TNF agents as well as tofacitinib.[21,49]

There are 2 available vaccines for herpes zoster worldwide including the recombinant zoster vaccine (Shingrix) and the live zoster vaccine (Zostavax). Zostavax is no longer available in the United States. Previously, expert recommendations were to administer the Shingrix vaccine to high-risk patients with IBD. Such patients include those who are at least 40 years of age with a history of herpes zoster infection, those receiving repeated steroid courses, those on combination therapy in addition to steroids, as well as patients being treated with tofacitinib. Also, patients of an Asian race or those with diabetes mellitus are considered high risk.[21,38,50] For the remainder of individuals, those older than 50 years should receive the recumbent zoster vaccine.

In October 2021, the ACIP recommended 2 doses of Shingrix for the prevention of herpes zoster and related complications in adults aged 19 years or older who are or will be immunodeficient or immunosuppressed because of disease or therapy.

COVID-19 vaccine

Patients with IBD are not at an increased risk for contracting the severe acute respiratory syndrome coronavirus 2 (SARS-CoV-2) virus.[14] Many studies also demonstrate that immunosuppressive medications do not increase the risk of contracting SARS-CoV-2.[51–53] Newer data from the SECURE-IBD confirmed these findings and reinforced the deleterious effects of corticosteroids that increase the risk of adverse events.[54] It is important that we encourage our patients with IBD to remain on their medications in an effort for maintain remission.

There are several vaccines that have been developed and others that are being developed against SARS-CoV-2. Currently in the United States, there are 2 approved messenger RNA (mRNA) vaccines, the Pfizer BioNTech and the Moderna vaccines. There is also an adenovirus viral vector COVID-19 vaccine from Johnson and Johnson that has been approved. Recommendations are that all patients with IBD receive vaccination against SARS-CoV-2 with any of the 3 inactive vaccines at the earliest opportunity possible.[55] Given the accumulating evidence of a decreased immune response to a single dose of the viral vector Johnson and Johnson vaccine, the authors believe that the mRNA vaccines at the current dose are preferred for patients with IBD. The FDA has recently approved a third dose of the Pfizer vaccine for select individuals who are at a high risk for severe COVID 19. These individuals include patients 18 through 64 years who are immunocompromised, individuals older than 65 years, and other individuals whose are at a high risk of exposure. It is anticipated that a third dose of the Moderna vaccine and second dose of the Johnson and Johnson will be approved in the near future.

Live Vaccines

Live vaccines should not be administered to immunosuppressed patients with IBD, and it is preferable to administer them 4 weeks before starting immunosuppressive therapy. There are some exceptions depending on the degree of immunosuppression and the need of receiving the vaccine where administration of live vaccines can be considered. Such decisions should be individualized and performed very cautiously in a multidisciplinary fashion by the treating gastroenterologist, infectious disease specialist, and patient consent.[20] Common live vaccines include the varicella, measles mumps and rubella, and the live influenza vaccine. There are number of live travel vaccines such as the cholera, yellow fever, and typhoid vaccines.

Cancer Prevention (Screening and Surveillance)

Colon cancer

Patients with IBD, namely ulcerative colitis involving more than the extent of their rectum and Crohn's disease involving at least one-third of the colon, are at an increased risk for the development of colon cancer after 8 years of symptoms. Surveillance for colon cancer starts at 8 years from diagnosis in these patients with frequency ranging between 1 and 5 years, based on risk factors for colorectal cancer including burden of inflammation, family history, and personal history of colon dysplasia.[56–58] Patients with concomitant primary sclerosing cholangitis (PSC) require a yearly colonoscopy from the time of their diagnosis of PSC due to their increased risk for the development of colon dysplasia and cancer.[59,60]

Cervical cancer

Most cervical cancer is caused by HPV 16 or 18.[44] Persistent HPV infection increases the risk of cervical cancer, and patients receiving immunosuppression have a higher rate of persistent HPV infection.[14] Studies have shown that the risk for the development of cervical dysplasia and cervical cancer is higher in patients on azathioprine, methotrexate, or combination therapy. There was a 30% increased risk for the development of cervical neoplasia among immunosuppressed patients with IBD compared with the general population.[44] Anti-TNF agents alone did not significantly increase this risk.[42,61,62] HPV vaccination has been shown to decrease the development of cervical cancers in more than 90% of the cancers that are caused by HPV. There is a consensus among the ACG preventive guidelines, the European Crohn's and Colitis Organization, and the American College of Obstetrics and Gynecology to perform cervical cancer screening and a Pap smear on an annual basis for immunosuppressed women with IBD.[14]

Skin cancer

IBD in itself increases the risk of melanoma and nonmelanoma skin cancers (NMSC).[63,64] Immunosuppressants further increase this risk. Thiopurines increase the risk of NMSC by 6 times.[7] Even after discontinuation of the thiopurine, the risk remains higher than that of patients who have not received a thiopurine. Of patients with Crohn's disease who have used ustekinumab, the risk of developing an NMSC was 0.2%.[65] As for the anti-TNF biologics, they increase the risk of melanoma by 2-fold.[66] Because of these increased risk, patients with IBD who are receiving immunosuppressive medications should be referred to a dermatologist who can better determine the frequency of periodic evaluations with many organizations recommending yearly examinations. Sunscreen use should be strongly encouraged for all patients with IBD, especially those who are immunocompromised.[67]

Bone Health

Patients with Crohn's disease have high rates of osteoporosis, even early after the diagnosis, before the start of immunosuppressive treatment. Reported rates of osteoporosis among patients with IBD are as high as 42%.[68–71] The cause of osteoporosis in patients with IBD is multifactorial and related to the use of medications, particularly corticosteroids, malabsorption, especially of vitamin D, the effect of disease on exercise, as well as dietary-related reasons. Based on the ACG preventive guidelines, it is recommended that all patients with IBD who have conventional risk factors undergo a bone mineral density at time of diagnosis and then periodically after that.[7] This recommendation applies to women 65 years and older, men 70 years and older, and patients with a preexisting fragility fracture. In addition, patients who have required multiple courses of steroids with a total exposure more than 3 months, those with malnutrition, and those with chronic inflammation are also recommended to have a baseline bone mineral density scan.[71,72] In addition to the aforementioned risk factors, the Crohn's and Colitis Foundation also considers patients with a low bone mass index, those who are smokers, and those with hypogonadism as high-risk patients and recommend they get a baseline DEXA scan of the hip and spine.[8] For patients whose DEXA scan returns normal, the recommendation is to repeat after 5 years, unless they have other risk factors to warrant more frequent follow-up.

Serial monitoring of vitamin D levels is also recommended.[9] The Cornerstones checklist also recommends that vitamin D and calcium supplementation be given to all patients who receive steroids.[9]

Mental Health Screening

Patients with IBD have been shown to have high rates of anxiety, depression, and fatigue when compared with the general population.[73,74] These conditions are underrecognized in lead to significant morbidity. It is crucial to identify and address these mental health issues early on to avoid progression. Depressive severity was found to be associated with suicidal ideation, and early psychiatric intervention is necessary among patients to prevent completed suicides.[75] All patients with IBD should be assessed for depression and anxiety in order to improve the outcomes of these patients.

Tobacco Use

Tobacco smoking is a very harmful habit with deleterious effects on the entire body. It has been linked to increase the risk for development of Crohn's disease as well as lead to a more complicated course with stricture development and the subsequent need for repeated surgical resections. In patients with Crohn's disease and intestinal resection, tobacco smoking has been associated with recurrence of postoperative Crohn's disease.[76,77] In addition, smokers with IBD have been found to have a higher risk of joint and skin extraintestinal manifestations.[78]

SUMMARY

Health care maintenance for patients with IBD is extremely important. Many patients with IBD receive immunosuppressive medications at a point during their time and being up to date with vaccinations as well as screening and surveillance of common cancers is crucial to provide them with the best care. All gastroenterologists who care for patients with IBD should be familiar with the health care maintenance recommendations and should take the initiative to ensure that their patients are current with all the recommendations. To facilitate this process, there are available checklists to guide and remind the treating physicians.[8,9]

AUTHORS' CONTRIBUTIONS

J.G. Hashash: drafting of the article. F.A. Farraye: critical review of the article.

CONFLICTS OF INTEREST/COMPETING INTERESTS

No conflicts of interest exist for any of the authors.

CLINICS CARE POINTS

- Inactive vaccines are safe for all patients regardless of immunosuppression status and can be administered irrespective of timing of immunomodulators, small molecules, or biologics.

- In general, live vaccines should not be administered to highly immunosuppressed patients but can be administered on a case-by-case basis to certain patients with low-level immunosuppression after discussion of the risk and benefits with the patient.

- Screening and surveillance for certain cancers, bone health, and mood disorders are underperformed, and increased awareness among treating physicians and patients can improve compliance and patient outcomes.

DISCLOSURE

J.G. Hashash has no financial disclosures. F.A. Farraye is a consultant for Arena, BMS, Braintree Labs, GI Reviewers, GSK, Innovation Pharmaceuticals, Iterative scopes, Janssen, Pfizer, and Sebela. He sits on a data safety monitoring board for Lilly and TheraVance.

REFERENCES

1. Mir FA, Kane SV. Health maintenance in inflammatory bowel disease. Curr Gastroenterol Rep 2018;20(5):1–6.
2. Marín AC, Gisbert JP, Chaparro M. Immunogenicity and mechanisms impairing the response to vaccines in inflammatory bowel disease. World J Gastroenterol 2015;21(40):11273.
3. Selby L, Kane S, Wilson J, et al. Receipt of preventive health services by IBD patients is significantly lower than by primary care patients. Inflamm Bowel Dis 2008;14(2):253–8.
4. Hashash JG, Farraye FA. On-site availability improves vaccination rates in patients with inflammatory Bowel Disease. J Crohns Colitis 2021;3(4):1–2, 360.
5. Gurvits GE, Lan G, Tan A, et al. Vaccination practices in patients with inflammatory bowel disease among general internal medicine physicians in the USA. Postgrad Med J 2017;93(1100):333–7.
6. Wasan SK, Coukos JA, Farraye FA. Vaccinating the inflammatory bowel disease patient: deficiencies in gastroenterologists knowledge. Inflamm Bowel Dis 2011; 17(12):2536–40.
7. Farraye FA, Melmed GY, Lichtenstein GR, et al. ACG clinical guideline: preventive care in inflammatory bowel disease. J Am Coll Gastroenterol 2017;112(2): 241–58.
8. Available at: https://www.crohnscolitisfoundation.org/sites/default/files/2019-09/Health%20Maintenance%20Checklist%202019-3.pdf. Accessed October 15, 2021.
9. Available at: https://www.cornerstoneshealth.org/wp-content/uploads/2020/08/NEW-IBD-Checklist-for-Monitoring-Prevention-526a.pdf. Accessed October 15, 2021.
10. Syal G, Serrano M, Jain A, et al. Health maintenance consensus for adults with inflammatory bowel disease. Inflamm Bowel Dis 2021;27(10):1552–63.
11. Bhat S, Caldera F, Farraye FA. Barriers to administering vaccines in inflammatory bowel disease centers. Inflamm Bowel Dis 2021;27(8):1356–7.

12. Available at: https://www.cdc.gov/travel/yellowbook/2020/travelers-with-additional-considerations/immunocompromised-travelers. Accessed October 15, 2021.

13. Visser L. The immunosuppressed traveler. Infect Dis Clin 2012;26(3):609–24.

14. Kucharzik T, Ellul P, Greuter T, et al. ECCO guidelines on the prevention, diagnosis, and management of infections in inflammatory bowel disease. J Crohns Colitis 2021;15(6):879–913.

15. Freedman MS, Ault K, Bernstein H. Advisory Committee on Immunization Practices Recommended Immunization Schedule for Adults Aged 19 Years or Older—United States, 2021. Morbidity Mortality Weekly Rep 2021;70(6):193.

16. Reich J, Wasan S, Farraye FA. Vaccinating patients with inflammatory bowel disease. Gastroenterol Hepatol 2016;12(9):540.

17. Dotan I, Werner L, Vigodman S, et al. Normal response to vaccines in inflammatory bowel disease patients treated with thiopurines. Inflamm Bowel Dis 2012;18(2):261–8.

18. Rahier J-F, Papay P, Salleron J, et al. H1N1 vaccines in a large observational cohort of patients with inflammatory bowel disease treated with immunomodulators and biological therapy. Gut 2011;60(4):456–62.

19. Desalermos A, Pimienta M, Kalligeros M, et al. Safety of Immunizations for the Adult Patient with Inflammatory Bowel Disease - A Systematic Review and Meta-analysis. Inflamm Bowel Dis 2021. izab266.

20. Croce E, Hatz C, Jonker EF, et al. Safety of live vaccinations on immunosuppressive therapy in patients with immune-mediated inflammatory diseases, solid organ transplantation or after bone-marrow transplantation–a systematic review of randomized trials, observational studies and case reports. Vaccine 2017;35(9):1216–26.

21. Caldera F, Hayney MS, Cross RK. Using number needed to harm to put the risk of herpes zoster from tofacitinib in perspective. Oxford University Press US; 2019.

22. Long MD, Gulati A, Wohl D, et al. Immunizations in pediatric and adult patients with inflammatory bowel disease: a practical case-based approach. Inflamm Bowel Dis 2015;21(8):1993–2003.

23. Kim DK, Bridges CB, Harriman KH. Advisory committee on immunization practices recommended immunization schedule for adults aged 19 years or older: United States, 2016. Ann Intern Med 2016;164(3):184–94.

24. Rubin LG, Levin MJ, Ljungman P, et al. 2013 IDSA clinical practice guideline for vaccination of the immunocompromised host. Clin Infect Dis 2014;58(3):e44–100.

25. Hashash JG, Picco M, Farraye FA. Health maintenance for adult patients with inflammatory bowel disease. Curr Treat Options Gastro 2021;19:583–96.

26. Tinsley A, Navabi S, Williams ED, et al. Increased risk of influenza and influenza-related complications among 140,480 patients with inflammatory bowel disease. Inflamm Bowel Dis 2019;25(2):369–76.

27. Stobaugh DJ, Deepak P, Ehrenpreis ED. Hospitalizations for vaccine preventable pneumonias in patients with inflammatory bowel disease: a 6-year analysis of the Nationwide Inpatient Sample. Clin Exp Gastroenterol 2013;6:43.

28. Launay O, Abitbol V, Krivine A, et al. Immunogenicity and safety of influenza vaccine in inflammatory bowel disease patients treated or not with immunomodulators and/or biologics: a two-year prospective study. J Crohns Colitis 2015;9(12):1096–107.

29. Andrisani G, Frasca D, Romero M, et al. Immune response to influenza A/H1N1 vaccine in inflammatory bowel disease patients treated with anti TNF-α agents: effects of combined therapy with immunosuppressants. J Crohns Colitis 2013;7(4):301–7.

30. Hagihara Y, Ohfuji S, Watanabe K, et al. Infliximab and/or immunomodulators inhibit immune responses to trivalent influenza vaccination in adults with inflammatory bowel disease. J Crohns Colitis 2014;8(3):223–33.

31. Melmed GY. Vaccinations while on thiopurines: some protection is better than none. Am J Gastroenterol 2012;107(1):141.

32. Cullen G, Bader C, Korzenik JR, et al. Serological response to the 2009 H1N1 influenza vaccination in patients with inflammatory bowel disease. Gut 2012; 61(3):385–91.

33. deBruyn JC, Hilsden R, Fonseca K, et al. Immunogenicity and safety of influenza vaccination in children with inflammatory bowel disease. Inflamm Bowel Dis 2012; 18(1):25–33.

34. Mamula P, Markowitz JE, Piccoli DA, et al. Immune response to influenza vaccine in pediatric patients with inflammatory bowel disease. Clin Gastroenterol Hepatol 2007;5(7):851–6.

35. Lu Y, Jacobson DL, Ashworth LA, et al. Immune response to influenza vaccine in children with inflammatory bowel disease. Am J Gastroenterol 2009;104(2):444.

36. Caldera F, Hillman L, Saha S, et al. Immunogenicity of high dose influenza vaccine for patients with inflammatory bowel disease on anti-TNF monotherapy: a randomized clinical trial. Inflamm Bowel Dis 2020;26(4):593–602.

37. Park JK, Lee YJ, Shin K, et al. Impact of temporary methotrexate discontinuation for 2 weeks on immunogenicity of seasonal influenza vaccination in patients with rheumatoid arthritis: a randomised clinical trial. Ann Rheum Dis 2018;77(6): 898–904.

38. Caldera F, Hayney MS, Farraye FA. Vaccination in patients with inflammatory bowel disease. J Am Coll Gastroenterol 2020;115(9):1356–61.

39. Long MD, Martin C, Sandler RS, et al. Increased risk of pneumonia among patients with inflammatory bowel disease. Am J Gastroenterol 2013;108(2):240.

40. Kantsø B, Simonsen J, Hoffmann S, et al. Inflammatory bowel disease patients are at increased risk of invasive pneumococcal disease: a nationwide Danish cohort study 1977–2013. Am J Gastroenterol 2015;110(11):1582–7.

41. Van Aalst M, Garcia Garrido HM, Van Der Leun J, et al. Immunogenicity of the currently recommended pneumococcal vaccination schedule in patients with inflammatory bowel disease. Clin Infect Dis 2020;70(4):595–604.

42. Marehbian J, Arrighi MH, Hass S, et al. Adverse events associated with common therapy regimens for moderate-to-severe Crohn's disease. J Am Coll Gastroenterol 2009;104(10):2524–33.

43. Li M, Yang Q-F, Cao Q, et al. High-risk human papilloma virus infection and cervical neoplasm in female inflammatory bowel disease patients: a cross-sectional study. Gastroenterol Rep 2019;7(5):338–44.

44. Kane S, Khatibi B, Reddy D. Higher incidence of abnormal Pap smears in women with inflammatory bowel disease. Official J Am Coll Gastroenterol ACG 2008; 103(3):631–6.

45. Available at: https://www.fda.gov/vaccines-blood-biologics/vaccines/gardasil-9. Accessed October 15, 2021.

46. Freedman MS, Bernstein H, Ault KA. Recommended adult immunization schedule, United States, 2021. Ann Intern Med 2021;174(3):374–84.

47. Meites E, Szilagyi PG, Chesson HW, et al. Human papillomavirus vaccination for adults: updated recommendations of the Advisory Committee on Immunization Practices. MMWR Morb Mortal Wkly Rep 2019 Aug 16;68(32):698–702.

48. Ning L, Liu R, Li S, et al. Increased risk of herpes zoster infection in patients with inflammatory bowel disease: a meta-analysis of cohort studies. Eur J Clin Microbiol Infect Dis 2020;39(2):219–27.
49. Nugent Z, Singh H, Targownik LE, et al. Herpes zoster infection and herpes zoster vaccination in a population-based sample of persons with IBD: is there still an unmet need? Inflamm Bowel Dis 2019;25(3):532–40.
50. Khan N, Patel D, Trivedi C, et al. Overall and comparative risk of herpes zoster with pharmacotherapy for inflammatory bowel diseases: a nationwide cohort study. Clin Gastroenterol Hepatol 2018;16(12):1919–27.e3.
51. Taxonera C, Sagastagoitia I, Alba C, et al. 2019 novel coronavirus disease (COVID-19) in patients with inflammatory bowel diseases. Aliment Pharmacol Ther 2020;52(2):276–83.
52. Allocca M, Fiorino G, Zallot C, et al. Incidence and patterns of COVID-19 among inflammatory bowel disease patients from the Nancy and Milan cohorts. Clin Gastroenterol Hepatol 2020;18(9):2134–5.
53. An P, Ji M, Ren H, et al. Prevention of COVID-19 in patients with inflammatory bowel disease in Wuhan, China. Lancet Gastroenterol Hepatol 2020;5(6):525–7.
54. Ungaro RC, Brenner EJ, Agrawal M, et al. Impact of Medications on COVID-19 Outcomes in Inflammatory Bowel Disease: Analysis of Over 6,000 Patients from an International Registry. Gastroenterology 2021;162(1):316–9.e5.
55. Siegel CA, Melmed GY, McGovern DP, et al. SARS-CoV-2 vaccination for patients with inflammatory bowel diseases: recommendations from an international consensus meeting. Gut 2021;70(4):635–40.
56. Murthy SK, Feuerstein JD, Nguyen GC, et al. AGA Clinical Practice Update on Endoscopic Surveillance and Management of Colorectal Dysplasia in Inflammatory Bowel Diseases: Expert Review. Gastroenterology 2021;161(3):1043–51.e4.
57. Lichtenstein GR, Loftus EV, Isaacs KL, et al. ACG clinical guideline: management of Crohn's disease in adults. Am J Gastroenterol 2018;113(4):481–517.
58. Long MD, Sands BE. When do you start and when do you stop screening for colon cancer in inflammatory bowel disease? Clin Gastroenterol Hepatol 2018; 16(5):621–3.
59. Bergeron V, Vienne A, Sokol H, et al. Risk factors for neoplasia in inflammatory bowel disease patients with pancolitis. Am J Gastroenterol 2010;105(11): 2405–11.
60. Trivedi PJ, Crothers H, Mytton J, et al. Effects of primary sclerosing cholangitis on risks of cancer and death in people with inflammatory bowel disease, based on sex, race, and age. Gastroenterology 2020;159(3):915–28.
61. Dugué PA, Rebolj M, Hallas J, et al. Risk of cervical cancer in women with autoimmune diseases, in relation with their use of immunosuppressants and screening: population-based cohort study. Int J Cancer 2015;136(6):E711–9.
62. Rungoe C, Simonsen J, Riis L, et al. Inflammatory bowel disease and cervical neoplasia: a population-based nationwide cohort study. Clin Gastroenterol Hepatol 2015;13(4):693–700.e1.
63. Singh S, Nagpal SJS, Murad MH, et al. Inflammatory bowel disease is associated with an increased risk of melanoma: a systematic review and meta-analysis. Clin Gastroenterol Hepatol 2014;12(2):210–8.
64. Singh H, Nugent Z, Demers AA, et al. Increased risk of nonmelanoma skin cancers among individuals with inflammatory bowel disease. Gastroenterology 2011; 141(5):1612–20.
65. Available at: https://www.medicalnewstoday.com/articles/326482#overdose. Accessed October 15, 2021.

66. Moran G, Lim A, Bailey J, et al. dermatological complications of immunosuppressive and anti-TNF therapy in inflammatory bowel disease. Aliment Pharmacol Ther 2013;38(9):1002–24.
67. Available at: https://55aa842f6e.nxcli.net/ibd-checklists/) wco. Accessed October 15, 2021.
68. Lichtenstein GR, Sands BE, Pazianas M. Prevention and treatment of osteoporosis in inflammatory bowel disease. Inflamm Bowel Dis 2006;12(8):797–813.
69. Hashash JG, Binion DG. Exercise and inflammatory bowel disease: insights into etiopathogenesis and modification of clinical course. Gastroenterol Clin 2017; 46(4):895–905.
70. Ali T, Lam D, Bronze MS, et al. Osteoporosis in inflammatory bowel disease. Am J Med 2009;122(7):599–604.
71. Bernstein CN, Leslie WD, Leboff MS. AGA technical review on osteoporosis in gastrointestinal diseases. Gastroenterology 2003;124(3):795–841.
72. Vestergaard P. Bone loss associated with gastrointestinal disease: prevalence and pathogenesis. Eur J Gastroenterol Hepatol 2003;15(8):851–6.
73. Hashash JG, Knisely MR, Germain A, et al. Brief behavioral therapy and bupropion for sleep and fatigue in young adults with Crohn's Disease: an Exploratory Open Trial Study. Clin Gastroenterol Hepatol 2020;20(1):96–104.
74. Hashash JG, Ramos-Rivers C, Youk A, et al. Quality of sleep and coexistent psychopathology have significant impact on fatigue burden in patients with inflammatory bowel disease. J Clin Gastroenterol 2018;52(5):423–30.
75. Hashash JG, Vachon A, Ramos Rivers C, et al. Predictors of suicidal ideation among IBD outpatients. J Clin Gastroenterol 2019;53(1):e41–5.
76. Hashash JG, Regueiro M. A practical approach to preventing postoperative recurrence in Crohn's disease. Curr Gastroenterol Rep 2016;18(5):25.
77. Hashash JG, Regueiro MD. The evolving management of postoperative Crohn's disease. Expert Rev Gastroenterol Hepatol 2012;6(5):637–48.
78. Severs M, van Erp SJ, Van Der Valk M, et al. Smoking is associated with extraintestinal manifestations in inflammatory bowel disease. J Crohns Colitis 2016; 10(4):455–61.